KU-021-286

COGNITIVE THERAPY FOR CHRONIC PAIN

COGNITIVE THERAPY FOR CHRONIC PAIN

A Step-by-Step Guide

Beverly E. Thorn

Foreword by Dennis C. Turk

THE GUILFORD PRESS
New York   London

© 2004 The Guilford Press
A Division of Guilford Publications, Inc.
72 Spring Street, New York, NY 10012
www.guilford.com

All rights reserved

Except as indicated, no part of this book may be reproduced, translated, stored in a retrieval
system, or transmitted, in any form or by any means, electronic, mechanical, photocopying,
microfilming, recording, or otherwise, without written permission from the Publisher.

Printed in the United States of America

This book is printed on acid-free paper.

Last digit is print number: 9 8 7 6 5 4 3 2 1

LIMITED PHOTOCOPY LICENSE

These materials are intended for use only by qualified mental health professionals.

The Publisher grants to individual purchasers of this book nonassignable permission to reproduce the therapist handouts, client handouts, and appendices. This license is limited to you, the
individual purchaser, for use with your own clients and patients. It does not extend to additional
clinicians or practice settings, nor does purchase by an institution constitute a site license. This
license does not grant the right to reproduce these materials for resale, redistribution, or any
other purposes (including but not limited to books, pamphlets, articles, video- or audiotapes,
and handouts or slides for lectures or workshops). Permission to reproduce these materials for
these and any other purposes must be obtained in writing from the Permissions Department of
Guilford Publications.

Library of Congress Cataloging-in-Publication Data

Thorn, Beverly E.
    Cognitive therapy for chronic pain : a step-by-step guide / by Beverly E. Thorn.
        p. cm.
    Includes bibliographical references and index.
    ISBN 1-57230-979-2 (pbk.)
    1. Chronic pain—Treatment.   2. Cognitive therapy.   I. Title.
    RB127.T499 2004
    616′.0472—dc22

                                                                                          2004004579

To my patients and my students,
who hold the keys to wisdom, if only I will listen

ABOUT THE AUTHOR

Beverly E. Thorn, PhD, is Professor of Psychology and Director of the PhD Program in Clinical Psychology at the University of Alabama, where she has been on the faculty since 1986. She received her PhD in bioclinical psychology from Southern Illinois University in 1980, satisfying the degree requirements for a doctorate in clinical psychology as well as physiological psychology. Dr. Thorn's research has included the investigation of descending pain-inhibitory systems in the brain using traditional behavioral neuroscience techniques, as well as psychological assessment and treatment outcome research in the area of pain management. Most recently, she has been involved in research investigating the important components of cognitive-behavioral treatment for chronic painful conditions, and, specifically, assessing and restructuring maladaptive cognitions associated with painful states. Dr. Thorn has held research grants from the National Institute on Drug Abuse and Roche Laboratories, and is presently funded by the National Institute on Neurological Disorders and Stroke. She is a Fellow of the Society of Behavioral Medicine and of the Division of Health Psychology of the American Psychological Association.

FOREWORD

Chronic pain is a prevalent and costly problem for its sufferers and for society in general. Estimates suggest that 25–30% of the U.S. population suffers from some chronic pain condition, and the costs of treating pain are astronomical—upward of $150 billion each year in direct medical expenditures, indemnity costs, legal costs, and loss of tax revenues (National Research Council, 2001; U.S. Bureau of the Census, 1996). Looking at pain in the abstract, however, is inadequate: It fails to consider the burden of pain and the incalculable human suffering of each affected individual, along with his or her significant others.

By definition, *chronic* pain extends over long periods of time—months, years, and even decades. Although people with acute pain can often receive significant relief from primary health care providers, people with persistent pain become enmeshed in the medical community as they travel on an often futile pilgrimage from doctor to doctor, laboratory test to laboratory test, and imaging procedure to imaging procedure, in a continuing quest to achieve an elusive diagnosis and to have their pain treated successfully.

Systematic attempts to treat pain have been closely aligned with how pain is conceptualized and evaluated. The traditional biomedical view of chronic pain considers it as a symptom of some underlying physical pathology, often in a specific body location (e.g., knee, shoulder, back). Extensive efforts are undertaken to identify the source of the pain—the "pain generator." The quest then is to identify the generator and either to eliminate it or, if this cannot be accomplished, to block the nociceptive signals from reaching the brain (where they are perceived as pain) by surgical, pharmacological, or physical means. In a sense, the view is that of the body as a machine. A body in pain is seen as the result of some broken or worn-out part that needs to be fixed or replaced.

Despite advances in the neurobiology of pain and the advent of new medications and sophisticated interventions, there appears to be no cure on the horizon for the diverse set of chronic pain conditions. Even the most advanced pharmacological preparations available appear to reduce pain by about 35% in fewer than 50% of pain sufferers (Turk, 2002), often with little accompanying improvement in physical or emotional functioning. Moreover, significant adverse events may prohibit continuation of medication. Much the same can be said for surgery, neuroaugmentative procedures, and other somatic modalities: A significant number of people do not experience elimination of their pain following invasive procedures, and some may experience iatrogenic complications requiring incremental treatment. In short, chronic pain is a generic term for a large, disabling set of conditions that no treatment currently available can eliminate or even palliate.

The traditional biomedical model that I have outlined focuses on the physical perturbations; it tends to neglect the fact that nociception is perceived and is being reported by a conscious individual, with a life history that preceded the onset of the pain, who lives in a social context. Moreover, when pain persists over extended periods of time, the symptom comes to be influenced by a range of affective, cognitive-behavioral, and environmental factors. The individual's interpretations of the noxious sensations are therefore based on prior learning history, sociocultural context, current life circumstances, and the availability of coping resources—internal, social, and spiritual, as well as financial. Negative interpretations of the meaning of the pain ("Will I ever be able to function like I did before the pain began?", "Will the pain persist and lead me to become an invalid?"), beliefs ("Physicians should be able to find and treat the cause," "I'm letting my family down"), and attitudes ("I should not have to live this way!") will contribute to negative mood (e.g., fear, despair, anger) and behavior ("If I perform household chores, it will make my pain worse and might even lead to increased injury; thus I should cease the activity").

Failure to consider the whole person within the biomedical model has resulted in assessment focused on identifying a physical cause for the pain. In the absence of a physical basis, inferences of psychological causation are often invoked. The traditional view is that pain has either a physical basis or a psychological one. Even though this dichotomous view has been shown to be inadequate, they are pervasive and persistent. There is no question that physical factors contribute to pain; nor is there any argument that psychological factors, including conscious motivation, may play a part in the symptom reporting of some patients. However, it has become equally evident that numerous psychosocial factors (including many of which the patient is unaware) contribute to the experience of pain and disability (Turk & Okifuji, 2002).

It is well to recall the comment of John Bonica, the seminal figure in the modern movement to understand pain better and to treat its sufferers, in the preface to the first edition of his volume *The Management of Pain* (1954), and repeated in the second edition some 36 years later (1990):

> The crucial role of psychological and environmental factors in causing pain in a significant number of patients only recently received attention. As a consequence, there has emerged a sketch plan of pain apparatus with its receptors, conducting fibers, and its standard function, which is to be applicable to all circumstances. But . . . in so doing, medicine has overlooked the fact that the activity of this apparatus is subject to a *constantly changing influence of the mind.* (p. 12, emphasis added)

People with chronic pain conditions reside in a complex and costly world that is also populated by their significant others, health care providers, employers, and third-party payers. Family members feel increasingly hopeless and distressed as medical costs, disability, and emotional suffering increase while income and available treatment options decline. Health care providers become frustrated as available medical treatment options are exhausted while the pain conditions do not abate or worsen, with accompanying disability. Employers and co-workers grow resentful as productivity declines because the employees with chronic pain are frequently absent from work and others must take over their responsibilities. Third-party payers stand by helplessly or react adversely as health care costs soar with repeated diagnostic testing and growing numbers of unsuccessful treatments. In time, those involved may question the legitimacy of the pain complaints, since often a medical basis for the reported symptoms seems inadequate or completely lacking. Some may suggest that the persons with pain are attempting to gain attention, to avoid undesirable activities, or to seek payments for disability compensation. Others may suggest that the pain is not real and is all "psychological."

Persistent pain therefore confronts people with a cascade of ongoing stressors that compromise all aspects of their lives. As they withdraw from society, they may alienate family and friends, relinquish their jobs altogether, engage in prolonged litigation, and become ever more isolated. For many, the pain becomes the central focus of their lives. Moreover, the experience of "medical limbo"—the presence of a painful condition that eludes diagnosis and that carries the implication of either psychiatric causation (or even malingering) on the one hand, or an undiagnosed life-threatening disease on the other—is itself a source of stress and can initiate psychological distress or aggravate a premorbid psychiatric condition. Thus it should hardly be surprising that such patients become preoccupied with feelings of anger, helplessness, hopelessness, frustration, isolation, depression, and pervasive demoralization.

How persons with chronic pain view their plight, more than the presence of physical pathology, will affect how they present themselves to others and how they respond to treatment. As a result of persistent pain, people often become emotionally distressed, experience major sleep disturbance, drastically alter their daily functioning, and worry about the future. These thoughts, feelings, and behaviors will amplify distress and instill inactivity and avoidance of activities that patients fear will produce further pain or harm, leading to even greater physical deconditioning and disability. Thus a vicious circle is initiated and perpetuated.

There has been growing recognition that pain is a complex perceptual experience influenced by a wide range of psychosocial factors—including emotions; social and environmental context; sociocultural background; the meaning of pain to the person; and beliefs, attitudes, and expectations—as well as biological factors (Turk & Monarch, 2002). Moreover, research has suggested that the social and familial context in which pain persists can play a central role in the amplification of pain and maintenance of disability. Consequently, the social context cannot be ignored in considering treatment and facilitating successful rehabilitation. The weighting or balance among various contributors may vary over time and across individuals. However, the psychosocial factors must be evaluated and treated in conjunction with the physical and predispositional psychological ones in order to ensure therapeutic success.

Proliferations of studies, systematic reviews, and several meta-analyses have confirmed the clinical utility and cost-effectiveness of cognitive-behavioral treatments, both alone and combined with more traditional methods (e.g., Guzman et al., 2001; McCracken & Turk, 2002; Morley, Eccleston, & Williams, 1999). In response to the results of this body of research, the role of mental health specialists has been noted in government publications and initiatives, such as that of the U.S. Department of Veterans Affairs. Governmental organizations in other countries (e.g., Canada, Australia, United Kingdom, Sweden) have also documented the important role of psychological factors and psychologists in the reports of pain and pain management. Private medical certifying agencies (e.g., the U.S. Joint Commission on the Accreditation of Healthcare Organizations, the U.S. Commission for the Accreditation of Rehabilitation Facilities) and professional organizations that have proposed practice guidelines (e.g., the American Academy of Neurology) likewise have recognized the importance and complexity of pain and the need to go beyond exclusive reliance on physical modalities to treat patients with pain. Moreover, the acknowledgment of the importance of psychological factors in pain has resulted in a large number of mental health providers' evaluating and treating such patients in specialized pain clinics, in a variety of medical settings, and in private practices. The American Psychological Association has designated psychological treatment of chronic pain as one of the 25 areas for which there is empirical validation for psychological intervention.

In recent years, there has been an explosion of research on psychological factors in pain (e.g., Turk & Okifuji, 2002). With the growth of such a research base, greater attention is now being given to a prescriptive approach, whereby psychologically supported treatments are "tailored" to patients with identified psychosocial characteristics that may be combined with medical interventions and rehabilitative programs (Turk, 1990). Although the research supports the importance of addressing psychological and behavioral factors as well as physical ones, few sources to date have indicated how this should be accomplished.

The challenge becomes how to help people cope with the presence of pain—how to help them live "with it" when their real desire is to live "without it." In this volume, Beverly E. Thorn takes on the challenge. She offers an insightful and informative critique of the role of cognitive processes in chronic pain and beautifully weaves together relevant research with her extensive clinical experience to provide a practical and useful description of a cognitive approach to the treatment of chronic pain. The volume's detailed discussion of the content of each treatment session is enlivened by the use of clinical dialogues and the inclusion of assessment instruments, integration of the assessment within the treatment, advanced organization for each session, summaries highlighting the key points contained in each session for both the clinician and patient, and clinical tips to address common problems encountered are particularly valuable. Following one group of patients throughout the treatment serves as a useful means of demonstrating the connections among the sessions and the incremental process incorporated. This wonderful volume by a master clinician offers important insights coupled with a "how-to-do-it" format. It will be an indispensable resource for those with experience in treating patients with chronic pain, as well as those who are new to treating this difficult population.

DENNIS C. TURK, PhD
University of Washington
School of Medicine

REFERENCES

Bonica, J. J. (1990). *The management of pain* (2nd ed.). Philadelphia: Lea & Febiger. (Original work published 1954)

Guzman, J., Esmail, R., Karjalainen, K., Malmivaara, A., Irvin, E., & Bombardier, C. (2001). Multidisciplinary rehabilitation for chronic low back pain: Systematic review. *British Medical Journal, 322,* 1511–1516.

McCracken, L. M., & Turk, D. C. (2002). Behavioral and cognitive-behavioral treatment for chronic pain: Outcome, predictors of outcome, and treatment process. *Spine, 27,* 2564–2573.

Morley, S., Eccleston, C., & Williams, A. (1999). A systematic review and meta-analysis of randomized controlled trials of cognitive behaviour therapy and behaviour therapy for chronic pain in adults, excluding headache. *Pain, 80,* 1–13.

National Research Council. (2001). *Musculoskeletal disorders and the workplace.* Washington, DC: National Academy Press.

Turk, D. C. (1990). Customizing treatment for chronic pain patients: Who, what, and why. *Clinical Journal of Pain, 6,* 255–270.

Turk D. C. (2002). Clinical effectiveness and cost effectiveness of treatments for chronic pain patients. *Clinical Journal of Pain, 18,* 355–365.

Turk, D. C., & Monarch, E. S. (2002). Biopsychosocial perspective on chronic pain. In D. C. Turk & R. J. Gatchel (Eds.), *Psychological approaches to pain management: A practitioner's guidebook* (2nd ed., pp. 3–29). New York: Guilford Press.

Turk, D. C., & Okifuji, A. (2002). Psychological factors in chronic pain: Evolution and revolution. *Journal of Consulting and Clinical Psychology, 70,* 679–690.

United States Bureau of the Census. (1996). *Statistical Abstract of the United States: 1996.* Washington, DC: Author.

PREFACE

My primary reason for writing this book is to provide a detailed, specific focus on the *cognitive* part of cognitive-behavioral therapy (CBT) for chronic pain. As I interpret the current research, focusing on a patient's cognitive processes will enhance treatment success. In this book, I translate the available psychosocial research into a practical, evidence-based treatment program. Any translation requires personal interpretation, and my book is no exception. Although I rely heavily on findings that have been replicated, some extrapolation is necessary in going from research to clinical application. I hope what I say will encourage practitioners to use the procedures, and will stimulate clinical researchers to further investigate the cognitive processes driving the experience of, and adjustment to, pain.

THE FRAMEWORK FOR COGNITIVE INTERVENTIONS

Although it is clear that behavioral change is a necessary component of adjusting to chronic painful conditions, *motivating* clients to change remains a challenge. I believe cognitive interventions are an important first step in treatment for many sufferers from chronic pain, especially those patients who have a tendency to hold negative distorted thoughts and beliefs about their pain (in traditional pain language, those patients who tend to catastrophize).

The clinician who conceptualizes clients with pain in cognitive terms understands the perspective from which these clients' appraisals, thoughts, and beliefs arise. This context is part biological, part psychological, part interpersonal, and part societal. The milieu shaping health-related cognitions involves the expectations we all have regarding our present-day health care delivery system. As medical technology continues to advance, and medicines become more and more specifically formulated and marketed, our society expects (if not demands) cures for any variety of illnesses, including chronic pain. Our culture also reinforces the belief that people are not responsible for their own bodies' functioning. These attitudes and beliefs prime the pump for seeking the "quick fix" and incite a greater reliance on medication. Perhaps the greatest therapeutic challenge regarding pain management, then, is the obstacle posed by our culture's promotion of the patient as a passive recipient of diagnosis, treatment, and cure. Cognitive interventions can help the clinician chip away at this societal barrier.

An important component of the cognitive conceptualization of pain involves understanding that clients' phenomenological experience of pain (i.e., their thoughts and feelings about the pain) provides the perceptual screen through which any physiological stimulus must pass. When we have pain, it is quite common to ask, "Why this pain? Why this time?" We are seeking an explanation that makes sense—one suggesting that the pain is temporary and not indicative of something much worse. Our self-explanations become beliefs about the nature of the pain, the way it should be treated, and the amount of control we have over the situation.

Pain has adaptive significance: It gets us to orient toward the stimulus causing the pain, appraise the stimulus as a potential threat, and remove ourselves from dangerous situations. Pain also causes withdrawal and reduction or cessation of activity in order to allow damaged tissue to heal, and motivates us to seek diagnosis and treatment. However, when escape from or avoidance of pain is impossible—as is the case in many chronic painful conditions— thoughts of helplessness, hopelessness, and catastrophic outcome often arise.

When medical diagnoses and interventions fail to provide the hoped-for information and treatments, patients still seek explanations and desire an end to their pain. As the patients continue to rest and seek diagnoses and cures, they may spiral downward into a disability syndrome difficult to escape. Subsequently, patients develop the identity of "disabled pain patients," and assume the role commensurate with such a core belief.

INTENDED READERS

This book is for practitioners already focusing on pain management, as well as for clinicians who have more general practices but occasionally treat patients with pain. For those with more general practices, I envision two possible audiences. One group might have a health background (e.g., nurses, health educators) and have some knowledge of the medical aspects of pain, but not be familiar with cognitive therapy. The other group might be mental health practitioners who have some familiarity with cognitive therapy, but not necessarily with pain. Because I expect an audience with varied backgrounds, throughout the text I point to relevant additional sources for readers less familiar with certain topics (e.g., traditional CBT approaches for pain, the basics of cognitive therapy, the pathophysiology of pain).

TERMS OF REFERENCE

You will notice that I interchange the terms "patient" with "client" and "he" with "she" throughout the book. Because the active involvement of the recipient of treatment is so important, and because the term "patient" often conveys that of a passive recipient of diagnosis and treatment, I personally prefer to use the term "client." Also, the term "patient" conveys an illness conceptualization that may not best serve the recipient of therapeutic services, even one with a chronic painful condition. On the other hand, I acknowledge that the use of the term "patient" is very common in clinical psychology as well as in behavioral medicine. Therefore, I have chosen to use both terms in this book. I have also made a choice to use the terms "he" and "she" interchangeably when referring to both the practitioner and the recipient of services. It may be easier to refer to all practitioners as "he" and all clients as "she," but the implication of doing that is obvious and unfortunate. To avoid the awkwardness of using "he/she," I will begin and end one patient example with the same reference (e.g., "she") and then exchange the reference for the next example.

BEVERLY E. THORN

ACKNOWLEDGMENTS

Thank you to my husband, who listened to endless drafts of each chapter, would not accept my catastrophic reactions to constructive criticism, and carried the family load for the duration of the book's writing. Thank you to my son, the "Energizer bunny," who lets me work and helps me play. Thank you also to Jim Nageotte and Barbara Watkins at The Guilford Press, who took great care with my drafts and my insecurities, and nurtured me along on my first book.

CONTENTS

PART II.
A Cognitive Treatment Program for Chronic Pain

Appendices

LIST OF FIGURES, TABLES, AND HANDOUTS

FIGURES

TABLES

THERAPIST HANDOUTS

CLIENT HANDOUTS

All pain is real enough to those who have it;
all stand equally in need of compassion.

—Andrew Miller, *Ingenious Pain*

PART I

RATIONALE, THEORY, RESEARCH, AND ASSESSMENT

CHAPTER 1

WHY FOCUS ON COGNITIONS
IN CHRONIC PAIN?

Our thoughts, usually automatic and often not immediately conscious, have a profound impact on both our short-term and long-term adjustment to pain. Cognitive therapy focuses specifically on the cognitive process and the assumptions and beliefs that underlie this process. Cognitive-*behavioral* therapy (CBT) is a wider approach, often based on a reinforcement (or "operant") model: Thoughts or behaviors that are rewarded increase, and thoughts or behaviors that are ignored decrease. Although all CBT now includes some cognitive interventions, descriptions of CBT approaches typically contain only passing mention or brief coverage of the cognitive components. Simply put, there is a shortage of specific information focusing on cognitive therapeutic interventions for pain management. And that brings us to this book.

WHY COGNITIVE APPROACHES ARE IMPORTANT IN PAIN MANAGEMENT

The multidisciplinary treatment of chronic pain has been the norm for several decades. Historically, the first pain clinics to include a psychological component to their treatment approach were based on the operant model of pain (Fordyce, 1976), and as such were strongly behavioral. In a strict operant model, behavior is determined by reinforcement, and cognitions are irrelevant to the prediction of behavior (Fordyce, Fowler, & DeLateur, 1968). Although the psychological treatment of chronic pain has since expanded to include the cognitive, its heritage is decidedly behavioral. Today's psychologically based interventions are grounded within a cognitive-behavioral model (Turk, Meichenbaum, & Genest, 1983) and do consider cognitive factors, including appraisals, beliefs, and expectations, as well as ongoing

3

cognitive processes, such as automatic thoughts and self-statements. However, the behavioral aspects of psychological treatment for pain have been around longer and are more thoroughly researched than the cognitive aspects. Thus there is more behaviorally based than cognitively based information available to the practitioner. This book tries to remedy that.

Although it is not always clear which components of CBT are the critical agents of change, it is fair to say that the cognitive components are crucial aspects of treatment—not only to reduce pain, but also to improve mood and decrease disability (see, e.g., Kerns, Turk, Holzman, & Rudy, 1986). CBT focused primarily on teaching behavioral self-management skills is less effective for patients who engage in high levels of negative automatic thinking about their pain (Geisser, Robinson, & Riley, 1999; Turk & Rudy, 1992b); therefore, these patients might be especially suited for a cognitive treatment focus. In addition, when offered first in a CBT program, cognitive treatment modules allow for greater cumulative improvement (Knapp & Florin, 1981). (See Chapter 3 for a more thorough discussion of the relevant research literature.)

For some patients, an unfortunate consequence of dealing with chronic pain may be that they come to develop a personal identity as "chronic pain patients." Such persons continue to seek diagnoses and medical cures, often "shopping" from doctor to doctor, to no avail. They also take on a "sick person" role, equating chronic pain with disability. The paradox is that patients who accept their pain as a chronic condition have *lower* perceived pain levels, *less* pain-related distress and depression, *less* avoidance of activities, *lower* levels of disability, and *greater* daily function (McCracken, 1998). "Acceptance" here is defined as recognizing that one has a chronic condition that cannot necessarily be cured, letting go of fruitless attempts to rid oneself of the pain, working toward living a satisfying life despite the pain, and not equating chronic pain with disability. In fact, it has been suggested that one of the main aims of CBT should be to facilitate patients' acceptance of their pain, and, in doing so, to broaden their identity beyond that of "disabled chronic pain patients" (Morley, Shapiro, & Biggs, 2004).

This goal, however, requires starting with a patient who is often a passive recipient of the biomedical "curative" approaches (surgery, medication); moving her toward being an active collaborator in pain self-management strategies (aimed not at eliminating the pain, but rather at increasing function in spite of the pain); and facilitating the ultimate goal of adopting a new identity as a person with pain. Obviously, patients will vary widely in terms of their level of motivation and commitment to take on a very new approach. The typical patient, though, has been well steeped in a medicalized approach to dealing with health-related problems, and thus may enter into CBT with little understanding of what is involved—or may assume that such approaches are for those without "real" pain. Thus it is probably unrealistic to expect typical patients with pain to adopt behavioral self-management strategies, without first helping them to change their mindset. Helping clients to become aware of and examine the thoughts, beliefs, and cognitive schemas that are shaping their coping attempts is an important first step in motivating them to take on a new set of strategies, and ultimately a new identity for themselves. Such cognitive motivational techniques are the essence of this book.

The father of operant treatment for chronic pain, Wilbert Fordyce, asserted that we must get patients with chronic pain to relinquish "ownership" of their pain, indicating that patients who "own" their pain have come to incorporate the pain/illness into their sense of personal identity (W. E. Fordyce, personal communication, October 22, 1999). This goal may be of immense therapeutic value, because many sufferers *do* experience chronic pain as "their pain."

Yet a key to successful treatment is the clinician's understanding and acknowledgment of each patient's pain experience. The challenge of cognitive therapy is to begin within the cognitive and emotional framework of the patient and gradually shape the patient's cognitions toward a different phenomenological experience. Regardless of the causes of the pain (and these are *always* multifaceted), it is the patient's *experience* of pain that is key to cognitive therapy. As we will see, there is clear evidence that the patient's cognitive experience of pain predicts adjustment to a greater extent than any other variable.

Bear in mind that a cognitive approach to pain does not imply a person's pain is not real. Many patients with chronic pain, upon being referred to a mental health practitioner, conclude that the physician believes their pain is psychogenic, functional, or psychologically based (in other words, not "real"). Indeed, when pain persists beyond the point at which an injury is declared to be healed, or when someone has pain but no physical etiology can be found, the patient is often assumed to be willfully exaggerating the pain or making it up to get out of something unpleasant. This is rarely the case. Although there are some few individuals who knowingly fake their pain symptoms, persons characterized as malingerers or those with factitious disorder make up a small percentage of the patients we are likely to see for pain management (Boothby & Thorn, 2002). But many sufferers from pain have had insult added to injury by these inferences. An unfortunate related misconception is that patients overreport the level of pain and distress they actually feel, and have more pain behaviors and greater dysfunction than are warranted by the physical aspects of the pain.

When patients feel that the reality of their pain has been delegitimized by medicine, they are less receptive to potential interventions by mental health practitioners. I have a favorite cartoon: a man sitting in a psychologist's office, who exclaims, "Of course the pain is in my head. It's a headache!" Pain is a perception, and like all perceptions, it is filtered through the brain. I often tell my clients that in a way, the pain *is* in their heads—not in the way that others have implied, but because all pain, even for a broken leg, is in the head. Pain is only perceived as pain because the brain interprets the stimulus as pain. Since the brain is the organ that processes cognitions and emotions, the brain is responsible for integrating sensory, cognitive, and emotional information as part of the interpretive process involved in pain perception. The patient's cognitive and emotional experience of his pain *is* the reality. To really *do* cognitive therapy, the practitioner must successfully "get into the patient's head" as it relates to his pain.

FROM THE BIOMEDICAL MODEL TO THE BIOPSYCHOSOCIAL MODEL

The biopsychosocial model of pain provides a conceptual rationale for including cognitive interventions in pain management strategies. First proposed by Engel (1977), the biopsychosocial model acknowledges biological processes, but also highlights the importance of experiential factors. Prior to the currently accepted biopsychosocial model, a biomedical model dominated all illness conceptualization for almost 300 years and still dominates in the popular imagination. The biomedical approach to pain was, and is, purely mechanistic and reductionistic. This approach sees a simple causal link between the amount of damage to the body and the amount of pain: The more damage, the more pain.

As we now know, the experience of pain does not correspond with amount of tissue damage. We have a wealth of research to support this fact, and here is just one example: In a study exploring the important predictors of disability in workers with low back injuries, researchers found that actual physical pathology accounted for only 10% of the disability 1 year after the evaluation. However, 59% of the disability was explained by psychosocial variables (Burton, Tillotson, Main, & Hollis, 1995). Unfortunately, despite evidence to the contrary, in many ways medicine still operates as if the physical source of the pain is the most important predictor of the experience of pain.

Another common misconception is that acute injury *always* produces pain. If you break your leg, everyone expects you to be in pain. The fracture can be seen on the X-ray; it is quantifiable; it is therefore considered "real," and pain is seen as justified. Nevertheless, the relationship between acute injury and the experience of pain is not as automatic as one might think. For example, during World War II, many U.S. soldiers as well as citizens were severely injured in a battle in Anzio, Italy. Frank Beecher, who was one of the medics there and later went on to become a pain researcher, observed that the meaning of the pain had a great deal to do with a person's experience of pain. Injury to the soldiers meant that they were going home, and many, even those with traumatic amputation of a limb, did not need pain medication. The citizens, on the other hand, had no means of escape; with similar injuries, they experienced fierce pain and required a great deal of analgesic medicine (Beecher, 1959). This example holds personal relevance for me, because my father was one of those who lost a limb at Anzio. Although he didn't remember being interviewed by Beecher, he did remember thinking, "This is my ticket home!"

In their now famous gate control theory of pain, Melzack and Wall (1965, 1982) proposed that the brain plays a *dynamic* role in pain perception, as opposed to simply being the passive recipient of pain signals. They originally hypothesized that a gating mechanism in the spinal cord can widen or narrow as a result of descending signals from the brain, thus allowing relatively more, or fewer, pain signals to ultimately reach the brain. They also suggested that psychological factors can inhibit or enhance the sensory flow of pain signals, and thus influence the way the brain ultimately responds to painful stimulation. If psychological processes can actually change the way the brain processes pain, this holds tremendous potential for psychological interventions. The gate control theory opened the door for pain to be included within the biopsychosocial model of illness.

There is growing research support for the idea that cognitive and emotional activity, such as hypervigilance to potential pain and fear of reinjury, can amplify pain signals and "rewire" the brain circuitry associated with pain perception, thereby increasing the experience of pain. (See Appendix A for more details on the pathophysiology of pain.) For example, in a study using functional magnetic resonance imaging (fMRI), researchers demonstrated that distinct areas of the brain are involved in pain processing versus pain anticipation (Ploghaus et al., 1999). More importantly, although the level of brain activation in the regions associated with sensory pain processing remained stable across time, the level of activation in the more cognitive–emotional pain anticipation regions *increased* over time. Thus it appears that cognitions, emotions, and pain experiences can actually change the way the brain processes input from pain receptors.

The example above involves psychological processes that *increase* brain signals associated with pain. It is even more intriguing to consider the possibility that adaptive cognitions and emotions can *reduce* pain signals and temper the perceptual experience of pain. With the advent of fMRI and other increasingly sophisticated neuroimaging technology, the future holds great promise in helping us quantify pain in a very different way, in-st(image)

cluding a greater appreciation of the importance of cognitive and affective mechanisms in the pain experience.

NOMENCLATURE USED FOR DEFINING, DIAGNOSING, AND TREATING PAIN DISORDERS

Taxonomies of pain, pain diagnoses, and pain treatment methods will not be covered in depth as part of this book. However, some brief information is provided below, as well as references to other resources.

Definitions of Pain

Consistent with the biopsychosocial model of pain, the International Association for the Study of Pain (IASP) defines "pain" as an unpleasant experience that accompanies both sensory *and emotional* modalities; may *or may not* be accompanied by identifiable tissue damage; and is influenced by multiple factors, *including cognitive, affective, and environmental* (Merskey, 1986; Merskey & Bogduk, 1994; emphasis added). Although the IASP does not provide definitions of "chronic pain," "acute pain," or "recurrent pain," since these terms are frequently used clinically and in the research literature, brief descriptions of these and other relevant terms are included in Table 1.1. (See Turk & Okifuji, 2001, for a fuller discussion of pain taxonomy.)

TABLE 1.1. Common Pain Terms

- *Pain*—"An unpleasant sensory and emotional experience associated with actual or potential tissue damage, or described in terms of such damage" (Merskey & Bogduk, 1994, p. 210).

- *Acute pain*—Pain that is elicited by injury and activation of pain receptors (e.g., trauma, surgery, disease), usually lasts a short time, and remits when tissue is healed. Health care intervention is typically sought and often effective (Turk & Okifuji, 2001).

- *Chronic pain*—Pain that is often (but not always) elicited by an injury but worsened by factors removed from the original cause, usually lasts a long time, and is not explained by underlying pathology. Health care intervention is frequently sought and rarely effective (Turk & Okifuji, 2001).

- *Chronic pain versus acute pain*—Distinction commonly defined via arbitrary chronological demarcations (3 months, 6 months), or based on subjective notions of whether the pain extends beyond the expected healing period (Turk & Okifuji, 2001).

- *Recurrent pain*—Pain that is episodic (usually brief), but occurring across an extended time period, thereby sharing characteristics of both acute and chronic pain. Because the problems extend over a long period of time, social and behavioral factors may be more influential over illness behavior than they are with acute pain (Turk & Okifuji, 2001).

- *Pain behaviors*—Verbal or nonverbal actions that communicate discomfort (sighing, grimacing), or are used in an attempt to ameliorate pain (rubbing, using prosthetic devices) (Prkachin, 1986).

- *Disability*—Restriction or loss of capacity to perform an activity in the normal manner (Turk & Okifuji, 2001).

Pain Diagnoses

There are two ways that patients in pain currently receive diagnoses: via the diagnostic system of the *International Classification of Diseases*, 10th revision (ICD-10; World Health Organization, 1992; see also *http://www.cdc.gov/nchs/icd9.htm* and *http://66.17.109/flashcode.home.jsp* for further information), which physicians use to classify physical health problems as well as mental disorders; or via the *Diagnostic and Statistical Manual of Mental Disorders*, 4th edition, text revision (DSM-IV-TR; American Psychiatric Association, 2000), which psychiatrists and psychologists use to classify mental disorders. It is certainly possible for patients to receive ICD diagnoses of physical health problems as well as DSM diagnoses of mental disorders, and comorbidity is not uncommon. Clinicians working with patients who have chronic pain can expect these individuals to carry either or both categories of diagnoses. The criteria and codes for a DSM-IV-TR diagnosis of pain disorder are listed in Table 1.2. See Appendix B for a critique of the ICD and DSM diagnostic systems as they pertain to pain.

Procedural Codes for Treatment

Under the Current Procedural Terminology (CPT) coding system, which provides reimbursement codes for mental health practitioners, activities that have been most frequently reimbursed include clinical interviews; psychological assessments; and individual, couple, and group therapy for patients diagnosed with mental disorders. In January 2002, six additional procedure codes called the Health and Behavior Codes were put in place, and they now provide the means for mental health practitioners to work with patients who have physical health problems but may not have mental illness diagnoses. These codes provide for assessment and intervention activities, including cognitive, behavioral, social, and psychophysiological procedures used for preventing, treating, or managing health problems. Appendix B provides further discussion of the CPT system, as well as a list of the Health and Behavior Codes.

TABLE 1.2. DSM-IV-TR Criteria and Codes for Pain Disorder

DSM-IV-TR criteria for pain disorder

- Pain is reported in one or more specific areas.
- Pain causes distress or functional impairment.
- Psychological issues play a significant role in pain.
- Pain is not purposely produced or feigned.
- Pain is not accounted for better by mood, anxiety, or psychotic disorder, and it does not meet criteria for dyspareunia (painful intercourse).

DSM-IV-TR codes for pain disorder

- 307.80 Pain disorder associated with psychological factors (specify acute or chronic)
- 307.89 Pain disorder associated with both psychological factors and a general medical condition (specify acute or chronic)

FROM THE BIOPSYCHOSOCIAL MODEL OF PAIN
TO THE STRESS–APPRAISAL–COPING MODEL

The biopsychosocial model underscores the important interactions among biological, psychological, and social variables regarding illness and pain. Although it provides an important general reference point, it does not focus on cognitive mechanisms in sufficient detail to be used as a guide for cognitive therapy. Cognitive therapy starts with conceptualizing the client's problems via the cognitive model. The cognitive model (Beck, 1976), is based on the understanding that patients' cognitions have an impact on other thoughts, emotions, behaviors, and even physiological processes. In order to apply the cognitive model to pain, research-based guidelines are needed on what specific patient behaviors, emotions, and especially cognitions are likely to affect the pain experience, and vice versa. For this reason, I have chosen to develop a stress–appraisal–coping model of pain based on the current psychosocial pain research literature, and to adapt Lazarus and Folkman's (1984) transactional model of stress as the structural foundation for the model.

Pain is included among a growing list of stress-related disorders (Humphrey, 1984), and its cognitive, emotional, physiological, and behavioral sequelae fit nicely within a transactional model of stress and coping. Several researchers have suggested conceptualizing chronic pain via a stress-and-coping model (Smith & Wallston, 1992; Thorn, Rich, & Boothby, 1999), but up to the present, it has not been developed to the point of actually applying it in a structured therapeutic approach. In a nutshell, the stress–appraisal–coping model of pain suggests that patients' cognitions have a direct impact on their adjustment to chronic pain through their appraisal of the pain and related stressors, their beliefs about their ability to exert control over the pain situation, and their choice of coping options. Focusing on the cognitive components, the stress–appraisal–coping model of pain provides the basis for the assessment and treatment methods detailed in this book.

OVERVIEW OF THIS BOOK

Following this first chapter, Chapter 2 presents the stress–appraisal–coping model of pain; it also provides the conceptual and organizational rationale for the assessment instruments suggested in the book, as well as the subsequent treatment sessions. Chapter 3 summarizes the research supporting the treatment approach in the rest of the book. Chapter 4 presents a description of assessment instruments relevant to cognitive therapy for pain. (Suggested assessment instruments, with scoring instructions, are included for your use in Appendices C–I.) Part II of the book presents a 10-module manualized treatment approach for the application of cognitive therapy techniques for chronic pain, organized around the stress–appraisal–coping model of pain. The modules are preceded by an introductory chapter that considers general therapeutic issues regarding the process of implementing cognitive therapy for pain management. Case vignettes and excerpts of session transcripts are included in each treatment module, to help illustrate the actual therapeutic issues that arise, and to help bring to life the therapeutic techniques used to deal with them. Each module also includes session outlines as well as homework worksheets, which can be reproduced and given to clients for their use.

CHAPTER SUMMARY

In this chapter, I have introduced the rationale for providing a book focused on cognitive interventions for pain management. The historical context of pain as a purely physical phenomenon (biomedical model) has been critiqued. Cognitive therapy as applied to pain management has been described, and placed within the context of CBT and the biopsychosocial model of pain. Current definitional, diagnostic, and treatment procedure nomenclature has also been reviewed. Finally, the conceptual and organizational framework for the assessment and treatment approach covered in this book, the stress–appraisal–coping model of pain, has been introduced. Chapter 2 will provide the details of this model.

A THEORETICAL MODEL OF COGNITIVE THERAPY FOR CHRONIC PAIN

Cognitive therapy is based on a rich theoretical tradition. The theory in this area is continually evolving and being sharpened, and at the same time, it provides a solid foundation for the research and clinical work that draws from it. However, in order to fruitfully apply cognitive theory and therapy to pain-related issues, clinicians need a detailed, research-based understanding of the interface between cognition and chronic pain. This chapter introduces a stress–appraisal–coping model of pain, which can provide this detailed understanding in a clinically useful way. It also provides the conceptual and organizational structure for the rest of the book.

I begin with Lazarus and Folkman's (1984) transactional model of stress, considering the elements of their model and developing them as they apply to pain. I use their model as an organizational base for several reasons:

1. It is multidimensional, incorporating temperament, biological factors, social considerations, thoughts, and behavior.
2. It considers cognitions at several levels, including immediate reactions to environmental changes, thought processes developed to sort and choose coping options, and beliefs developed over time.
3. It is a model of stress, and I view chronic pain as stress-related.
4. It provides for cognitive treatment approaches.

Others have suggested that a transactional model of stress could be used for understanding chronic pain, but until now this conceptualization has not been developed sufficiently from the standpoint of understanding pain, nor has it been used to formulate an integrated treatment approach. Unless this is done, the stress model is just an interesting theory, but with no direct application to pain. In this chapter, I take a transactional stress model and develop each construct as it relates to the psychosocial pain literature, focusing on cognitions.

According to Lazarus and Folkman's (1984) model, dispositional variables such as personality, stable social roles, and/or biological parameters can affect a person's interaction with a stressor. In addition, people engage in a series of dynamic appraisal processes that influence their response to the stressor, including whether coping responses will be attempted, and which ones, if so. Appraisal processes are thoughts (cognitions), and they involve cognitive interpretations of events or stimuli. "Primary appraisals" are those relating to judgments about whether a potential stressor is irrelevant, benign/positive, or stressful. Beliefs about coping options, and their possible effectiveness, are called "secondary appraisals" in the transactional model of stress. Finally, coping responses, which involve both cognitive and behavioral efforts to manage stress, ultimately influence important adaptational outcomes such as social functioning, morale, and somatic health.

It is clear that the demands of a stressor do not remain static, but are constantly changing. As the demands change, appraisals change, and coping responses are subsequently altered. It has been noted that appraisal and coping often occur in "episodes" of encounter and retreat in response to the changing demands of the stressor (Hewson, 1997). Unfortunately, for patients with chronic pain, the changing demands of the stressor, and the episodes of interaction between appraisal and coping efforts, often reflect a downward spiraling of adaptation and functioning—ultimately leading to a syndrome of disability.

A stress–appraisal–coping model of pain provides an ideal framework for organizing the assessment and cognitive treatment of chronic pain. The model is represented in Figure 2.1.

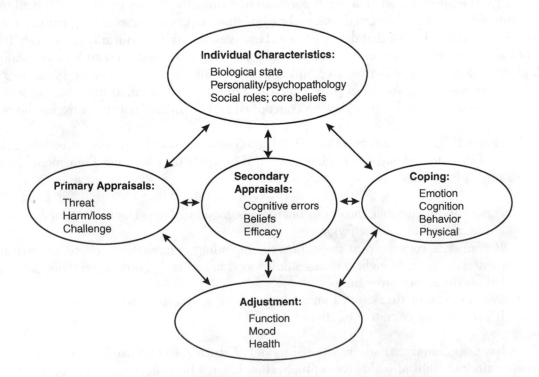

FIGURE 2.1. The stress–appraisal–coping model of pain.

INDIVIDUAL CHARACTERISTICS

A cognitive perspective of pain does not negate the importance of individual variables, such as temperament, biological aspects, and social issues. Such factors are important in formulating the case conceptualization. However, a cognitive conceptualization of pain suggests that cognitions interact with these variables in an important way, and that cognitive therapy can influence cognitive processes.

Biological Factors

As we continue to learn more about the body's complex physiological response to the stress associated with pain, knowledge about pain/stress physiology and about the biological state of the patient becomes increasingly important. For example, we now know that short-term stress responses include constriction or dilation of various blood vessels, which can have a direct impact on muscular or visceral pain. Furthermore, chronic stress responses include a variety of endocrine reactions that compromise immune function. Particular disease states are also important to consider. Some disorders associated with pain (e.g., lupus) may have widespread and devastating physiological consequences, which are often degenerative. Other disorders (e.g., fibromyalgia), although recognized disease states, are poorly understood in terms of pathophysiology or course of illness. Viewing pain from a cognitive perspective does not discount the importance of physiological mechanisms associated with stress and pain. However, the cognitive perspective suggests that the thoughts and feelings associated with one's physical state can have a profound impact on functional adaptation to the disease. In Appendix A, I provide a brief overview of the pathophysiology of pain, stressing how the most recent biomedical findings may help explain the role of the nervous system in chronic pain.

Chronic pain disorders often co-occur with psychological disorders, particularly anxiety and depression, and psychological conditions further complicate the treatment of chronic pain. It is quite common for patients with pain to be prescribed psychotropic medications in addition to pain medications. Since cognitive therapy has been shown to be an evidence-based treatment for mood disorders, the interventions detailed in this book may have the added benefit of helping with clients' depression and anxiety. However, at times it may also be important to have a patient evaluated for a trial of psychotropic medication in conjunction with therapy. Particularly when we consider the long-term efficacy of combination pharmacotherapy and psychotherapy for depression (Keller, McCullough, & Klein, 2000), combined treatments may frequently have merit.

Extensive knowledge regarding pathophysiology and disease states is the purview of physicians, which means that part of any health care provider's comprehensive understanding of a patient with pain will come via communication with one or more physicians involved in the patient's care. This will include information regarding physical assessment procedures, diagnostic information, and physical interventions such as surgery and medication. As I have stated above, since patients with pain are often prescribed a variety of medications, and the need for these medications often changes over time, it is important to establish and maintain a collaborative relationship with each patient's primary physician. At the end of Appendix B, I provide a sample summary note that can be copied to a collaborating physician as a guide for initiating such a relationship.

Social Roles

Although pain experts recognize that the experience of pain is influenced by biological, psychological, *and social* factors, the social context of pain has received relatively little attention. Since social roles have an important influence on the way we all behave, it makes sense that they would merit consideration in the comprehensive evaluation of potentially disabling states, such as chronic pain (Fordyce, 1998). Social roles are multidimensional and cover a diverse range of contexts, such as personal roles (including gender roles), family roles (including couple roles), societal roles, occupational roles, and roles within the health care system (including patient roles). Although family context has received some consideration in the pain literature, its coverage typically involves interpersonal interactions between patients and spouses or partners. Patient roles adopted by sufferers from chronic pain have received virtually no research attention, and future research in this area would be a welcome contribution to our knowledge base. (For a more complete discussion of the importance of social context in understanding pain, see Ranjan, 2001.)

Gender role issues have received more research attention than any other social roles in the area of pain. "Gender role" refers to a society's generally accepted set of characteristics for each sex. As this pertains to pain, the male gender role ("masculinity") is stereotypically that of stoicism, whereas the female gender role ("femininity") is stereotypically that of increased sensitivity (Fillingim, 2001).

It is well known that women are more likely than men to report high levels of pain (Hasvold & Johnson 1993; Verbrugge, 1990), show higher rates of health care utilization (Taylor & Curran, 1985), and display more pain behavior (Keefe et al., 2000; Sullivan, Tripp, & Santor, 2000) (see Unruh, 1996, for a review). The factors responsible for sex differences in pain are still not completely understood, although differences in physiology have historically been given more weight than psychosocial variables (Lautenbacher & Rollman, 1993; Levin & DeSimone, 1991; Unruh, 1996). Several studies have shown that the extent to which one takes a traditional gender role (i.e., the level at which one adopts stereotyped notions of "masculine" and "feminine") is associated with pain responsiveness (Hochstetler, Rejeski, & Best, 1985; Otto & Dougher, 1985; Sanford, Kersh, Thorn, Rich, & Ward, 2002). Furthermore, when researchers statistically control for gender role, the sex differences commonly found between men and women tend to disappear (Thorn et al., in press).

Differences in the socialization of male and female children with regard to pain are apparent very early in life. For example, in an observational study of preschool children, although boys and girls did not differ in the frequency or severity of pain-causing incidents, adult caregivers provided more physical comfort to girls who were expressing distress. In addition, girls were much more likely than boys to react to pain by crying, screaming, or showing anger (Fearon, McGrath, & Achat, 1996). This increased attention toward girls may have a detrimental impact in the long run. If female children are habitually responded to with greater concern and caregiving than male children, it is possible that they are being shaped into individuals with a greater propensity toward dependence and a personal sense of emotional vulnerability.

Personality Factors

Personality characteristics, such as a tendency toward certain styles of thinking, are also individual variables that belong in a cognitive conceptualization of pain adaptation. In a diathesis–stress model of chronic pain, Turk (2002b) has proposed that certain predispositional factors, including temperamental tendencies toward negative affectivity, increase one's risk for becoming disabled following exposure to physical trauma. There is a body of research evidence demonstrating an association among personality characteristics such as neuroticism (Affleck, Urrows, Tennen, & Higgins 1992; Martin et al., 1996), negative affectivity (Crombez, Eccleston, Van den Broek, Van Doudenhove, & Goubert, 2002), and emotional vulnerability (Thorn et al., in press) on the one hand, and the experience of pain on the other. These dispositional tendencies are seen as less changeable than are cognitive processes such as automatic thoughts, or mood states such as anxiety.[1] Nevertheless, they may be important to understand, particularly when making predictions about prognosis for a particular patient. Since psychologists often provide these types of assessments, other health care professionals, including physicians, may expect to confer with psychologists during the process of case conceptualization and treatment planning for patients with pain. Additional information regarding personality assessment is provided in Chapter 4.

Core Beliefs

Dysfunctional attitudes (often referred to as negative "core beliefs" or "schemas"; Beck, 1976) could also be included under the individual-differences category in the proposed model of pain. In the cognitive therapy literature, core beliefs are seen as the most deeply held processes—underlying "worldviews" about the self. Negative core beliefs and negative schemas are not necessarily activated unless negative life events trigger them. However, they are thought to create a cognitive vulnerability that interacts with negative life events to lead to a variety of emotional disorders (Haaga, Dyck, & Ernst, 1991; Henriques & Leitenberg, 2002). If negative core beliefs (negative schemas, temperamental diatheses) create a cognitive vulnerability that makes sufferers from chronic pain more predisposed toward dysfunction and disability, then these core beliefs need to be assessed and addressed as part of the cognitive therapeutic process. Since chronic pain and associated stressors are certainly interpreted as negative life events by clients, it is reasonable to expect that they will activate negative core beliefs, and these beliefs must therefore be addressed in therapy. In addition to general core beliefs, patients with pain develop beliefs about themselves as persons in pain (e.g., "disabled," "pain patient"). These deeply held pain-related beliefs can also have an impact on a patient's ultimate adaptation, and therefore must be considered in therapy. Suggestions for the assessment of general dysfunctional attitudes/core beliefs are made in Chapter 4.

Table 2.1 summarizes the discussion above regarding individual characteristics and associated adjustment to pain.

PRIMARY APPRAISALS

In a transactional model of stress, "stress" is not an event or stimulus. Rather, it is the judgment that an event or stimulus taxes or exceeds one's resources, thereby endangering one's well-being. According to this conceptualization, something not appraised as stressful is not

---

[1]This is not to say that patients with chronic pain have a disorder of personality. It is important not to equate personality tendencies with the strongly pejorative label of "personality disorder." Personality disorders are specific diagnostic entities characterized by, among other things, long-standing and notable relationship difficulties.

TABLE 2.1. Individual Characteristics Associated with Adjustment to Pain

- *Biological factors*: Disease state (e.g., type and course) does not predict dysfunction, but provides a context for understanding the types of medical treatment the patient may have (e.g., surgery, medication).

- *Social roles*: Gender roles and cultural expectations have an impact on beliefs about the cause and "appropriate" treatment of pain, thus influencing choice of coping options.

- *Personality factors*: Temperamental characteristics such as neuroticism, negative affectivity, and emotional vulnerability increase risk of disability.

- *Core beliefs*: Deeply held beliefs about the self as a person in pain may evolve over the course of illness, but are grounded in early formulations about the self.

considered a stressor. In terms of pain, then, in the absolute sense neither the pain stimulus itself nor the biological response to the stimulus is considered "stress."[2] The cognitive process that translates the stimulus and response into "threatening" and "unmanageable" is the root of stress. "Pain," then, would only be considered a stressor when and if a person judges the perceptual experience as taxing or exceeding his ability to manage it.

Lazarus and Folkman (1984) identified three types of primary appraisals of an event or stimulus: "threat" (perception that the danger posed by the situation outweighs the individual's ability to cope); "harm/loss" (perception that damage has occurred as a result of the stimulus); and "challenge" (perception that the ability to cope is not outweighed by the potential danger of the stimulus). Appraisals regarding potential harm produce negative emotions such as fear and anxiety, whereas appraisals regarding damage done produce grief, sadness, and depressive emotions. Furthermore, appraisals that pain is stressful, harmful, and threatening have been associated with psychological dysfunction (Regan, Lorig, & Thoresen, 1988). On the other hand, appraisals focusing on the challenging aspects of the event(s) might produce feelings of commitment or conviction, or possibly even eagerness or excitement—particularly when the person believes that effective coping responses are possible. I will discuss the assessment of primary pain appraisals in Chapter 4. In the paragraphs below, each of the primary appraisal categories is considered and discussed as it relates to the experience of pain.

Threat Appraisals and Pain

If a pain stimulus is appraised as threatening, it probably engenders a particular type of cognitive processing—that is, a focus of attention toward the stimulus—as well as giving rise to certain emotional responses. Patients with chronic pain frequently complain of poor memory and inability to concentrate. In the field of cognitive psychology, the divided-attention theory suggests that people have a limited capacity for attention (Kahneman, 1973). If someone is overfocused on one stimulus, there is less attention available for other stimuli or cognitive

[2]The sensory stimuli associated with pain usually elicit some type of withdrawal or aversive response, but may not do so under certain conditions. The most dramatic example may be the cultural hook-hanging ceremony still practiced in some societies today, where a "celebrant" is chosen to represent the gods and bless the children and crops. Steel hooks are embedded in the man's back, from which he swings freely at the climax of the ceremony. Rather than eliciting "pain" or "stress," these nociceptive stimuli instead elicit euphoria (Kosambi, 1967).

tasks. There is support for this model as it relates to pain and memory (Kuhajda, Thorn, & Klinger, 1998; Kuhajda, Thorn, Klinger, & Rubin, 2002). Thus a hypervigilant focus on pain stimuli (or *anticipated* pain stimuli) may be a culprit in reducing a patient's ability to concentrate and attend to other tasks, as well as remembering important information. In addition to reducing one's available attention for other tasks, threat appraisals may give rise to emotional responses (e.g., anxiety, worry, fear of pain or reinjury) and behavioral responses (e.g., discontinuance or avoidance of activities that may be associated with pain). Fear of pain may further increase the patient's focus of attention on pain-related stimuli (Asmundson, Kuperos, & Norton, 1997; McCracken, 1997) and increase reluctance to engage in activities that might produce discomfort (Crombez, Vervaet, Lysens, Baeyens, & Eelen, 1998). Avoidant behaviors, of course, add to the physical deconditioning of the patient, thus compounding the disability associated with the pain condition.

Loss Appraisals and Pain

The perception of the pain stimulus itself is not the only aspect of chronic pain that is perceived as stressful. Patients rarely maintain the level of activity they enjoyed previous to the chronic pain condition, often do not work, usually experience a significant loss of income and economic quality of life, and frequently exhibit associated relationship difficulties. Whereas the pain stimulus itself is likely to elicit a threat appraisal, the environmental challenges associated with chronic pain are likely to bring forth a primary appraisal of loss. There is some qualitative research supporting the hypothesis that patients with chronic pain often experience a sense of loss surrounding their circumstances (Walker, Holloway, & Sofaer, 1999). In addition, interviews with patients often reflect a perception of loss—for example, "I did a lot of hiking. I did a lot of camping. I did a lot of wrestling with the kids. And when the back injury happened, a lot of that was taken away" (Rhodes, McPhillips-Tangum, Markham, & Klenk, 1999, p. 1200). Depressed affect, a perceived sense of helplessness, and a reduced likelihood of engaging in adaptive coping behaviors are likely to be related to this sense of loss. Thus the primary appraisal of loss is also associated with affective and behavioral responses that do not bode well for ultimate adjustment. Each of these losses may contribute to the stress of a person with chronic pain, and each is thus an appropriate target for cognitively based pain therapy.

Challenge Appraisals

As it turns out, patients with chronic pain don't seem to use challenge appraisals very much in appraising the stress associated with their pain. In a telephone survey of individuals experiencing troubling pain in the past 2 weeks, only 14% of the sample appraised their most recently experienced pain as a challenge, even to a slight degree. By far, this sample appraised recent pain experiences as a threat to their well-being (Unruh & Ritchie, 1998). There is some evidence that in acute pain situations, men appraise pain as a challenge more often than women do. In this particular experiment, the level of threat appraisal accounted for the differences between the sexes in tolerance time in a laboratory-induced pain situation (Sanford et al., 2002).

Table 2.2 summarizes this discussion of primary appraisal processes and their pain-related sequelae.

TABLE 2.2. Three Kinds of Primary Appraisals and Their Sequelae

- **Threat:** The perception that danger outweighs coping ability.
  - *Emotion:* Produces negative emotions such as fear and anxiety, which can be psychologically debilitating.
  - *Cognition:* Narrows and fixates focus of attention toward pain or potential pain stimulus—thus lessening ability to shift attention to other stimuli, distorting a more realistic appraisal, and resulting in poor concentration and memory.
  - *Behaviors:* Reduces engagement in activities that might increase discomfort, and increases avoidance behaviors—leading to physical deconditioning, and thus exacerbating the disability.

- **Harm/loss:** The perception that damage has occurred/resulted from stimulus.
  - *Emotion:* Produces grief, sadness, and depressive emotions—all associated with psychological dysfunction.
  - *Cognition:* Increases thoughts of loss and helplessness—thus distorting a more realistic appraisal of the stressful situation.
  - *Behaviors:* Increases passivity, and reduces physical activity and other activities of daily living— leading to loss of work, income, and economic quality of life, as well as relationship difficulties.

- **Challenge:** The perception that ability to cope is not outweighed by potential danger.
  - *Emotion:* Produces feelings of commitment or conviction, and in certain situations even eagerness or excitement.
  - *Cognition:* Leads to belief that effective coping responses are possible, and to perception of some pain-related stimuli as a challenge. Stressors are perceived more realistically. Self-identification as a "well person with pain."
  - *Behaviors:* Increases likelihood of pain self-management, as well as engagement in independent activities of daily living—leading to lessened disability.

SECONDARY APPRAISALS

Secondary appraisals, like primary appraisals, are considered cognitive processes that can elicit emotions and influence one's choice of coping options. Acquired beliefs about the pain condition, and automatic thoughts that arise in anticipation of or in response to the pain, are considered secondary cognitive appraisal processes. A "belief" is a mental appraisal (cognition) regarding a situation, another person, or oneself. Beliefs can range from very global reflections of one's philosophy about the world or the self to highly specific appraisals of a particular circumstance (Lazarus & Folkman, 1984). Whereas a belief has been described as a cognitive understanding of a condition or event (Wrubel, Benner, & Lazarus, 1981), "automatic thoughts" are cognitions that arise somewhat mechanistically in response to a circumstance. Automatic thoughts can be likened to a running stream of semiconscious thought processes associated with the experience of pain or anticipated pain. Certainly, beliefs and automatic thoughts interact and mutually influence each other, and both influence coping and adaptation. Since a cognitive conceptualization of chronic pain assumes that patients' cognitive activity is central to their adjustment and recovery, it is imperative to be able to assess and treat the patients' thoughts, both general and specific. For the purposes of this book, the term "belief" is used to reflect relatively more strongly held assumptions about the self, the world, or a situation, and "automatic thoughts" to refer to cognitions that arise somewhat unconsciously in response to a particular event. When these acquired beliefs or automatic thoughts are negatively distorted, they are considered to be cognitive errors. Assessment of pain-related automatic thoughts and of intermediate beliefs is discussed in Chapter 4.

Acquired (Intermediate) Beliefs

People experiencing chronic pain develop a set of beliefs about their pain and their ability to cope with the pain. Perhaps in order to help make sense of their condition, they formulate ideas about the cause of the pain and the way it should be treated. They acquire certain viewpoints about appropriate and inappropriate responses to their pain (e.g., "I should rest and avoid reinjury," "Others should be solicitous of my pain"). They also hold beliefs about how much control they have over their condition, whether they can execute certain coping responses, and whether particular coping responses will have any impact on their pain.

Beliefs about the cause, meaning, and ability to influence pain roughly correspond to the cognitive therapy terminology of "intermediate beliefs." Intermediate beliefs often have an underlying "should" or "must" message behind them.

Beliefs about Pain

Patients with chronic pain hold numerous beliefs about the cause, meaning, and appropriate treatment of their pain. These beliefs are not only personally formed, but also can be culturally shared. Many of these commonly held beliefs are erroneous as well as maladaptive. For example, a large survey study in Belgium found that many people—whether they had low back pain or not—believed that such pain is a direct result of injury, that movement is likely to exacerbate the condition, and that rest and pain medications are the best treatment options (Szpalski, Nordin, Skovron, Melot, & Cukier, 1995). Such beliefs undoubtedly influence the type of treatment persons with back pain will seek, as well as their willingness to engage in treatment approaches that are counterintuitive to their beliefs. In addition, since people without back pain conditions were also found to hold these beliefs, the significant others of people with back pain are likely to reinforce and strengthen these beliefs in the sufferers.

A patient's belief about the cause of pain—independent of distinct differences in physical pathology—has an impact on the amount of distress and disability the patient has, and also influences the treatment approach taken by physicians. In a study of patients with heterogeneous chronic pain, patients associating the onset of pain with trauma reported higher pain severity, and showed more emotional distress and greater life interference, than patients reporting a more ambiguous onset. However, there were no objective differences in physical pathology between the patients who attributed the onset of their pain to a specific trauma and those who did not. Also, patients reporting a traumatic onset to pain were more likely to be prescribed opioid medication, nerve blocks, and transcutaneous electrical nerve stimulation by physicians than those patients who did not report a traumatic onset (Turk & Okifuji, 1996; Turk, Okifuji, Starz, & Sinclair, 1996). Thus, regardless of distinct differences in physical pathology, one's belief about the cause of pain affects the treatment approach taken by physicians and can make the pain even more difficult to cope with.

Beliefs about One's Control over Pain

The concepts of "locus of control" (LOC), "self-efficacy," and "outcome expectancy" were derived from social learning theory (Bandura, 1986), which states that on the basis of their history of reinforcement, individuals develop patterns of expectancies and beliefs about the level of control they have over their environment. It is not really known whether the concepts of LOC and self-efficacy are different from each other. Some researchers have suggested that these concepts share a great deal of commonality and may be markers of some higher-order construct, such as neuroticism or self-esteem (Judge, Erez, Bono, & Thoreson, 2002). Since LOC and self-efficacy have extensive coverage as separate entities in the research literature, and since each has been associated with treatment outcome, they are worth discussing separately.

LOC refers to beliefs about whether certain outcomes in life are the results of one's efforts (internal) or the results of luck, fate, or the actions of others (external). Patients endorsing high internal LOC report lower pain intensities and less frequent pain than those endorsing low internal LOC; they also gain more from multidisciplinary pain treatment, learn their exercises better, and perform the exercises more frequently following treatment (Harkapaa, 1991; Harkapaa, Jarvikoski, Mellin, Hurri, & Luoma, 1991). In addition, successful multidisciplinary treatment is associated with large decreases in patients' attribution of pain control to luck, fate, or the actions of others, and moderate increases in their sense of personal control over their pain (Lipchik, Milles, & Covington, 1993).

Self-efficacy is the belief that one can actually perform a certain behavior, and outcome expectancies are judgments regarding the consequences of such behavior. It is clear from numerous research studies that perceived self-efficacy operates as an important cognitive factor in adaptation to chronic painful states. For example, in a study of inpatients with chronic pain, patients' beliefs about their ability to carry out a particular therapeutic activity were strongly related to their efforts to cope, although patients' beliefs about the consequences of their coping efforts (outcome expectancy) were generally unrelated to their coping efforts (Jensen, Turner, & Romano, 1991). Thus patients' beliefs about what they can do in an effort to cope may be more important than their beliefs about whether or not these coping efforts actually work! Why might this be the case? Perhaps it doesn't matter too much whether I believe that a certain coping strategy will work if I don't believe that I can carry out the therapeutic activity in the first place. At the very least, if I know that I can carry out certain coping options, there is at least a chance that *something* will work.

Automatic Thoughts/Cognitive Errors

In the cognitive therapy literature, automatic thoughts are considered to be the easiest to identify and change of the potential cognitive errors. Automatic thoughts are so named because they happen without effort and occur almost reflexively, making them seem preprogrammed. As such, patients may not be consciously aware of the thoughts. Automatic thoughts seem to occur with great frequency, taking place as an ongoing dialogue of thought processes associated with a specific environmental event or circumstance. Automatic thoughts, like core beliefs and intermediate beliefs, may or may not be factual; when factually distorted, they are considered to be cognitive errors. Beck (1976) and others have written a great deal about the association of cognitive errors (i.e., disorders in thinking) with disorders of emotion. With pain disorders as well, there is substantial research evidence that the greater the tendency to display overly negative, distorted automatic thoughts, the greater a patient's report of pain, dysfunction, depression, and overall maladjustment to the pain condition (Jensen, Turner, Romano, & Karoly, 1991). In addition, several studies have shown that the association between cognitive distortions and maladjustment is specific to pain-related cognitive errors and not to more general cognitive errors (Flor & Turk, 1988; Smith, Follick, Ahern, & Adams, 1986; Smith, Peck, Milano, & Ward, 1988).

Catastrophizing

Without question, the cognitive thought process labeled "catastrophizing" has been studied more than any other cognitive variable thought to influence pain perception and adjustment to pain. Pain researchers first using the term "catastrophizing" agreed that the construct involves negative pain-related cognitions, but they differed in their descriptions regarding the kinds of negative thoughts they observed. For example, Chaves and Brown (1987) asked persons undergoing a stressful dental procedure to report the thoughts and images they experienced, or the strategies they engaged in, during the procedure. Participants characterized as "catastrophizers" were described as individuals who had a tendency to *magnify or exaggerate the threat value* or seriousness of the pain sensations (e.g., "I wonder whether something serious may happen"). Spanos, Radtke-Bodorik, Ferguson, and Jones (1979) interviewed subjects about their pain experience following an experimental cold-pressor task (ice-water immersion of the hand). Individuals who reported thought content reflecting *worry, fear, and the inability to divert attention away from pain* were classified as "catastrophizers" (e.g., "I kept thinking, 'I can't stand this much longer; I want to get out' "). In developing the Coping Strategies Questionnaire, Rosenstiel and Keefe (1983) included a Catastrophizing subscale in their measure. The items on the Catastrophizing subscale reflected elements of *helplessness and pessimism* in relation to one's ability to deal with the pain experience (e.g., "It's terrible and it's never going to get any better"). What is important from our perspective as practitioners is that this construct we refer to as "pain-related catastrophizing" is most definitely a cognitive process associated with maladaptive, distorted thinking.

The conceptualization of "catastrophizing" as it is used in the pain literature denotes a much broader range of concepts than the term in traditional cognitive therapy literature. Whereas in conventional cognitive therapy, the term has been used to denote very specific cognitive errors (i.e., making negative predictions about future outcomes that may not be realistic—Beck, 1976; or focusing on and exaggerating the negative aspects of a particular experience—Burns, 1980), in the pain literature, "catastrophizing" refers to a variety of negative automatic thoughts.

Pain-related catastrophizing has been variously conceptualized as a primary appraisal process, a secondary appraisal process, and a coping strategy (Sullivan, Thorn, et al., 2001; Thorn, Rich, & Boothby, 1999). Although I have chosen to introduce the concept of catastrophizing under the category of secondary appraisals (specifically, automatic thoughts), catastrophic thoughts can occur as part of the primary appraisal process, as part of automatic thoughts, or as part of acquired belief systems. In the treatment modules of this book, I will be introducing techniques that target catastrophic thought processes (or any cognitive distortions, for that matter) as they occur in primary appraisal as well as in secondary appraisal (automatic thoughts, intermediate beliefs) processes.

Other Cognitive Errors

It is clear that patients with chronic painful conditions have other types of negative, distorted thoughts in addition to catastrophizing, even when the concept of catastrophizing is broadly defined, as above. For example, during clinical interviews, such patients have made statements reflecting a negative sense of self (e.g., "I am useless"), negative thoughts about interactions with others (e.g., "No one wants to hear about my problems"), and self-blame regarding their pain problems (e.g., "It's my own fault that I hurt like this") (Gil, Williams, Keefe, & Beckham, 1990). From these interviews, an assessment instrument was constructed regarding negative thoughts in response to pain flare-ups (the Inventory of Negative Thoughts in Response to Pain [INTRP]; Gil et al., 1990). In three different populations with chronic pain (patients with sickle cell disease, rheumatoid arthritis, and mixed chronic pain), responding to a pain episode with negative self-statements and negative thoughts about interactions with others was found to be associated with more severe pain and psychological distress during a pain flare-up.[3] In addition, it was found that patients with chronic daily pain had more frequent negative thoughts during a pain episode than patients having intermittent pain (Gil et al., 1990). We do not know how closely these types of negative thoughts overlap with depressive thoughts, but it is clear that in addition to paying attention to clients' negative catastrophic automatic thoughts in response to pain, we should attend to what patients say about themselves and their interactions with others in response to pain, particularly during a pain flare-up. It is also important to be aware that unremitting daily pain is a risk factor for the types of negative thoughts discussed above, and that these negative automatic thoughts make it even more difficult for a patient to cope.

Table 2.3 summarizes the preceding discussion of secondary appraisal processes and associated adjustment to pain.

TABLE 2.3. Categories of Secondary Appraisals and Associated Implications

- *Intermediate beliefs:* Acquired attitudes arising from personal, cultural, and environmental factors, often characterized by "should," "must," and "ought."

  - *Beliefs about pain*: Attitudes about the nature of pain, the cause of pain, and/or the appropriate treatment for pain; these influence both distress and disability.

  - *Beliefs about one's control over pain*: Attitudes based on sense of self-efficacy (belief in ability to carry out a relevant task) and LOC (self—internal, or others—external); these influence willingness to engage in pain self-management.

- *Automatic thoughts/cognitive errors*: Frequently occurring, situation-driven thoughts that can occur without conscious awareness, and that influence ultimate selection of coping strategy.

  - *Catastrophizing*: A negatively distorted orientation to pain or anticipated pain. A robust predictor of perceived pain levels, disability, and adaptation to chronic pain conditions.

  - *Other cognitive errors*: Negative sense of self, negative interpretation of interaction with others, and self-blame. All are associated with greater distress and dysfunction.

---

[3]By "pain flare-up," I am referring to an episode of pain exacerbation, which is usually the most difficult for a client to deal with. Patients with chronic pain may or may not have constant, unremitting pain; some will have intermittent pain. However, all such patients deal with episodes of pain, which are often called "pain flare-ups."

COPING

Coping responses include both cognitive and behavioral efforts to lessen perceived stress (Lazarus & Folkman, 1984). By "cognitive" coping, I am referring to techniques that might influence one's pain, or the impact of stressors related to pain, via one's thoughts. "Behavioral" coping techniques, on the other hand, modify overt behavior in an effort to alleviate pain or pain-related stressors. Although coping strategies are often categorized as "behavioral" or "cognitive," the lines drawn between the two categories of coping are not rigid, and they should be considered relative rather than fixed categories.

It is important to acknowledge that for patients with chronic pain, the pain stimulus itself is not the only thing with which they must cope. As I have noted earlier, chronic pain has a number of associated stressors, and each requires (possibly different) coping efforts. Coping with chronic pain encompasses all of the efforts made to deal with the multiple physical, emotional, and behavioral ramifications of a chronic pain condition, and each stressor may require a different kind of coping effort.

Coping is not necessarily linked with mastery or with adaptive outcome. For example, even if relaxation exercises do not result in pain reduction (or some other anticipated outcome), they are still considered coping attempts because they are efforts to reduce the impact of a chronic painful condition (Keefe, Lefebvre, & Smith, 1999). On a related note, some coping efforts (such as expressive pain behaviors to solicit emotional support) may actually be maladaptive or unhelpful, but if they are employed in an attempt to manage demands that are judged to tax or exceed the resources of the person, they are nonetheless considered under the category of coping (Hewson, 1997).

Within a cognitive conceptualization of pain, it is assumed that the necessary preconditions for a client to engage in any sort of adaptive coping (behavioral or cognitive) include the cognitive processes (primary and secondary appraisals) conducive to those coping efforts. For example, if a patient views your treatment goal of increased exercise as having great potential for exacerbating his pain condition (primary appraisal—threat), and he believes the best treatment for his back pain is inactivity (secondary appraisal—intermediate belief about pain), he is unlikely to comply with the treatment. Or if another patient believes her fibromyalgia has taken her away from the activities that previously brought her satisfaction (primary appraisal—loss), she may also be less likely to believe that she can have an impact on her pain or even successfully carry out the treatment tasks expected of her (secondary appraisal—intermediate belief about control over pain), and she too is unlikely to comply with treatment. Thus patients' primary and secondary appraisals certainly interact with their selection and implementation of potential coping responses, and this is why the cognitive therapy techniques presented in this book focus on these appraisal processes.

Table 2.4 presents a summary of the concept of coping as it relates to chronic pain.

TABLE 2.4. Summary of Coping and Its Relation to Chronic Pain

- Includes behavioral and cognitive efforts.
- Represents attempts to reduce pain *or* stress related to pain.
- May *or may not* be related to mastery or adaptive outcome.

ADJUSTMENT

The last component of the stress–appraisal–coping model of pain is the adjustment component. The concept of "adjustment" is multidimensional, and should not be equated with the unidimensional notion of reduced or eliminated pain as *the* measure of success. Successful adjustment is measured along a variety of domains, including, among others, affective, behavioral, and perceptual. Lazarus and Folkman (1984) conceptualize adjustment along three dimensions: social functioning, morale, and somatic health. Particularly for patients with chronic pain, positive adjustment does not simply refer to psychological well-being, but also encompasses physical and social functioning. The aspects of adjustment most relevant to these patients include pain severity, pain behaviors, activity level, physical strength, mobility, medication use, health services utilization, employment status, and affective variables such as depression and anxiety (Jensen, Turner, Romano, & Karoly, 1991). These variables have been further categorized into three separate components of adjustment to chronic pain: activity level, psychological functioning, and utilization of medication/professional services (Jensen & Karoly, 1991). Although the focus of this book is on cognitive assessment and interventions, bear in mind that our ultimate goal as practitioners is to influence the various markers of adjustment mentioned above. As you will read in Chapter 3, measures of treatment success are often made with specific reference to these markers of adjustment. Table 2.5 presents a summary of the concept of adjustment as it relates to chronic pain.

So far in this chapter, I have proposed a stress–appraisal–coping model of pain. The final part of this chapter provides an overview of the cognitive treatment program for chronic pain presented in this book. As shown in Table 2.6, it integrates standard cognitive treatment techniques into the stress–appraisal–coping model of pain.

WHAT IS COGNITIVE THERAPY AS APPLIED TO PAIN MANAGEMENT?

Early in his formulation of the cognitive model, Beck (1976) theorized that at the core of various mental disorders (particularly anxiety and depression), there is a disorder in thinking. He posited that this thinking disorder involves an idiosyncratic but systematic bias in information

---

TABLE 2.5. Summary of Adjustment and Its Relation to Chronic Pain

- Involves more than an elimination of pain.
- Is multidimensional, involving physical, social, and psychological functioning.
- Is often quantified using these measures:.
  - Perceived pain (including intensity and unpleasantness).
  - Psychological function (especially distress, depression).
  - Activity level (including work status, disability markers).
  - Medication intake (sometimes separated into sedative/hypnotics, nonopioid analgesics, and opioid analgesics).
  - Health care utilization (number of physician contacts, number of hospitalizations, or number of surgeries).

TABLE 2.6. Integration of the Elements of the Stress–Appraisal–Coping Model of Pain with Associated Cognitive Techniques Offered in This Book

- *Individual variables (core beliefs)*: Acquired, deep-seated belief systems about the self, acquired in part during childhood. Also, core beliefs about the self as a person in pain, which develop partly from general core beliefs acquired in childhood. Core beliefs often give rise to intermediate beliefs.
  - *Intervention*: Identifying Beliefs and Changing Beliefs (for general, non-pain-specific, core beliefs— Module 5)
  - *Intervention*: Identifying Pain Beliefs and Changing Pain Beliefs (for pain-specific core beliefs— Module 6)

- *Primary appraisals*: Initial judgments regarding pain or potential pain, and related environmental demands. These shape secondary appraisals and selection of potential coping options.
  - *Intervention*: Recognizing the Stress–Pain–Appraisal Connection (Module 1)

- *Secondary appraisals*: Automatic thoughts and acquired intermediate beliefs regarding pain, anticipated pain, and related environmental demands.
  - *Automatic thoughts*: Frequently occurring cognitions in reaction to various environmental demands.
    - *Intervention*: Identifying Automatic Thoughts (Module 2)
    - *Intervention*: Evaluating Automatic Thoughts (Module 3)
    - *Intervention*: Challenging Automatic Thoughts and Constructing Alternative Thoughts (Module 4)
  - *Intermediate beliefs*: Acquired attitudes toward how the world "ought" to be, and toward one's chronic pain condition. These often give rise to automatic thoughts.
    - *Intervention*: Identifying Beliefs and Changing Beliefs (Module 5)
    - *Intervention*: Identifying Pain Beliefs and Changing Pain Beliefs (Module 6)

- *Coping*: Cognitive, affective, and behavioral attempts to manage pain and associated environmental demands. Cognitive coping involves thoughts, or thought techniques, used in an attempt to mitigate the stress (including emotional distress) associated with chronic pain.
  - *Intervention*: Constructing Coping Self-Statements (Module 7)
  - *Intervention*: Using Expressive Writing (Module 8)
  - *Intervention*: Learning and Using Assertive Communication (Module 9)

processing, recall, and interpretation of events and experiences. I am not proposing that chronic pain is caused by a disorder in thinking. Rather, as shown in this chapter and detailed in the next chapter, there is evidence that chronic pain is often associated with particular information-processing styles and characteristic themes regarding interpretation of events and experiences. As we will see, there is evidence that although many pain-related thoughts and appraisals contain some truth, they are distorted to some extent, causing unnecessary suffering. The brain is the interpretive agent, and thoughts and feelings are situated in the brain. If patients' brains say that they are in pain, that assertion is the reality. This contention, of course, renders the organic–psychogenic distinction obsolete. Moving beyond the physiological (nociceptive) stimulus, to understanding the cognitive and emotional implications of an individual client's pain, is the essence of a cognitive conceptualization.

The stress–appraisal–coping model of pain asserts that patients' cognitions impact their adjustment to chronic pain through a variety of mechanisms, including appraisal of the pain and related stressors; thoughts and beliefs about pain and about the self as a person in pain; and the coping options patients ultimately choose. Thus understanding patients' pain requires understanding their appraisals, thoughts, and beliefs about the pain. As we develop an understanding of clients' phenomenological experience of pain by considering their appraisals, thoughts, and beliefs, we can then begin to help them evaluate these cognitions and systematically construct alternative thoughts that will better serve them. The cognitive therapy technique used to help clients evaluate, challenge, and construct alternative thoughts and beliefs is called "cognitive restructuring," and this procedure receives considerable attention in this book.

TREATMENT RATIONALE

The 10-module cognitive treatment program presented in Part II of this book is intended to be integrated with other multidisciplinary approaches to chronic pain, including behavioral components. It is offered as a self-contained set of interventions, because I recommend it as initial preparation for any further self-management. But it can be adapted to particular settings and for particular clients.

The program begins with a psychoeducational approach to the concept of pain as a stress-related disorder—pain as real, but nonetheless stress-related. Helping patients conceptualize chronic pain as a stress-related disorder begins the process of understanding the cognitive part of the multifaceted nature of pain. This sets the stage for presenting the concept of primary appraisals as they relate to pain: pain as threat, challenge, or loss. Treatment Module 1 introduces clients to the concept of appraisals of stressors associated with pain. Exercises helping clients see the importance of their initial judgments regarding pain and associated stressors underscore the importance of cognitions as they relate to pain. Furthermore, in teaching clients that the judgments they make about a stressful situation (i.e., threat, loss, or challenge appraisals) influence the way they cope with pain, the practitioner gives clients a tool for reevaluating certain stressful events. Although I do not label the initial exercises as cognitive restructuring exercises, teaching clients to observe and categorize their judgments regarding primary stress appraisals sets the stage for the more structured, step-by-step cognitive restructuring exercises found later.

A substantive component of cognitive therapy for pain involves working with patients' automatic thoughts and beliefs, categorized as secondary appraisals in the cognitive model of pain. The technique of cognitive restructuring is used to help clients recognize their thoughts and beliefs; examine their validity; and, if their cognitions are distorted in the negative direction, construct more realistic alternative cognitions. Virtually all cognitive therapy approaches include the technique of cognitive restructuring. Whereas automatic thoughts are considered to be reflexive and initially not consciously available to a client, helping her to recognize these cognitions as they occur, and to evaluate their authenticity, allows the client to gain more control over these thought processes. In addition, constructing alternative adaptive responses, though initially effortful, becomes more automatic as the client continues to practice the technique of cognitive restructuring. Although cognitive restructuring is a common tool for all cognitive therapists, the level of detail covered may be quite variable. Since I view this technique as central to a cognitive therapy program for pain management, I spend three modules (Treatment Modules 2–4) covering cognitive restructuring. When clients are first learning to apply the cognitive restructuring techniques to their own pain management, it is helpful to slow down and take a more methodical approach than in later sessions, after they have experienced some success with cognitive restructuring. Devoting three treatment sessions to cognitive restructuring of automatic thoughts will help you really drive home these principles for clients early in the treatment program.

In Treatment Modules 5 and 6, I introduce the concept of evaluating and challenging intermediate and core beliefs. Although intermediate beliefs are not thought to be as fixed as core beliefs, they are nonetheless considered more difficult to change than automatic thoughts (Beck, 1995). Therefore, the treatment of intermediate and core beliefs is deferred until after a client has achieved success with challenging automatic thoughts. Treatment Module 5 covers general acquired attitudes and beliefs (intermediate beliefs, core beliefs). Treatment Module 6 helps the client examine his pain-specific intermediate and core beliefs—beliefs about the cause, appropriate treatment of, and ability to manage or control the pain, and beliefs about the self as a person in pain. I apply Burns's downward-arrow technique (Burns, 1980) to help clients examine general intermediate and core beliefs, as well as pain-specific intermediate beliefs and core beliefs about the self as a person in pain.

In Treatment Module 7, I offer a treatment session teaching coping self-statements. Positive self-statements are conceptually tied to cognitive restructuring techniques, because as part of cognitive restructuring, we practitioners help our clients construct more realistic, adaptive thoughts to replace the original distorted thoughts. However, coping self-statements are also more generally aimed at increasing clients' overall sense of personal empowerment (internal LOC and sense of self-efficacy) than they are specific rejoinders to individual automatic thoughts.

A final aspect of the cognitive intervention program offered in this book involves teaching expressive writing exercises and assertiveness training. Expressive writing exercises (Treatment Module 8) are given to provide an outlet for a client to process her emotions regarding the chronic pain, without overwhelming others who have close interactions with the client (e.g., her spouse or partner, physicians). Assertiveness training (Treatment Module 9) gives the client a tool to ask directly for what she wants and needs, without inadvertently increasing the use of expressive pain behaviors in the process of doing so.

Table 2.6 presents an integration of the elements of the stress–appraisal–coping model of pain with the associated cognitive techniques offered in this book.

CHAPTER SUMMARY

The stress–appraisal–coping model of pain presented in this chapter takes the philosophical stance that chronic pain is a stress-related disorder and employs a transactional stress approach to organize the various concepts presented. Each component of the model (individual differences, primary appraisals, secondary appraisals, and coping) has been presented as part of the interactive process that shapes a person's ultimate adaptation to a chronic painful condition. I have also tried to show that this model is a clinically useful structure for organizing both the research and the treatment of cognition-related chronic pain mechanisms. As will be discussed in Chapter 4, the specific pain-related appraisals and other factors in Tables 2.2, 2.3, 2.4, and 2.5 are likely targets for cognitive assessment. Findings from the assessment can guide therapists in individualizing the intervention techniques mentioned above.

The next chapter will review the research supporting the relative importance of cognitive interventions for chronic pain, and will also provide specific information supporting the treatment approach detailed in this book. Certainly, clinicians want to be convinced that there is an empirical basis for the treatment they are offering. In addition, managed care panels and quality assurance boards may require evidence of a scientific basis for treatment programs they are being requested to fund. Chapter 3 provides the research literature necessary to demonstrate the evidence basis for this treatment.

THE RESEARCH FOUNDATION
FOR COGNITIVE TREATMENT OF PAIN

Although cognitive-behavioral therapy (CBT) has become a widely accepted treatment for chronic pain, researchers have not yet clearly specified the active ingredients of successful treatment. Studies comparing treatment approaches are often difficult to evaluate (as well as difficult to conduct), but they offer promise in determining the crucial components to treatment success. The first section of this chapter reviews the findings of treatment outcome studies evaluating the overall importance of cognitive interventions, but does not compare the relative worth of individual cognitive techniques. This general review examines the literature comparing the behavioral components of CBT with the cognitive components of CBT.

The individual components offered in cognitive treatment often include cognitive restructuring techniques as well as cognitive coping skills training. It is therefore important to review the evidence base for each of these components of cognitive treatment, and this is done in the next two sections of this chapter. Clearly, the research establishes that successfully changing patients' distorted thinking results in changes in their pain reports as well as associated distress, which provides support for cognitive restructuring techniques. The research regarding cognitive coping skills training is more difficult to interpret, for a variety of methodological reasons, but the technique labeled "positive coping self-statements" has shown consistent empirical support. This research is reviewed in some detail, particularly since the literature regarding cognitive coping skills training has served as a source of confusion for clinicians regarding what techniques they should actually teach.

In addition to a review of the empirical basis for cognitive restructuring and cognitive coping techniques, other treatment components offered in this book require empirical justification. Expressive writing instruction and assertiveness training are not categorized as cognitive restructuring techniques, nor are they strictly *cognitive* coping skills; nevertheless, I base their inclusion on a cognitive case conceptualization. Empirical support for these techniques, as well as their place in pain management, is covered in later sections of this chapter.

EVALUATION OF THE GENERAL IMPORTANCE OF COGNITIVE INTERVENTIONS

CBT is the common standard of psychosocial intervention for pain (Morley, Eccleston, & Williams, 1999). Treatment outcome studies of patients with pain have shown that cognitive-behavioral interventions not only reduce pain, but also increase adaptive coping responses, self-efficacy, and physical functioning, and decrease maladaptive cognitions (Gil et al., 1996; James, Thorn, & Williams, 1993; Johansson, Dahl, Jannert, Melin, & Andersson, 1998; Kropp, Gerber, Keinath-Specht, Kopal, & Niederberger, 1997; Turner & Clancy, 1986; Turner & Jensen, 1993). Furthermore, CBT is cost-effective relative to medication and/or hospitalization (Turk, 2001, 2002a), and CBT is associated with returning previously disabled patients to work (Cutler et al., 1994).

Much of the literature describing CBT implies that this treatment approach is clearly operationalized and implemented in a standardized fashion. In fact, many different interventions are employed under the general rubric of CBT. Clinical researchers frequently fail to describe the exact components utilized in their CBT protocol—and even when these components are described, they differ widely across studies, making it difficult to determine the crucial components of treatment success. This lack of clarity in the literature leads to the assumption that all cognitive-behavioral interventions are equally efficacious; however, there is no empirical basis for this thinking. There is actually a relative scarcity of studies comparing the efficacy of CBT components, although careful examination of those available offers some intriguing clues regarding the potential agents of change in CBT, and the evidence appears to indicate that cognitive components are an important element of treatment.

When we are evaluating conclusions made by the authors of CBT outcome studies, several caveats are in order. First, sample size often dictates the power with which differences can be detected. If a study is examining relatively subtle differences between treatments, the sample size will need to be large enough to detect small effects. Many clinical treatment outcome studies are based on sample sizes too small to detect the kinds of differences we might be looking for. Second, outcome measures differ across studies, making generalization difficult. Although meta-analyses are useful in helping to incorporate and analyze the effects of multiple related studies, out of necessity they limit their evaluation of outcome to those measures that are utilized in all of the studies they are comparing (Morley et al., 1999). Thus the outcome measures evaluated in meta-analyses are most often the typical, overarching outcomes (such as pain self-report and affective distress), rather than specific measures that might shed light on the mechanism of change with treatment. Third, as stated earlier, the details of the treatment protocol are often poorly specified even in treatment outcome research, making it difficult to determine the exact nature of the intervention. With these cautionary constraints in mind, let us examine the available evidence.

Most comparison studies of CBT for pain treatment have compared "behavioral" components with "cognitive" components. Relaxation, biofeedback, and behavioral pacing strategies are most often categorized as behavioral components of CBT, whereas cognitive restructuring and cognitive coping skills training are usually referred to as the major cognitive components of CBT. Cognitive coping skills training for pain includes (but is not limited to) attention diversion strategies, reinterpreting pain sensations, positive self-statements, and imagery techniques. Cognitive restructuring includes the identification and modification of dysfunctional thinking. When applied to the treatment of pain, cognitive restructuring typically focuses on identifying and decreasing dysfunctional pain-related cognitions.

Several studies have examined the efficacy of behavioral components of CBT (biofeedback and/or relaxation training) as compared to cognitive components (cognitive coping skills training or cognitive restructuring). One study compared treatment success for patients with pain who received cognitive treatment alone, biofeedback alone, or no treatment. Although both treatment groups showed decreases in medication use, only the cognitive treatment produced a significant decrease in pain flare-ups (Holroyd, Andrasik, & Westbrook, 1977). A similar study compared treatment success for patients with headache who received cognitive therapy, biofeedback, or both treatments combined (Knapp & Florin, 1981). All treatments reduced headache activity; however, the cognitive intervention also resulted in lower depression, less irritability, and more positive self-evaluation. Moreover, the researchers noted that in the groups receiving combined cognitive and biofeedback treatments, those patients receiving the cognitive component *before* the biofeedback component reported less affective distress in the follow-up phase. The authors speculated that the group receiving cognitive therapy first had more time to consolidate the skills introduced in the cognitive procedure, and thus made greater gains overall. It is also possible that intervening at the cognitive level prior to intervening at the behavioral level increases patients' receptivity to future behavioral interventions by changing their appraisals, beliefs, and attitudes about coping options.

Other studies have evaluated treatment results for relaxation alone compared to a combination of relaxation with other cognitive techniques. One group of researchers found that relaxation training resulted in decreases in headache activity, but that patients receiving the combined intervention including cognitive components showed even greater headache reduction (Mitchell & White, 1977). Another group showed that relaxation training decreased pain and depression, although patients receiving the combined relaxation/cognitive intervention showed comparatively greater pain reduction as well as decreases in daily life stress (Tobin, Holroyd, Baker, Reynolds, & Holm, 1988). One study specifically examining the differential efficacy of cognitive restructuring versus relaxation and imagery training did not find expected differences: Mildly disabled patients with low back pain who received either cognitive restructuring or relaxation/imagery showed equal reductions in reports of pain intensity, compared to those of a wait-list control group. However, neither of the groups showed greater improvements than the wait-list control group in depression, cognitive errors, pain behavior, or self-reported disability following treatment (Turner & Jensen, 1993). Two problems associated with this study were that the participants were not particularly dysfunctional at the onset of treatment (thus creating a ceiling effect, for which it is difficult to demonstrate significant improvements) and that the sample size was small (making the study less likely to detect relatively small, subtle differences in treatment outcome). A similar study using more severely impaired patients with pain compared cognitive interventions (which in this study included relaxation instruction) to an operant behavioral treatment program (Kerns, Turk, Holzman, & Rudy, 1986). Although both treatments reduced patients' use of the health care system and increased progress on individually defined treatment goals, only the patients receiving the treatment containing the cognitive components showed improvements on pain severity, affective distress, and other psychosocial measures.

Taken together, the available research suggests that the cognitive components of CBT are an important element of the CBT package for pain management, providing pain-specific as well as non-pain-specific benefits. In addition, offering cognitive treatment modules to patients who engage in relatively greater levels of cognitive distortion, particularly early in the CBT regimen, may enhance overall treatment success.

Another way to examine the potential importance of the cognitive components of pain treatment is to determine what factors predict positive treatment outcome. If cognitive factors have an important role in predicting successful adaptation to pain, this lends credence to the hypothesis that cognitions are key treatment variables. The next section reviews the importance of cognitive variables in predicting outcome. As we will see, distorted pain-related thoughts and beliefs have a negative impact on adaptation to chronic pain, and successfully changing distorted thinking has a positive impact on outcome.

EVALUATION OF THE IMPORTANCE OF COGNITIONS IN PAIN ADAPTATION

Without question, positive outcome in pain treatment, whether it is primarily behavioral, primarily cognitive, or mixed and multidisciplinary, is predicted by changes in attitudes, beliefs, and cognitions. For example, Jensen and Karoly (1991) evaluated a large sample of patients with heterogeneous pain who participated in multidisciplinary treatment to determine which psychosocial variables predicted favorable outcome. Changes in beliefs and cognitive coping strategies were strongly associated with improved function and decreased health care use following treatment, but posttreatment improvements were only very weakly associated with changes in behavioral coping strategy use. The researchers concluded that improvement following multidisciplinary pain treatment is more strongly related to changes in what patients *think* about their pain than to changes in what they actually *do* about it. A similar conclusion was reached by Holroyd and colleagues (1984), who examined the mechanisms associated with electromyographic (EMG) biofeedback treatment success in patients with headache. Ironically, the actual change in EMG level was not associated with treatment success. However, patients' *belief* in the success of the training, and subsequent increases in patient self-efficacy and internal locus of control (LOC) *were* associated with pain reduction.

It certainly follows, then, that interventions aimed at changing patients' appraisals, beliefs, and other cognitions (especially those that are negatively distorted) could have a powerful impact on positive adaptation to chronic pain states. The negative cognition that we know the most about, in terms of pain management, falls under the general term "catastrophizing."

The Association of Negative Cognitions with Pain Adaptation

Catastrophizing has been shown to be a robust predictor of pain, disability, and adaptation to chronic painful conditions—and it does so over and above other factors, such as disease, pain intensity, depression, anxiety, fear of pain, and neuroticism (Flor, Behle, & Birbaumer, 1993; Geisser, Robinson, Keefe, & Weiner, 1994; Gil, Thompson, Keith, Tota-Faucette, Noll, & Kinney, 1993; Jacobsen & Butler, 1996; Keefe, Brown, Wallston, & Caldwell, 1989; Martin et al., 1996; Robinson et al., 1997; Sullivan & Neish, 1999; Sullivan, Rouse, Bishop, & Johnson, 1997). Clearly, individuals who catastrophize about their pain function more poorly than persons who do not catastrophize.

Although most of the research on catastrophizing has been correlational, the view that catastrophizing is causally related to pain is certainly implied in the pain literature. Although it is impossible to "prove" cause without experimentally manipulating catastrophizing, some studies have shown the predictive ability of catastrophizing for later pain ratings. For example, catastrophizing assessed 1 week (Sullivan & Neish, 1999) or 10 weeks (Sullivan, Bishop, & Pivik, 1995) before a painful procedure predicted pain ratings in response to the procedure. In another study, catastrophizing prospectively predicted pain ratings in patients with arthritis 6 months later, even when the investigators controlled for initial pain ratings (Keefe et al., 1989). Of course, it is also necessary to consider the possibility that the experience of pain may cause catastrophic thinking. The fact that catastrophizing scores in asymptomatic undergraduates or patients undergoing dental procedures (Sullivan & Neish, 1998) are lower than those seen in patients with chronic pain (Sullivan, Stanish, Waite, Sullivan, & Tripp, 1998) suggests that the experience of pain certainly contributes to catastrophic automatic thoughts. It makes sense then, that catastrophizing influences pain, and that the experience of pain influences catastrophizing.

It is interesting to note that women tend to score higher than men on measures of catastrophizing. These sex differences have been found in patients with a wide variety of pain types, including musculoskeletal pain (I. Jensen, Nygren, Gamberale, Goldie, & Westerholm, 1994) and osteoarthritis of the knee (Keefe et al., 2000); in undergraduates exposed to a cold-pressor task (Sullivan, Tripp, Rodgers, & Stanish, 2000; Sullivan, Tripp, & Santor, 2000); and in junior high school students (Gil, Abrams, Phillips, & Keefe, 1989). No study has reported higher levels of catastrophizing in men.

There also appear to be some differences in catastrophizing based upon age. In a university dental clinic, older age was associated with lower levels of catastrophizing (Sullivan & Neish, 1998), and older women undergoing breast cancer surgery demonstrated less catastrophic thinking than did younger women (Jacobsen & Butler, 1996). Perhaps related is the finding by some depression researchers that the incidence of depression in older adults is 1–4%, a lower range than that found in a younger population (Blazer, 1994).

The research on sex differences and age differences in catastrophizing is quite relevant to us as clinicians. It is important to understand that women (and perhaps young women) may be more vulnerable to catastrophic cognitive errors than men, and thus targeted treatment of catastrophizing thoughts may be particularly useful for clients with chronic pain who are women and relatively young. Although we certainly should not assume that all of our younger female clients will be high on catastrophic cognitive errors, at this point it is fair to consider them an "at-risk" group.

Are Changes in Cognitions Responsible for Pain Adaptation?

Certainly, it is now clearly established that specific cognitive factors targeted for change in pain management (e.g., pain-related catastrophizing) are associated with positive outcome (e.g., reduced disability, reductions in pain severity, improved mood). However, the vast majority of the available treatment outcome research is correlational, and one could rightfully argue that the converse is true: that positive changes in outcome (e.g., fewer pain episodes, lower perceived pain intensity, less disability) cause decreases in maladaptive cognitions.

In order to support the idea that cognitive change is responsible for positive outcome, we must be able to show that changes in cognitions occur *before* changes in outcome (DeRubeis & Feeley, 1990). In cognitive research on depression, which is further advanced than cognitive research on pain, investigators have constructed research designs that allow them to determine the correlation between early treatment changes in maladaptive cognitions and later treatment changes in outcome. These are compared with the correlations obtained between early treatment changes in outcome and later treatment changes in maladaptive cognitions (a "cross-lagged panel" design). The strength of the correlations, when compared with each other, determines the casual direction. Several depression researchers have shown that early treatment changes in cognitive factors accounted for later treatment changes in depression, but that the converse was not true; these findings provide support for the hypothesis that cognitive change is a crucial process variable in the successful treatment of depression (DeRubeis & Feeley, 1990; Feeley, DeRubeis, & Gelfand, 1999; Jacobson et al., 1996).

Although the type of research design discussed above does not provide absolute proof that the key therapeutic element is cognitive, results from cross-lagged panel designs provide a stronger test of the model than simple correlational designs. To date, one published study has examined the question of whether cognitive change is the process through which positive treatment outcome occurs for patients with chronic pain. Using the cross-lagged panel design described above, researchers were able to show that changes in catastrophic thinking and perceived helplessness early in treatment were significantly correlated with later treatment changes in pain severity and functioning, but that early treatment changes in pain severity and functioning were not correlated with later treatment changes in catastrophizing and perceived helplessness (Burns, Kubilus, Bruehl, Harden, & Lofland, 2003). It is important to note that these findings were obtained with the impact of depression statistically controlled; thus the cognitive change associated with positive outcome for pain is unique to pain, and not simply a by-product of treating depression in patients with chronic pain.

Based on the available literature, it is fair to say that above and beyond simple correlational studies, there is empirical support for the importance of changing negatively distorted cognitions in patients with pain. The research reviewed above makes a compelling argument that reductions in maladaptive cognitions drive subsequent decreases in perceived pain and increases in function. It certainly follows, then, that interventions aimed at changing negative cognitions could have a powerful impact on positive adaptation to chronic pain states. And the treatment technique most commonly associated with this process is cognitive restructuring.

Since it is apparent that cognitive variables are critical to pain management, it makes sense that clinicians would be interested not only in eliminating negatively distorted pain-related cognitions, but also in enhancing the use of adaptive cognitions. Certainly, part of the process of cognitive restructuring involves teaching patients to replace negatively distorted thoughts with alternative, more realistic thoughts. Thus, in a sense, cognitive restructuring involves teaching adaptive cognitions. Nevertheless, the pain literature has given considerable attention to the potential efficacy of a wide variety of specific adaptive cognitive coping techniques. There is a large and complicated literature on the issue of coping techniques associated with positive adaptation to chronic pain, and some of the relevant studies are reviewed below. Although the available research often considers behavioral as well as cognitive coping, I will confine my discussion to the cognitive coping literature whenever possible.

EVALUATION OF COGNITIVE COPING STRATEGIES

Many models of pain and illness consider coping responses to be central to our understanding of how one adjusts to chronic medical conditions (cf. Arathuzik, 1991; Tunks & Bellissimo, 1988; Turk, Meichenbaum, & Genest, 1983; Unruh, 1996; Weir, Browne, Roberts, Tunks, & Gafni, 1994), and a great deal of research has been devoted to identifying the kinds of coping that predict positive adaptation to chronic painful states. However, there are many inconsistencies in the findings, making conclusions about coping strategies quite difficult to interpret. Part of the problem associated with the coping research is that many researchers have used composites of various coping strategies, rather than investigating the efficacy of individual coping strategies. A problem associated with using general coping categories or composites of coping is that it does not tell us how individual coping strategies are related to functioning. Another problem is that researchers have mixed the concepts of appraisals (both primary and secondary) into their investigations of "coping" processes, which also serves as a cause for confusion. A third problem is that different researchers have used different labels for what seems to be the same coping strategy, thus confounding the issue further. For example, the re-interpretation of pain sensations (e.g., "I don't think of it as pain, but rather a dull or warm feeling," and "If my pain feels shooting, I try and pretend that it is only tingling") has been variously referred to as "emotional distancing from pain," "dissociation," "focused sensory at-tention," and "somatization" (Boothby, Thorn, Stroud, & Jensen, 1999; Fernandez & Turk, 1989). And finally, researchers have combined cognitive coping strategies with behavioral coping strategies, thus making it difficult to determine the relative importance of either.

The majority of the early research on pain coping strategies used rationally derived cate-gories, such as "emotion-focused" versus "problem-focused" (Lazarus & Folkman, 1984), "passive" versus "active" (Brown & Nicassio, 1987), and "illness-focused" versus "wellness-focused" (Jensen, Turner, Romano, & Strom, 1995). Most of the research using rationally de-rived categories concluded that the use of "active," "problem-focused," and "wellness-focused" coping strategies (e.g., exercise, activity despite the presence of pain, positive cop-ing self-statements) is associated with better psychological and physical functioning. On the other hand, "maladaptive" coping strategy composites often include types of strategies de-scribed as "passive," "emotion-focused," or "illness-focused" (e.g., pain-contingent rest, seek-ing solicitous responses from others, catastrophizing, medication use), and the use of these types of coping attempts often predicts poorer functioning. The predictive abilities of these "adaptive" and "maladaptive" composite measures have frequently been compared, and it is interesting to note that although maladaptive strategies are strongly related to negative out-come, adaptive strategies show only modest correlations with positive outcome. (For reviews of the pain coping literature, see Jensen et al., 1991, and Boothby et al., 1999.) Some re-searchers have noted that patients with chronic pain actually use very little problem-focused coping in managing their pain problems (Turner, Clancy, & Vitaliano, 1987). Thus a *lack* of maladaptive pain-related cognitions is much more robustly predictive of poor outcome than the *presence* of adaptive pain-related cognitions is predictive of positive outcome (Geisser, Robinson, & Riley, 1999).

In early work on categories of cognitive coping strategies, one listing included the fol-lowing: (1) imagining pleasant events, (2) focusing on other things, (3) dissociating oneself from the pain, (4) imagining the affected area as numb, and (5) concentrating on sensations other than pain (Scott & Barber, 1977). A later text classified cognitive coping strategies into two broad categories: those used primarily to change one's appraisal of the painful situation, and those used mostly to divert one's attention away from the pain stimulus (Turk et al., 1983).

A meta-analysis of 51 experimental pain studies comparing a variety of cognitive strate-gies to no-treatment controls or placebo (expectancy) conditions revealed a strong positive ef-fect for cognitive strategies compared to no treatment in enhancing pain tolerance or reduc-ing pain ratings. However, no significant differences in efficacy were found among the various strategies (Fernandez & Turk, 1989). Since this review involved studies using mostly acute, experimentally induced pain, it is not known whether the same findings would hold true in studies of chronic pain. However, it is important to consider the fact that in clinical populations, we are unlikely to restrict our treatment to one single cognitive strategy. Thus almost all of the true experimental manipulation studies comparing the efficacy of particular cognitive strategies are likely to come from the laboratory, rather than from clinical populations.

In a study conducted after this meta-analytic review, other researchers found that no one particular cognitive coping strategy seemed to be better than the others, although giving experimental subjects the choice to use their preferred coping strategy made a great deal of difference in how long they were willing to tolerate experimental pain (and how high their pain intensities were) (Rokke, al Absi, Lal, & Klein, 1993). So, although we still don't know whether specific cognitive coping strategies are better than others, we do know that giving individuals the option to select from a smorgasbord of choices is potentially beneficial.

Another meta-analysis of cognitive coping strategies is also relevant to our discussion. This review compared distraction strategies with attentional strategies used to cope with stress (almost all the studies reviewed included pain-related stressors, and most, but not all, involved experimentally induced pain). In the first analysis, it appeared that distraction strategies (e.g., asking the participant to name biographical facts, distraction via slides, proofreading tasks, diversion imagery) were superior to attentional strategies. However, when attentional strategies were further divided into attention to the objective sensations of the stimulus[1] versus attention to one's emotional reaction to the stimulus, attention to sensations were clearly superior to attending to one's emotional response *or* to distraction strategies (Suls & Fletcher, 1985).

It is interesting to note that other researchers have found that certain individual variables (i.e., sex, level of pain severity) and appraisals (i.e., health or pain-related anxiety, catastrophizing) influence the utility of distraction, sensory focus, or emotional focus techniques. For example, one study reported that the coping strategies of diverting attention, ignoring pain, and coping self-statements have all been positively associated with level of physical activity in patients with chronic pain, but only for patients reporting relatively low levels of pain severity (Jensen & Karoly, 1991). In another study, males reported less pain when instructed to focus on the sensory qualities of the stimulus, and females showed greater pain response when told to focus on the emotional aspects of the experience (Keogh & Herdenfeldt, 2002). Yet another study showed that individuals scoring high on catastrophizing did not do well with distraction strategy training, but showed better pain tolerance when taught how to monitor the pain stimulus and manipulate their thoughts in relation to the pain stimulus (Heyneman, Fremouw, Gano, Kirkland, & Heiden, 1990). Finally, for patients scoring high on measures of health anxiety, distraction techniques were not effective in reducing pain during physical therapy, but when patients were instructed to focus on their physical sensations, their reports of pain and anxiety went down (Hadjistavropoulos, Hadjstavropoulous, & Quine, 2000).

Research investigating the interactions between individual personality or appraisal variables and coping strategies may provide the most precise answers regarding the efficacy of particular coping strategies. That is, a more effective approach may be assessing which coping strategies work with which kinds of patients, rather than globally assessing the efficacy of coping strategies without considering patients' temperament or appraisal processes. Thus the

---

[1]Note that this type of attention to the sensory qualities of the stimulus has been variously labeled "somatization," "focused attention," "distancing," and "dissociation."

more research we do, the more we discover that individual and appraisal variables interact with treatment variables to influence their ultimate effectiveness.

Although analysis of coping strategy efficacy at the detailed level suggested above may become the norm for the future, the presently available research is based mostly on evaluating the efficacy of cognitive coping strategies independent of individual or appraisal variables. In fact, *numerous* studies have tried to determine whether certain cognitive coping strategies are relatively more useful than others for patients with chronic pain. Although the findings are rather inconsistent, some generalizations can be made. As I have emphasized above, the use of negative, distorted cognitions (catastrophic thinking, as well as negative self-statements and negative reflections regarding social interactions with others) can be considered an "anticoping" cognitive strategy. Numerous studies have found strong and consistent relationships between cognitive errors and maladjustment to pain. Likewise, the use of wishful thinking, praying,[2] and hoping (at least as these concepts are currently defined) has been associated with greater dysfunction, although the findings are not nearly as strong as with cognitive errors (Dozois, Dobson, Wong, Hughes, & Long, 1996; Geisser, Robinson, & Henson, 1994). Examples of these cognitive strategies are "I wish that the situation would go away, or somehow be over," "I pray for the pain to stop," and "I have faith in doctors that someday there will be a cure for my pain," respectively. Furthermore, cognitive strategies involving distraction or diverting attention (e.g., "I watch TV to distract myself from the pain") have not been found to be particularly useful techniques for patients with chronic pain. Although some studies have found a relationship between distraction strategies and positive outcome, many have not found any relationship, and recent reports indicate that distraction strategies may actually serve an anticoping function in patients with chronic pain (Hill, 1993; Riley, Robinson, & Geisser, 1999; Robinson et al., 1997). Although research regarding sensory focusing and emotional distancing strategies shows promise, particularly in pointing out that the efficacy of certain strategies may interact with individual personality or appraisal variables, the evidence base for these strategies is not yet robust enough to be considered well established. A final generalization that can be made is this: The use of positive coping self-statements (e.g., "I concentrate on convincing myself that I will deal with the pain and that it will get better in the near future") has been associated with better adjustment in patients with chronic pain, and since this finding has been consistent across various studies, it can be considered to be empirically justified (Hill, 1993; Riley et al., 1999; Van Lankveld, Van't Pad Bosch, Van De Putte, Naring, & Van Der Straak, 1994).

Table 3.1 summarizes my interpretation of the potential utility of teaching specific cognitive coping strategies to help patients better manage chronic pain. Of all the cognitive coping strategies listed in this table, I view positive coping self-statements as having sufficient empirical justification for including them as part of a cognitive treatment package. At first glance, you might regard such self-statements as merely the alternative, more realistic responses patients have already learned to construct in order to combat the emotional impact of cognitive errors. However, I view coping self-statements as something more broadly representative of positive coping; I consider them to be cognitive cues, or shortcuts, to a positive cognitive process that can be used in a variety of situations to facilitate adaptive coping re-

---

[2]In my opinion, there are two kinds of praying: one that asks God to cure or remove the pain, and another that asks God to give the person strength to do what is needed to cope with the pain. Although there is no research currently available on this, I hypothesize that the latter type of prayer would be similar to coping self-statements in terms of serving an adaptive function.

TABLE 3.1. Utility of Cognitive Coping Strategies for Chronic Pain Management

Category	Description	Example	Potential Utility
Focused attention	Attending to the sensory qualities of the pain	"I think of myself as being interested in pain and wanting to describe it to myself in detail."	Some support
Distancing	Reinterpreting pain sensation in an emotionally detached way	"I try not to think of it as my body, but rather as something separate from me."	Some support
Positive self-statements	Telling oneself that one can manage the pain	"I 'psych' myself up to deal with the pain, perhaps telling myself that it won't last much longer."	Good
Ignoring pain	Disregarding or overlooking the pain	"I don't pay any attention to it."	Equivocal
Praying/hoping/wishing	Calling upon God or luck to cure and end the pain	"I pray for the pain to stop."	Not helpful
Imagery distraction	Imagining a scene incompatible with pain	"I use my imagination to develop pictures that help distract me."	Not helpful
Mental distraction	Distraction through mental activity	"I describe objects in the room to myself."	Not helpful
Catastrophizing	Focusing on the negative emotional component of the pain	"I find myself expecting the worst."	Anticoping

sponses. Because there is empirical support for their use, and because they fit nicely within the theoretical framework presented by the stress–appraisal–coping model of pain, I offer a treatment module focused on coping self-statements.

Theoretically, I view coping self-statements as fitting under the categories of self-efficacy and locus of control (LOC). In Chapter 2, I have organized self-efficacy and LOC under the secondary appraisal category of intermediate (acquired) beliefs, specifically beliefs about one's control over pain (or the stress associated with the pain). Recall that in general, LOC refers to beliefs about an individual's sense of personal control over his environment (including pain and pain-related stressors), and that an internal LOC is associated with better adjustment to chronic pain. Self-efficacy relates to the belief that an individual can actually accomplish a certain goal—typically, perform a certain behavior. However, self-efficacy as it relates to pain can be broadened to include a person's belief in his ability to reduce the perception of pain intensity, belief in his ability to reduce the frequency of pain flare-ups, or even belief in his ability to use the cognitive techniques he has been taught. These self-efficacy beliefs are also associated with better adaptation to chronic pain.

The next two sections of this chapter examine two interventions (expressive writing and assertiveness training) that have a well-established evidence base in populations without pain, but have received less research attention in populations with pain. Both interventions have some empirical support for use with pain, but their research base is richer in other populations. Writing exercises and assertiveness exercises can certainly be construed as more behavioral than cognitive, and the reader may question why they are included in a book about cognitive therapy. Recall that the distinction between the "cognitive" and the "behavioral" is not always clear-cut, and that the conceptualization process, more than a technique itself, guides our categorization of the technique as behavioral or cognitive. Because I conceptualize the use of these techniques from a cognitive basis, and because I think they offer a unique approach that complements the rest of the treatment, I include them as treatment modules and review their efficacy below. In these next sections, I also provide the cognitive conceptualization for including these treatment modules. Briefly, I view expressive writing exercises as the therapeutic link between thoughts and emotions, while I conceptualize assertiveness exercises as focusing on the connection between pain-related thoughts and verbal (as well as nonverbal) pain behaviors. Thus, while expressive writing and assertiveness techniques are in some ways supplementary to cognitive therapy, aimed at affect and behavior, they are also directly related to a cognitive conceptualization of patients with chronic pain. I further explain these rationales in the sections below.

RATIONALE FOR AND EVALUATION OF EXPRESSIVE WRITING EXERCISES

Expressive writing exercises have been used as a tool for facilitating emotional disclosure in a variety of populations; they involve having patients write about their deepest thoughts and feelings regarding trauma, loss, or illness. These exercises have been empirically validated as beneficial to survivors of trauma, patients with cancer, those with asthma, people with HIV, and some populations with chronic pain (D'Souza et al., 2003; Gillis et al., 2003; Kelley, Lumley, & Leisen, 1997; Norman, Lumley, Dooley, & Diamond, 2004; Pennebaker, Mayne, & Francis, 1997; Smyth, 1998; Smyth, Stone, Hurewitz, & Kaell, 1999). It is important to note that some of the research reports an initial worsening of mood after emotional disclosure, followed by more delayed beneficial effects on other measures such as pain, physical disability, and even health care utilization (Lumley, in press).

Since the instructions for most expressive writing exercises ask patients to write their deepest thoughts and feelings, this exercise specifically targets emotions as well as thoughts, and encourages their expression. Remember that earlier in this chapter I have reviewed the research literature regarding coping with pain, which has consistently suggested that emotion-focused coping strategies are related to negative outcome. Furthermore, the empirical literature on coping with stressful experiences has concluded that emotion-focused coping is maladaptive (Kohn, 1996; Moos & Schaefer, 1993).

Although it is true that the stress and pain literature has generally concluded that emotion-focused coping is maladaptive, further examination of the studies may offer a different interpretation. Looking closely at the research criticizing emotion-focused coping for pain and stress, we find that "emotion-focused" coping measures often contain combinations of items reflecting more than just the use of emotional expression. Emotion-focused coping composites often contain denial/avoidance items, as well as items reflecting distress and/or self-deprecation. Thus the way pain researchers have measured emotion-focused coping could have confounded it with other concepts. Furthermore, there is a rich literature showing that emotional processing and emotional expression are useful to people confronting serious health-related issues, such as heart attack and cancer (Pennebaker et al., 1997; Stanton et al., 2002). These studies generally use different assessment techniques aimed at removing mixed concepts such as denial, distress, and self-deprecation from their measures of emotion-focused coping. The pain literature really hasn't progressed to the point of using these types of assessments.

It has been suggested that long-term efforts to suppress intense emotions may lead to increases in perceived stress over time, with associated disruptions in a variety of self-regulatory processes, including immune response function (Pennebaker & Beall, 1986; Schwartz & Kline, 1995). Furthermore, the discharge of emotions may be important to promote optimal psychological and physical adaptation to long-term stress (Schwartz & Kline, 1995). Since the various challenges of coping with chronic pain can easily be viewed as long-term stressors, it is probably important to provide some mechanism for the expression of intense emotions.

Because expressive writing exercises include writing about one's thoughts as well as emotions, they obviously involve cognitions. At a conceptual level, though, I see expressive writing exercises to be an important bridge between cognitions and subsequent emotions, as well as between emotions and subsequent cognitions. Similar to the way people can be unaware of their cognitions, patients can have emotions or feelings about their pain and pain-related stressors that they may not have an immediate awareness of. In addition, people can experience emotions in a diffuse way that is not easy to process without self-clarification. Expressive writing may be a process by which to facilitate patients' recognition of strong emotions, so that they can then process those emotions. Emotional processing requires integration of the cognitive as well as the emotional. Finally, it is not uncommon for clients to be afraid of their negative emotions, and fearful that expressing them will somehow "unleash the monster." Expressive writing gives clients an opportunity to identify and clarify emotions, as well as to discover that they have some level of control over their emotions.

Actually, there is one more reason why I suggest teaching expressive writing to patients with chronic pain. Some clinical researchers have proposed that catastrophic thinking, and subsequent expression of negative thoughts and feelings to loved ones, may serve a communal coping function; that is, expression of negative thoughts and feelings to others may be undertaken to get loved ones to pay attention and offer support. The next section of this chapter will discuss whether expressing negative thoughts and feelings actually accomplishes the goal of getting support and attention from loved ones, but for now consider the possibility that for some patients, or under certain circumstances, expressions of negative thoughts and emotions serve a cathartic role. If this is the case, expressive writing exercises may provide an appropriate outlet for discharging negative thoughts and emotions without risking criticism or rejections from others.

There are two very interesting studies in the pain literature related to expressive writing and catastrophizing, and they both found that expressive writing was more beneficial for patients who endorsed more catastrophic pain-related thoughts than for patients who did not score high on the measure of catastrophizing. One study reported that emotional processing via expressive writing was useful in reducing dental anxiety and pain reports in patients undergoing a scaling and root-planing procedure (i.e., removing hard and soft deposits from the surface of teeth, above and below the gum line; Sullivan & Neish, 1999). In this study, patients were classified as "catastrophizers" if they scored above the median (i.e., over 16) on the Pain Catastrophizing Scale (PCS; Sullivan et al., 1995), and as "noncatastrophizers" if they scored below the median. Prior to undergoing the dental hygiene procedure, half of the catastrophizers and half of the noncatastrophizers were asked to write about the thoughts and feelings they typically experienced during dental treatment, focusing on the aspects they found most distressing. Their control counterparts were simply asked to write about their activities from the previous day. In the control condition, catastrophizers reported more pain and distress than their noncatastrophizing counterparts. However, providing the catastrophizers with a single 5-minute opportunity to disclose their emotions reduced their pain and distress levels to those of the noncatastrophizers. It is interesting to note that patients scoring high on the PCS did not become "noncatastrophizers" as a result of this single exercise; they still endorsed high levels of catastrophic thinking and dental anxiety even after the treatment. Nevertheless, the expressive writing exercise helped them cope with the aversive dental experience much better than their control counterparts did. Incidentally, although dental hygiene is not commonly considered to be that painful, this study showed that at least for those high in catastrophic thinking, the pain ratings were similar in magnitude to those provided by patients suffering from chronic pain (Rosenstiel & Keefe, 1983; Sullivan & D'Eon, 1990).

In another study, women with chronic pelvic pain (CPP) were given instruction regarding writing about the stress associated with their CPP for 3 days, compared to controls, who were told to write about positive events in their lives unrelated to the CPP. Expressive writing resulted in lower overall affective ratings of pain compared to the control condition. Furthermore, for patients with higher scores on catastrophizing, negative affect, and/or ambivalence over emotional expression, expressive writing led to less disability and increased positive affect than for patients who did not have high scores on these measures (Norman et al., 2004).

The final area of research reviewed in this chapter involves the use of assertiveness training for pain management. As you will see, assertiveness training is not aimed at pain reduction per se, but focuses more on the issue of whether expression of negative thoughts and emotions to others in order to secure emotional and instrumental support is a maladaptive strategy that causes interpersonal relationship stress. Assertiveness exercises are seen as a way to help patients with pain express their wants and needs in a direct manner that does not involve the expression of their deepest negative thoughts and feelings—often an overwhelming experience for significant others.

RATIONALE FOR AND EVALUATION OF ASSERTIVENESS TRAINING

Although assertiveness training has a long therapeutic heritage, and although it is often included as part of the treatment regimen for patients with chronic pain, there are very few studies examining its specific efficacy with this population. As I have mentioned earlier, it is uncommon for interventions using bona fide patients to contain only one or two specific interventions to be compared; it is far more typical for the treatment to include multiple interventions. For example, in a description of a structured treatment program offered to veterans experiencing chronic pain, Fedoravicius and Klein (1986) included assertiveness training as part of a multimodule treatment package aimed at improving social skills, but they did not examine the relative efficacy of the specific modules. One study that did examine the differential efficacy of assertiveness training, progressive muscle relaxation, social reinforcement, and functional pain behavioral analysis found that relaxation and social reinforcement of increased activity had the most impact on pain intensity and "up time," while functional pain behavior analysis and assertiveness training had minimal impact (Sanders, 1983). However, the total number of participants in this study was 4, which limits meaningful conclusions. In another study of patients with duodenal ulcers, anxiety management training components and assertiveness training components were given to 11 patients, while 11 comparatively similar patients served as attention placebo controls. At a 60-day follow-up, patients receiving the active treatment experienced less ulcer-related pain, reported less severe ulcer symptoms, and consumed less antacid medication. The most impressive aspect of this study was that it also included an extended follow-up period, and after 3½ years, the treatment group was found to have significantly lower rates of ulcer recurrence (Brooks & Richardson, 1980).

What follows is a cognitive conceptualization of the utility of assertiveness training for patients with chronic pain. As I have noted in Chapter 2, chronic pain has many associated stressors, and relationship stress is certainly an important issue to consider. Beyond the obvious strain that any chronic illness places on close interpersonal relationships, there is some interesting research suggesting that interpersonal factors may promote or maintain disability in patients with chronic pain. If this is the case, we would certainly want to target these factors in our treatment.

Research examining the interpersonal relationships of patients with chronic pain has focused on spousal interactions, and generally finds that there is an association between "solicitous" spouse behaviors (i.e., expressions of concern, support, and provision of assistance) and poor pain outcomes. For example, several studies have shown that when patients perceive their spouses as solicitous in response to their expressions of pain, this perception is a strong predictor of heightened pain, lower activity levels, and increased disability (Flor, Kerns, & Turk, 1987; Flor, Turk, & Scholz, 1988; Williamson, Robinson, & Melamed, 1997). In an interesting twist on this research, another study found that if the spouses of patients with chronic pain perceived themselves as solicitous to their mates' pain, the spouses' perception was also predictive of increased patient pain and shorter walking duration on a treadmill when the spouses were present (Lousberg, Schmidt, & Groenman, 1993).

Studies actually observing patient–spouse interactions have also reported negative consequences of spousal solicitousness. For example, Romano, Jensen, Turner, Good, and Hops (2001) found that patients with pain increased their rate of pain behaviors following spousal solicitous behavior. Similarly, patients with chronic back pain who underwent a cold-pressor task reported increased pain intensity and shorter duration of arm immersion in cold water when solicitous spouses were present (Flor, Breitenstein, Birbaumer, & Fuerst, 1995).

The relation between solicitous spouse behaviors and increased pain behaviors has been explained via the principles of operant conditioning (Romano et al., 1992). The idea here is that patients' expressions of pain are aversive to spouses, who respond with decreased demands (e.g., fewer household responsibilities) in order to reduce the patients' pain behaviors. Decreased demands may result in a temporary reduction in pain, but this is likely to contribute to a cycle in which pain behaviors are reinforced over time.

Some researchers have proposed that patients' catastrophic thinking, and the subsequent expression of those negative thoughts and feelings to loved ones, may serve a communal coping function; that is, the patients use "expressive pain behaviors" in an attempt to gain emotional support from significant others (Sullivan, Tripp, & Santor, 2000; Sullivan et al., 2001). Expressive pain behaviors are those that communicate pain and distress to others (Sullivan, Adams, & Sullivan, 2004), such as verbal expressions of negative emotions (e.g., "I just can't take this pain any more!"), as well as nonverbal pain expressions (e.g., sighing, grimacing, moaning, etc.). The communal coping model of pain suggests that pain reduction may not always be the primary goal for patients, and that for some people or in certain situations, gaining emotional support via interpersonal relationships may be more primary (Thorn, Ward, Sullivan, & Boothby, 2003).

If negative thinking and expressive pain behavior are not necessarily aimed at reducing pain, but rather aimed at increasing social support, one would think that patients using this strategy would perceive their loved ones as more emotionally supportive. Although there isn't much research examining this hypothesis, we do know that patients with chronic pain who tend to catastrophize—even those who rate the quality of their relationships as good—perceive their partners as responding to their pain in a *punitive* fashion (i.e., responding with irritation, frustration, and anger), rather than being supportive or solicitous toward them (Boothby, Thorn, Overduin, & Ward, 2004). In a related study of patients with cancer, individuals who tended to catastrophize judged their spouses to be instrumentally helpful, but they did not judge their spouses to be emotionally supportive (Keefe et al., 2003).

Regardless of the reason why some patients with chronic pain tend to express their negative thoughts and feelings more than others, the results are not necessarily positive. As I've stated before, patients who engage in negative thinking report higher pain levels, more distress, and more dysfunction. Furthermore, they perceive their partners as punitive, rather than supportive, in response to their pain expressions. And in the study by Keefe and colleagues (2003) of patients with cancer and their spouses, patients who catastrophized were also judged more negatively by their spouses than patients who did not catastrophize. In addition, spouses of patients who catastrophized reported more caregiver stress than spouses of patients who did not catastrophize.

Expressing negative thoughts and emotions to significant others (e.g., spouses/partners, physicians), particularly in chronic situations, is thus probably perceived negatively by the recipients and may *reduce*, rather than increase, the patients' receipt of emotional support. With this in mind, the treatment module on assertiveness offers clients an assertive rather than a "pain-expressive" method of communication.

SUMMARY OF RESEARCH FINDINGS

My interpretation of the available research is that it is clearly supportive of cognitive interventions as a key element in CBT for pain. Although there is variability in terms of what particular techniques actually constitute "cognitive" versus "behavioral" interventions, cognitive interventions are typically categorized as cognitive restructuring techniques or cognitive coping strategy techniques. In the most convincing research to date, sophisticated methodology applied to cognitive interventions for pain has shown that positive changes in cognitions occur *before* reductions in distress and pain occur (Burns et al., 2003), thus providing supportive evidence for cognitive interventions in pain management. The literature regarding specific cognitive coping techniques is less clear, but the employment of positive coping self-statements has been consistently shown to be associated with more positive outcome. Practically speaking, cognitive restructuring techniques and training in positive coping self-statements lead to similar outcomes; that is, they lead to a reduction in maladaptive cognitions and an increase in adaptive cognitions. Although expressive writing exercises and assertiveness training are not strictly considered "cognitive" interventions, they fit within the cognitive conceptualization used in this book.

I have used aspects of this treatment approach in my clinical research with a mixed group of patients with chronic pain (Johnson & Thorn, 1989); in a specific-treatment-component analysis study of patients with headache (James, Thorn, & Williams, 1993); in a treatment study of patients with fibromyalgia (Kuhajda & Thorn, 2002); and in a National Institutes of Health–supported clinical trial for patients with headache (Thorn, 2002). Each of these clinical research studies has provided an opportunity for me to revise and refine the treatment manual, so that it will be easier to use and understandable to practitioners who may be less familiar with cognitive therapy.

CHAPTER SUMMARY

In this chapter, I have reviewed the literature regarding the importance of cognitive variables in CBT for chronic pain. Comparative treatment outcome studies suggest that cognitive variables are a critical component in successful CBT. The wealth of research on catastrophizing provides strong support for the important impact of distorted negative cognitions on patients' ability to cope with pain. Although the research exploring specific adaptive cognitive coping strategies is less clear-cut, it is nonetheless suggestive that certain cognitive coping strategies are worth teaching (e.g., positive coping self-statements) to patients with chronic pain, and that others do not merit instruction (e.g., distraction techniques). The research regarding expressive writing and assertiveness training as useful techniques for patients with chronic pain is also reviewed. Within these sections, I offer a rationale for including expressive writing and assertion training in a cognitive treatment program.

The next chapter provides an overview of psychometrically sound assessment instruments related to the cognitive treatment of chronic pain. Clinicians need empirically sound, yet efficient, instruments for assessing both process and outcome in their pain management programs (Morley, Shapiro, & Biggs, 2004). Although it is not feasible or useful to cover all of the available psychosocial instruments relevant to the cognitive treatment of pain, certain instruments are included because they are short, cognitively focused, and conceptually grounded in the stress–appraisal–coping model of pain. By the end of Chapter 4, you will have a battery of tools that you can incorporate into your initial assessment of each patient, treatment planning, and evaluation of the treatment as it progresses.

CHAPTER 4

ASSESSMENT ISSUES AND INSTRUMENTS RELEVANT TO COGNITIVE THERAPY FOR PAIN

Pain is a subjective experience, but this fact does not make it any less real. It does, however, make it difficult to measure. The problem of measuring pain has been the source of much controversy and probably some patient mismanagement. Asking a patient about her pain (patient self-report) has been regarded with suspicion, and pain researchers continually strive to come up with a better mechanism of measuring pain. Try as we might, we cannot express pain in terms of centimeters, or types of cells, or markers in the blood. There are people with terminal cancer who are debilitated and suffering terribly because of pain, and there are people with the same type of malignancy, same progression of disease, and so forth, who experience little if any discomfort because of pain. Thus our assessment of pain relies heavily on self-report measures, and it often includes questions regarding the ramifications of the pain, rather than simply the pain level per se.

In this chapter, I focus on the cognitive assessment of the pain experience. The psychosocial instruments most relevant to a cognitive therapeutic approach are those assessing patients' beliefs, attitudes, cognitions, and cognitive coping. As I have emphasized in Chapter 3, patients' cognitions, especially negative thought processes, predict poor patient adaptation to pain better than any other variable—including disease state, pain severity, sex, age, or depression. Thus we have come to realize just how important a person's thought processes are when it comes to treatment planning and treatment success.

AN INTRODUCTION TO PSYCHOSOCIAL PAIN ASSESSMENT

A useful psychosocial pain assessment ought to highlight specific problem areas unique to the individual, and should provide a road map for intervention. Furthermore, instruments used in psychosocial assessments should be reliable, be valid, and have some prognostic value (i.e., point to those who are likely vs. not likely to benefit from a particular type of treatment). In the ideal world, psychosocial pain assessments would provide a means for tracking the treatment progress of patients, and they could be compared pre- and posttreatment to document treatment success.

So what's the reality? Although psychosocial assessment may be a standard part of any multidimensional treatment program, and is usually covered by medical insurance, the assessments we typically conduct may or may not be particularly useful in treatment planning. Once an assessment is completed, the diagnosis made, and the report written, those materials are commonly filed away, and clinicians rarely refer to them again. Why might this be?

When psychologists first began working in the pain field, their assessments focused almost exclusively on the evaluation of traditional psychopathology, particularly depressive disorders. In many cases, psychologists and other clinicians continue to rely on standard measures of psychopathology (e.g., the Minnesota Multiphasic Personality Inventory–2 [MMPI-2]; Hathaway et al., 1989) or measures of pathological mood state (e.g., the Beck Depression Inventory–II [BDI-II]; Beck, Steer, & Brown, 1996). There are good reasons for doing so: Many of us are quite familiar with the traditional psychological assessment tools, since these are the ones we may have learned the most about in our training. Furthermore, these traditional assessment tools have strong empirical support, have a long history of use, provide accessible manuals for interpretation of results, and often have computerized interpretive reports available to the clinician, saving valuable time during the assessment phase. However, the general personality and psychopathology assessment tools were designed for psychiatric patients, not patients with pain, and the latter clients often react negatively to being given such measures. Furthermore, the most commonly administered personality test, the MMPI-2, consists of 567 items, which represents a considerable time investment for our patients.

Present-day pain assessment has been gradually shifting away from the traditional measures of personality and psychopathology and toward pain-specific psychosocial measures. When clinicians treating patients with pain go looking for pain-specific psychosocial instruments to include in their assessment battery, they will find a surplus of options; unfortunately, many of them are too lengthy to be practical in the clinical setting, too restricted in focus, and not readily interpretable. The plethora of psychosocial pain instruments now available has served as a cause for confusion rather than clarity: Do they measure separate or overlapping constructs? Which are the most important to use as pre-and posttreatment outcome measures? Is it really necessary to use a 60-item instrument, or will an abbreviated version adequately measure the issue of interest?

As a researcher, I have gotten caught up in the desire to design the "perfect" scale that fully captures whatever domain I am most interested in—one that demonstrates excellent internal consistency and validity, as well as predictive ability. In doing so, I am likely to restrict the focus of my scale and make it fairly long in order to make it psychometrically robust. Certainly, these scales have advanced our conceptual understanding of the psychosocial importance of pain, but the proliferation of psychosocial pain scales may be bewildering and not particularly useful to the clinician. As a clinician, I want a manageable number of items, presented in a user-friendly manner, that cover the important concepts and help me plan and evaluate treatment. Furthermore, if I can incorporate a client's responses to certain assessment questions within the treatment program itself, as a psychoeducational tool to illustrate the concept I am trying to get across in therapy, the instrument becomes invaluable.

In this chapter, I provide suggestions for the cognitive assessment of individual differences, primary appraisals, secondary appraisals, and coping processes for people struggling with chronic pain. Presenting an overview of all available cognitive and coping instruments is beyond the scope of this book, although I will introduce and briefly critique some of the more commonly used measures. The interested reader can also refer to a book on the assessment of pain (Turk & Melzack, 2001), and especially to the chapter in that book by DeGood and Tait (2001). In addition to providing a synopsis of commonly used measures, I present more in-depth coverage of certain instruments specifically useful for implementing the cognitive therapy regimen described in the present book. These instruments and their scoring keys are included as Appendices C–I, and can be reproduced by the reader and used with clients. The questionnaires I suggest (and include in these appendices) can be used to provide guidance regarding tailoring the basic treatment regimen to fit individual needs. More uniquely, they can be incorporated into the treatment itself and used as educational tools for the client, to emphasize the importance of cognitions and pain response. Included in Table 4.1 is a listing of the instruments I recommend using in conjunction with this book's cognitive treatment program. If you were to administer all of the suggested measures, you would be asking the client to respond to a total of 166 items, taking about 1 hour; this would represent a considerable time savings, compared to traditional personality measures such as the MMPI-2. In addition, these measures directly assess cognitions, are theoretically grounded in the stress–appraisal–coping model of pain, and can be used as psychoeducational tools within the treatment program itself.

TABLE 4.1. Suggested Measures to Be Used with This Book's Cognitive Treatment Program

- *Dysfunctional Attitude Scale–24 items* (DAS-24; Power et al., 1994): Global measure of core beliefs/dysfunctional attitudes.

- *Pain Appraisal Inventory* (PAI; Unruh & Ritchie, 1998): 16 items measuring primary pain appraisals of threat/loss and challenge.

- *Pain Beliefs and Perceptions Inventory* (PBPI; Williams & Thorn, 1989): 16 items measuring secondary appraisals (beliefs) about the cause and nature of pain.

- *Survey of Pain Attitudes—Revised* (SOPA-R; Jensen, Turner, & Romano, 2000): 35 items measuring secondary appraisals (beliefs) about the appropriate treatment of pain, and about one's ability to control pain.

- *Pain Catastrophizing Scale* (PCS; Sullivan, Bishop, & Pivik, 1995): 13 items measuring secondary appraisals (automatic thoughts) reflecting a negative cognitive set brought to bear during actual or anticipated painful experiences.

- *Cognitive Coping Strategies Inventory—Revised* (CCSI-R; Thorn, Ward, & Clements, 2003): 32 items measuring cognitive coping strategies reported to be used to manage pain.

- *Coping Strategies Questionnaire—Revised* (CSQ-R; Riley & Robinson, 1997): 27 items measuring behavioral and cognitive strategies reported to be used to manage pain.

ASSESSING INDIVIDUAL VARIABLES

As proposed in Chapter 2, individual differences cover physiological processes, personality or temperament, social factors, and more cognitively specific issues (such as core beliefs or general dysfunctional attitudes).

Biological State

Certainly, part of the initial assessment of a person presenting for pain management includes gathering information about the individual's physiological condition. Information regarding results of diagnostic testing, past or ongoing medical interventions (i.e., medication, surgeries), and presumed etiology as well as progression of the problem is important in formulating an understanding of the individual presenting for treatment. Some of this information can be obtained through interviewing the client, while some should be received from the patient's primary physician. It is generally very helpful for you to establish a line of communication with the patient's primary physician, and brief follow-up contacts with the physician regarding your treatment plan, as well as outcome, are usually very much appreciated.

Health Insurance Portability and Accountability Act (HIPAA) requirements signed into law in August 1996 have added a layer of protection to the client regarding transfer of health records and communication between health care providers. With an individual experiencing chronic pain, you will want to be able to receive pertinent health information from the patient's other health care providers (and, when necessary, exchange information regarding the patient). You will therefore need to be familiar with HIPAA and state regulations regarding health care information exchange.

During the initial intake session, I have clients bring in all the medications (pain and otherwise) they are taking on a daily or as-needed basis. I ask them to bring all these in a brown paper bag, and in their original prescription bottles if possible. I have an assistant who does nothing else during the intake session but write down all of the medications a client is taking, the dose, the date of the prescription, and the prescribing physician. She then makes a chart of the patient's medications, and I ask the patient for permission to share the medication chart with all of the physicians caring for him. I have never had a patient refuse permission, and I have received calls from a number of surprised and grateful physicians.

Appendix B provides a sample assessment summary note that can be copied to the referring physician.

Other Individual Variables

Assessment of Personality and Psychopathology

Personality factors may be an important component of assessing certain pain patients, and psychologists have historically provided such evaluations. This section is not meant to prepare you to conduct a personality evaluation, but it gives the context for this kind of assessment. A number of multidimensional inventories have been designed to assess both state and trait issues of personality, and the MMPI-2 (Hathaway et al., 1989) is often included as a standard part of any assessment battery.

Using the MMPI-2 for patients with chronic pain has certainly received its share of criticism, particularly since the advent of more narrowly defined pain inventories. Although it is not appropriate to use the MMPI-2 to determine the cause of the pain or to establish the supposed underlying personality pathology "explaining" the pain, it may nonetheless be a useful tool for determining the general level of distress, and for screening personality issues or comorbid psychopathology that might complicate treatment (Vendrig, 2000). As noted earlier, the MMPI-2 is quite lengthy (567 items); also, since it is not specific to pain, but assesses more general personality issues, patients with pain often question its relevance and/or object to the content of some items. In addition, the MMPI-2 has been noted to overpathologize patients with pain, who often receive similar profiles (Vendrig, 2000). Furthermore, MMPI-2 profiles have not been consistent in predicting treatment outcome (Bradley & McKendree-Smith, 2001).

Certainly, questions regarding a patient's personality structure or general psychopathology are relevant, and in some cases a formal assessment of these issues is merited. If a personality evaluation is considered important for a particular patient, referral to a psychologist comfortable with these diagnostic procedures, and subsequent communication with the psychologist, can enhance your general understanding of the patient. However, various other tools are more pain-specific and easier to administer and interpret; these are thus of more immediate relevance to your treatment planning and implementation.

Comprehensive Assessment of Social and Psychological Variables

A comprehensive pain-specific instrument that has been used a great deal in clinical research is the West Haven–Yale Multidimensional Pain Inventory (WHYMPI; Kerns, Turk, & Rudy, 1985). At 62 items, it provides a relatively efficient assessment of a broad range of individual psychosocial variables relevant to the chronic pain experience, and it is theoretically linked to the cognitive-behavioral therapy (CBT) approach. Although the WHYMPI does not exclusively assess cognitions, the questions are posed in terms of patients' perceptions of their pain problems, and thus it provides indirect information regarding appraisals, beliefs, and cognitions. The WHYMPI is organized into three sections, with a total of 12 subscales covering, for example, Pain Severity, Affective Distress, and self-report of participation in common daily activities. The items are presented with a 0–6 rating response format. Examples of WHYMPI items include "In general, how much does your pain problem interfere with your day-to-day activities?", "Rate your overall mood during the past week," and "How much has your pain changed your friendships with people other than your family?"

A unique feature of the WHYMPI is that one section assesses patients' perceptions of how their partners respond to them when they are in pain, and these items are organized into Solicitous, Distracting, and Punitive subscales. This section thus provides information regarding relationship issues that might interact with patients' experience of pain as well as their ultimate adjustment. Although individual subscale interpretation of the WHYMPI is generally not conducted, profile analyses have proven fruitful. Three reliable profiles of patients with pain have been identified and are labeled "dysfunctional," "interpersonally distressed," and "adaptive copers" (Turk & Rudy, 1990, 1992a). Patients identified as having interpersonally distressed profiles have been considered to be potential candidates for conjoint, as well as individual, therapy regarding their pain problems (Turk & Rudy, 1990, 1992a).

Although I don't use the WHYMPI with every patient, it can be a useful additional assessment tool as a pre–post outcome measure, or when questions arise about relationship issues that might complicate the treatment picture. A copy of the WHYMPI and of its scoring key is included in Jacob and Kerns (2001), or it can be obtained directly from Kerns via e-mail at *Robert.kerns@med.va.gov*. In addition, computer scoring of the WHYMPI is available (Rudy, 1989).

Assessment of Cognition-Specific Individual Variables: Core Beliefs and Dysfunctional Attitudes

Within a cognitive conceptualization, a person's core beliefs are also considered under the category of individual differences. As a reminder, core beliefs are considered to be more global (i.e., cross-situational) and more deeply held than cognitive processes like automatic thoughts. Individuals are thought to have both positive and negative core beliefs (also referred to as "schemas"—Beck, 1976); it is thought that negative core beliefs or schemas are activated by aversive life events (such as chronic pain).

The measure most closely associated with assessing core beliefs is the Dysfunctional Attitude Scale (DAS; Weissman & Beck, 1978). The DAS is a self-report measure that examines global, rather than situation-specific, cognitive errors and distortions. The scale was designed to test a prediction based on Beck's cognitive theory of depression: that extreme and negative general attitudes and beliefs might reflect an individual's predisposition toward depression. It was hypothesized that deeply held attitudes and beliefs might represent a cognitive vulnerability that, when coupled with negative life events, might trigger an emotional disorder. The original 100-item DAS was shortened to two 40-item scales (DAS-A and DAS-B; Weissman, 1979), and the DAS-A is now frequently used in cognitive therapy practice and research. An even shorter (24-item) DAS has since been developed, and it contains three subscales (Achievement, Dependency, and Self-Control) rather than providing a global measure of dysfunctional attitudes (Power et al., 1994). All of the scales use a 7-point rating response format, ranging from "totally disagree" to "totally agree." Some examples of items from the DAS-24 include "If I fail partly, it is as bad as being a complete failure" (Achievement), "If others dislike you, you cannot be happy" (Dependency), and "I should always have complete control over my feelings" (Self-Control).

It is not known whether the DAS is a useful adjunct to the assessment of chronic pain, because there is very little research on the use of this measure for patients with chronic pain. In one study using nondepressed patients with chronic pain, DAS scores were comparable to those of nonpatient controls, suggesting that the patients did not hold an inordinate number of dysfunctional attitudes (Binzer, Almay, & Eisemann, 2003). In another study using outpatients at a pain management clinic, DAS scores were shown to account for more than 50% of the variability in treatment outcome (Dyck & Agar-Wilson, 1997). This finding is even more impressive, because initial depression and pain severity scores were controlled for before the analysis of the impact of DAS scores. Thus, at least in the latter study, neither depression nor pain severity explained why DAS scores predicted treatment outcome. This means that DAS scores are not simply a reflection of depression or of pain, but may be a sign of a more general tendency toward dysfunctional thinking. These two studies suggest that patients with pain *on the average* may not score higher on the DAS than persons without pain, but that patients with higher DAS scores will have a poorer response to pain treatment. Thus intervening at this level of cognition may be an important aspect of treatment, particularly with individuals scoring high on the DAS.

Although there is no research available examining the differential predictive ability of the three DAS-24 subscales (Achievement, Dependency, Self-Control) for patients with chronic pain, I am particularly interested in the Dependency scale. A relatively high score on the Dependency scale may be predictive of a particular patient's need to receive emotional support based on his pain, and may be related to higher levels of pain-expressive behavior as well as higher levels of pain catastrophizing. At this point, these suggestions are merely speculative, because the research has not been conducted. An example of how such a patient might fill out the Dependency scale on the DAS-24 (with the associated DAS-24 item numbers) is given in Figure 4.1.

Because the DAS is intended to measure global beliefs and attitudes, it may be a helpful tool to consider using, especially the short (24-item) version. In my clinical practice, I have begun to use the DAS-24 as part of my pretreatment assessment battery; later, during the treatment module introducing core beliefs, I have the patient examine what he initially endorsed as a means of understanding what is meant by "core beliefs" (see Treatment Module 5). The DAS-24, plus a scoring key, is included in Appendix C. Score comparisons between formerly depressed psychiatric patients and nondepressed undergraduates are also included in a table as part of Appendix C. Since there are no comparative DAS-24 scores available for patients with pain, I suggest that if you use it, initially do so on an exploratory basis to develop your own local norms of reference.

Table 4.2 summarizes this section discussing assessment of individual differences in patients with pain, and provides a synopsis of the assessment instruments discussed within each category.

Attitudes	Totally Agree	Agree Very Much	Agree Slightly	Neutral	Disagree Slightly	Disagree Very Much	Totally Disagree
2. If others dislike you, you cannot be happy.		×					
5. My happiness depends more on other people than it does on me.	×						
8. What other people think about me is very important.	×						
11. I am nothing if a person I love doesn't love me.		×					
14. If you don't have other people to lean on, you are bound to be sad.		×					
17. I can find happiness without being loved by another person.						×	
20. I do not need the approval of other people in order to be happy.					×		
23. A person doesn't need to be well liked in order to be happy.					×		

FIGURE 4.1. DAS-24 Dependency scale: Hypothetical endorsements reflecting high Dependency score. For the DAS-24 itself, copyright 1994 by Michael J. Power. Reprinted by permission.

TABLE 4.2. Assessment of Individual Variables

- *Biological*—Diagnoses of physical health problem(s); medications; hospitalizations; surgeries; other invasive medical procedures. Obtained through patient interview and from physician.

- *Personality/psychopathology*—Basic personality structure, as well as psychopathological diagnoses. Usually assessed by psychologist.
  - *MMPI-2* (Hathaway et al., 1989) is commonly used, although not pain-specific, may be objectionable to patients with pain, contains many items and scales, and can overpathologize patients with pain.

- *Comprehensive psychosocial*—Multidimensional self-report of social and psychological variables of relevance to pain and outcome.
  - *WHYMPI* (Kerns et al., 1985) is reliable, valid, and widely used. 62 items, three sections, and 12 subscales, with three reliable patient profiles ("adaptive copers," "interpersonally distressed," "dysfunctional"). Items are not specific to cognitions, but relevant to appraisals, beliefs, and cognitions.

- *Cognitively focused*—Specific assessment of global thinking patterns, especially those deemed dysfunctional.
  - *DAS-24* (Power et al., 1994), abbreviated from the original 100-item DAS, targets general dysfunctional attitudes in three domains: Achievement, Self-Control, and Dependency. Use of DAS for patients with pain is limited, but predicts pain treatment outcome, and does not overlap with depression. DAS-24 may be clinically useful, especially when one is introducing the concept of core beliefs.

ASSESSING PRIMARY PAIN APPRAISALS

As discussed in Chapter 2, another important aspect of a client's thought processes is her primary appraisal of stimuli and environmental events. The transactional model of stress (Lazarus & Folkman, 1984) proposes three main types of primary appraisals: threat, harm/loss, and challenge. Each of these primary appraisal types is relevant to actual or anticipated pain stimuli, as well as environmental circumstances associated with chronic pain.

The Pain Appraisal Inventory (PAI; Unruh & Ritchie, 1998) was specifically designed to assess the primary appraisal processes of people experiencing troubling pain. This 16-item measure combines the primary appraisal categories of threat and harm/loss into one factor labeled the Threat/Loss scale and includes a second factor labeled the Challenge scale. Examples of Threat/Loss items on the PAI include "The pain seems threatening," and "I am concerned that the pain might become more than I can manage." Examples of Challenge items include "I think the pain makes me a stronger person," and "I think of this pain as a challenge." Although the originators of the PAI found that very few individuals experiencing troubling pain endorsed challenge appraisals, the instrument was nonetheless reliable in distinguishing threat/loss from challenge appraisals. It is interesting to note that individuals who responded with the highest level of challenge appraisals reported pain due to a recent medical procedure. This finding may suggest that when pain is predictable, particularly if it is associated with an expected positive outcome (i.e., "cure"), the pain may be considered less threatening.

When one is examining scores on the PAI, it may be useful to determine the relative emphasis of the patient's appraisals as threat/loss versus challenge, being aware that the norm is for people experiencing pain to focus more on threat and loss than on challenge appraisals. There is no treatment outcome research currently available using the PAI, but patients with very high scores on the Threat/Loss scale may need individually tailored interventions to calm their fears prior to introducing behavioral strategies such as increased exercise. Because these patients are likely to perceive exercise and other behavioral assignments as having a high potential for causing reinjury or triggering a pain episode, they may benefit from relaxation exercises with graded exposure techniques, for example (see Vlaeyen & Linton, 2000), in addition to cognitive interventions aimed at correcting maladaptive threat appraisals.

Although the PAI does not specifically do this, I find it important to help the client distinguish between threat appraisals and loss appraisals. You will note in Treatment Module 1 that clients receive specific instruction in all the primary appraisal processes, including threat, loss, and challenge. This is done by providing vignettes illustrating each of the different appraisals, as well as by using the clients' original PAI answers as a discussion guide. Once a client has learned to distinguish among these appraisals, the crucial next step is helping the client understand the connection between the primary appraisal and other cognitive, emotional, and behavioral responses (e.g., threat → avoidance or anxiety; loss → helplessness or depression; challenge → determination and perseverance).

Finally, I think it is important to use the PAI to help clients understand that appraisals of the stressors associated with their pain condition are not unitary or global judgments, but rather specific to particular situations or environmental events. Clients often begin treatment with the judgment that *any* pain stimulus (or potential for pain) is a red flag signaling danger and leading to avoidance, and that the pain has robbed them of *all* pleasurable aspects of life. They usually cannot conceive of an aspect associated with their pain that could be judged as a challenge or an opportunity for growth. When clients begin to separate out their pain-related stressors, and to make more differentiated appraisals regarding their potential as threats, losses, or challenges, they are on their way to taking some control over aspects of their pain situation.

In addition to using the PAI as a discussion guide, it can be used as part of your pre- and posttreatment assessment battery. Successful treatment would ideally result in lower Threat/Loss scores and higher Challenge scores. An example of how a beginning patient might fill out the PAI (first six items) is included in Figure 4.2. The PAI, along with a scoring key, is included in Appendix D.

Strongly Disagree	Moderately Disagree	Slightly Disagree	Slightly Agree	Moderately Agree	Strongly Agree	
1	2	3	4	5	6	

1. I am concerned that the pain might mean something is wrong with me   1 2 3 4 5 **6**

2. I think the pain is a chance to prove myself   1 **2** 3 4 5 6

3. I am concerned that the pain might become more than I can manage   1 2 3 4 5 **6**

4. I think the pain is a test of my strength and ability   1 2 **3** 4 5 6

5. I think something good might come out of having the pain   **1** 2 3 4 5 6

6. I am worried about getting things done   1 2 3 4 **5** 6

FIGURE 4.2. PAI (first six items): Hypothetical endorsements reflecting high Threat/Loss and low Challenge scores. For the PAI itself, copyright 1998 by Anita Unruh. Reprinted by permission.

TABLE 4.3. Assessment of Primary Pain Appraisals

- *Threat*—Judgment that the pain stimulus or potential pain stimulus poses a danger outweighing one's ability to cope; produces emotions such as fear and anxiety, and avoidance/escape behaviors.

- *Harm/loss*—Judgment that pain and pain-related stressors have caused damage; produces emotions such as grief, sadness, and depression, and a helpless, passive stance toward self-management.

- *Challenge*—Judgment that one's ability to cope is not outweighed by the pain or pain-related stressor; produces feelings of commitment, conviction, and eagerness, and an active stance toward pain self-management.
  - *PAI* (Unruh & Ritchie, 1998) assesses judgments of threat/loss or challenge associated with pain. Challenge appraisals are not commonly associated with pain, but decreasing threat/loss appraisals and increasing challenge appraisals are logical treatment goals. PAI does not distinguish between threat and loss, and when one is introducing primary appraisals, it may be clinically useful to do so.

Table 4.3 summarizes this section discussing assessment of primary pain appraisals, and provides a synopsis of the PAI.

ASSESSING SECONDARY APPRAISALS: ACQUIRED BELIEFS AND AUTOMATIC THOUGHTS

In Chapter 2, I have noted that secondary pain appraisals include acquired beliefs about one's pain and automatic thoughts that arise in response to pain-associated cues. Within the stress–appraisal–coping model of pain, beliefs and automatic thoughts interact and influence each other, and both have an impact on coping and adaptation. Acquired or intermediate beliefs include beliefs about pain and beliefs about one's ability to control pain. Automatic thoughts include a variety of cognitions arising in response to pain-related stressors, and negative automatic thoughts are often discussed in terms of catastrophic thinking.

Acquired (Intermediate) Beliefs

Beliefs about Pain

There are a wide variety of attitudes and beliefs[1] about the cause and meaning of the pain experience, and such acquired cognitions influence self-report of pain severity, level of dysfunction, and the type of treatment patients expect. Acquired beliefs about the way pain (and people in pain) should be treated also influence the adjustment process. The two most widely used measures to assess beliefs about the cause, meaning, and appropriate treatment of pain are the Pain Beliefs and Perceptions Inventory (PBPI; Williams & Thorn, 1989) and the Survey of Pain Attitudes (SOPA; Jensen, Karoly, & Huger, 1987). I advise using both the PBPI and the revised version of the original SOPA (SOPA-R; see below) as pre- and posttreatment measures, for several reasons: (1) They have been shown to be predictive of treatment outcome; (2) they are both relatively short; and (3) they measure somewhat different aspects of

---

[1]"Attitudes" are technically distinguished from "beliefs" in the following way: Attitudes are said to stem from a person's feelings toward a subject, and beliefs are said to arise from a person's information about a subject (Ajzen & Fishbein, 1977; Fishbein & Ajzen, 1975).

pain beliefs, as described below. I use these scales as pre- and posttreatment measures, but I also use them in session during Treatment Module 6, where pain-related beliefs are examined. In addition to calculating the scale scores, I suggest doing an item analysis of each client's responses. Visual inspection of the actual items endorsed by the client will give you a more complete sense of the patient's belief than a simple calculation of the scale scores will.

Patients' responses to these measures will help you understand what beliefs they have acquired over time regarding their pain, and their responses to the various items will help you determine the general content category of those beliefs. For example, if a patient scores high on the Medication scale of the SOPA-R, he is likely to believe that pain medications are the best way to manage his pain, and he may resist interventions aimed at reducing his reliance on them. The patient's beliefs regarding the importance of pain medications—including his perceptions of their long-term efficacy, and his fears regarding reductions or discontinuation—may need to be explored before he becomes willing to adopt other pain self-management behaviors. Another example, taken from the PBPI, involves a patient's responses on the Pain as Mystery scale. If a patient scores high on this scale, she may persist in trying to find physical "proof" of her pain in order to justify her level of distress and disability. The patient's beliefs regarding the one-to-one correspondence of pain perception with tissue damage may have to be addressed before she becomes ready to engage in pain self-management behaviors.

In the paragraph above, I have alluded to a patient's willingness to engage in pain self-management behaviors. Assessing a patient's acquired pain-related beliefs with the PBPI or the SOPA-R provides a means of generating hypotheses about his motivation to do so. Before describing the PBPI and the SOPA-R, I introduce a relatively newly developed (and still developing) measure of patients' readiness to adopt pain self-management behaviors: the Multidimensional Pain Readiness to Change Questionnaire (MPRCQ; Nielson, Jensen, & Kerns, 2003). I do not provide it as a measure in this book because it is still in the validation/revision stage, but I see it as an exciting development in the cognitive assessment of pain beliefs.

Multidimensional Pain Readiness to Change Questionnaire. Consideration of patients' motivation to engage in CBT or adopt related pain self-management behaviors has been given very little attention in the research literature (Jensen, Nielson, & Kerns, in press). Based on a theoretical model proposing stages in the process of change (precontemplation, contemplation, action, and maintenance; Prochaska & DiClemente, 1984), Kerns and colleagues developed a 30-item questionnaire, the Pain Stages of Change Questionnaire, to assess patients' general readiness to adopt pain self-management behaviors (Kerns, Rosenberg, Jamison, Caudill, & Haythornthwaite, 1997). This more general measure has been revised to incorporate the view that an individual's "readiness for change" may be different for the various facets of adaptive coping. For example, an individual may be at a high level of readiness to adopt relaxation skills, but at a low level of readiness to adopt exercise as a pain self-management behavior. The revised measure is called the MPRCQ (Nielson et al., 2003). Patients are asked to respond, on a 1–6 scale, regarding how ready they are to use various coping behaviors (e.g., exercise, task persistence, relaxation, cognitive coping, etc.). These motivational subscales show promise in tapping a dimension of cognitions different from what is assessed via other measures of acquired pain beliefs. The MPRCQ is still undergoing validation studies as well as revision of the scale itself (Nielson, Maleus, Jensen, & Kerns, 2004), and thus immediate application of this instrument for the pain practitioner is not possible. However, it may prove useful to follow the literature on the future development of this scale.

Pain Beliefs and Perceptions Inventory. The PBPI is a 16-item scale with four factors, measuring Pain as Mystery (patients' view of pain as a mysterious, aversive event that is poorly understood), Self-Blame (patients' belief that they are the appropriate target to blame for their pain experience), Pain as Permanent, and Pain as Constant. The PBPI has strong psychometric grounding, as well as proven relevance to patient behavior. However, since patients do not typically endorse much self-blame related to their pain, that particular scale may be limited in terms of usefulness. Some examples of PBPI items include "No one's been able to tell me exactly why I am in pain" (Pain as Mystery), "If I am in pain, it is my own fault" (Self-Blame), "I am continuously in pain" (Pain as Constant), and "My pain is here to stay" (Pain as Permanent). Research has shown that if a patient reports that he does not understand his pain condition (Pain as Mystery), he is likely to report greater psychological distress than if he understands the nature of his pain. Furthermore, higher scores on the Pain as Mystery scale are associated with appraisals of harm and threat. The belief that pain is a permanent condition is associated with anxiety, and patients who believe they are to blame for their pain problems are likely to be more depressed than patients who do not blame themselves. Patients who perceive their pain as constant report higher pain intensity levels than patients who perceive their pain to be intermittent. In addition, these sorts of beliefs (the view of pain as constant, permanent, or mysterious, or the belief that one is to blame for the pain condition) have negative associations with treatment compliance in physical therapy and health psychology interventions (Williams & Thorn, 1989). An example of how a patient might fill out the PBPI is provided in Figure 4.3.

Survey of Pain Attitudes—Revised. The original SOPA has undergone a number of revisions, the most recent of which is shorter (35 items) than an earlier 57-item version. The 35-item SOPA-R (Jensen, Turner, & Romano, 2000) assesses somewhat different beliefs and attitudes than the PBPI does. Its subscales (and a sample item from each) include the following:

	Strongly Disagree	Disagree	Agree	Strongly Agree
1. No one's been able to tell me exactly why I'm in pain.	−2	−1	1	**2**
2. I used to think my pain was curable, but now I'm not so sure.	−2	**−1**	1	2
3. There are times when I am pain–free.	**−2**	−1	1	2
4. My pain is confusing to me.	−2	−1	1	**2**
5. My pain is here to stay.	−2	−1	**1**	2
6. I am continuously in pain.	−2	−1	1	**2**
7. If I am in pain, it is my own fault.	**−2**	−1	1	2
8. I don't know enough about my pain.	−2	−1	**1**	2
9. My pain is a temporary problem in my life.	−2	**−1**	1	2
10. It seems like I wake up with pain and I go to sleep with pain.	−2	−1	1	**2**
11. I am the cause of my pain.	**−2**	−1	1	2
12. There is a cure for my pain.	−2	−1	**1**	2
13. I blame myself if I am in pain.	**−2**	−1	1	2
14. I can't figure out why I'm in pain.	−2	−1	1	**2**
15. Someday I'll be 100% pain–free again.	−2	**−1**	1	2
16. My pain varies in intensity but is always with me.	−2	−1	1	**2**

FIGURE 4.3. PBPI: Hypothetical endorsements reflecting high Pain as Mystery and Pain as Constant scores, moderate Pain as Permanent score, and low Self-Blame score.

Solicitude—belief in the appropriateness of solicitous responses from one's family when in pain (e.g., "My family needs to learn to take better care of me when I am in pain").

Medication—belief that medications in general are appropriate for chronic pain problems (e.g., "Medicine is one of the best treatments for chronic pain").

Disability—belief in oneself as unable to function because of pain (e.g., "My pain problem does not need to interfere with my activity level," reverse-scored).

Emotion—belief in a relationship between emotions and pain; (e.g., "Depression increases the pain I feel").

Medical Cure—belief that a medical cure exists for one's pain problem (e.g., "I trust that doctors can cure my pain").

Harm—belief that pain signifies damage and that exercise and activity should therefore be restricted (e.g., "If I exercise, I could make my pain problem much worse").

Patients holding these types of beliefs adjust more poorly to their painful condition, and specific types of beliefs are associated with particular outcomes. For example, believing that one is disabled, and that activity should be avoided because pain signifies damage, is associated with higher levels of physical disability; the belief that chronic pain is best managed with medications is associated with a greater number of pain-related emergency room visits; and the belief that others should be solicitous in response to one's pain is associated with poorer psychological adjustment (M. P. Jensen, Turner, Romano, & Lawler, 1994). An additional SOPA-R scale measures belief in one's personal control over pain (e.g., "I can control my pain by changing my thoughts"), and is labeled the Control scale. Patients holding high control beliefs, or those who increase their control beliefs with treatment, have been shown to have better overall adjustment to chronic pain (M. P. Jensen et al., 1994). I return to the Control scale in the section below, which discusses beliefs about one's control over pain. An example of how a patient might fill out the SOPA-R (first 10 items) is included in Figure 4.4.

Response key: 0 = This is very untrue for me.
1 = This is somewhat untrue for me.
2 = This is neither true nor untrue for me (or it does not apply to me).
3 = This is somewhat true for me.
4 = This is very true for me.

1. The pain I feel is a sign that damage is being done	0	1	2	3	**4**
2. I will probably always have to take pain medications	0	1	2	3	**4**
3. When I hurt, I want my family to treat me better	0	1	2	**3**	4
4. If my pain continues at its present level, I will be unable to work	0	1	2	3	**4**
5. The amount of pain I feel is out of my control	0	1	2	3	**4**
6. I do not expect a medical cure for my pain	0	**1**	2	3	4
7. Pain does not have to mean that my body is being harmed	**0**	1	2	3	4
8. I have had the most relief from pain with the use of medications	0	1	2	3	**4**
9. Anxiety increases the pain I feel	0	1	**2**	3	4
10. There is little that I can do to ease my pain	0	1	2	3	**4**

FIGURE 4.4. SOPA-R (first 10 items): Hypothetical endorsements reflecting low Control score; high Disability, Harm, and Medication scores; moderate Solicitude and Medical Cure scores; and neutral Emotion score. For the SOPA-R itself, copyright 1994 by Mark P. Jensen and Paul Karoly. Reprinted by permission.

The PBPI and the SOPA-35, including scoring keys, are reproduced in Appendices E and F, respectively.

Beliefs about One's Control over Pain

Various measures of locus of control (LOC) and self-efficacy are available to health care providers; some are very specific to a particular problem, and some are meant to be more global measures. Rather than suggesting that you use a separate measure to assess patients' LOC and self-efficacy, I suggest that you focus on the clients' responses to the Control scale of the SOPA-R, which pertains to belief in one's personal control over pain. This subscale can be used to measure a person's sense of self-efficacy in regard to controlling the pain problem. In addition, three other SOPA-R subscales offer indirect information regarding a person's LOC. The extent to which patients believe in a medical cure for their pain problem (Medical Cure), believe that medications are appropriate for chronic pain (Medication), and believe that significant others should be solicitous in response to their experience of pain (Solicitude) offer information regarding the patients' LOC—either directed internally, or directed toward the medical profession or significant others. Ideally, positive treatment outcome would be reflected in an increased score on the Control scale, and decreased scores on the Medication, Medical Cure, and Solicitude scales. An example of how a patient before treatment might fill out the Control scale of the SOPA-R (with the associated SOPA-R item numbers) is included in Figure 4.5.

Automatic Thoughts

As I have stated in Chapter 2, the term "automatic thoughts" refers to cognitions that arise, independent of one's immediate awareness, in response to a pain-related event. Distorted automatic thoughts have also been referred to as "cognitive errors." Although the Cognitive Errors Questionnaire (CEQ; Lefebvre, 1981) provides for the assessment of specific cognitive errors occurring in patients with low back pain, it has not been used much in research or clinical practice because of its length and format. Specifically, the CEQ contains 48 separate vignettes that are followed by one of four types of illogical or distorted inferences, in

Response key: 0 = This is very untrue for me.
　　　　　　　　1 = This is somewhat untrue for me.
　　　　　　　　2 = This is neither true nor untrue for me (or it does not apply to me).
　　　　　　　　3 = This is somewhat true for me.
　　　　　　　　4 = This is very true for me.

5. The amount of pain I feel is out of my control	0 1 2 3 **4**
10. There is little that I can do to ease my pain	0 1 2 **3** 4
21. I can control my pain by changing my thoughts	**0** 1 2 3 4
24. I have learned to control my pain	0 1 2 **3** 4
29. I am not in control of my pain	0 1 2 3 **4**

FIGURE 4.5. SOPA-R Control scale: Hypothetical endorsements reflecting low Control score. For the SOPA-R itself, copyright 1994 by Mark P. Jensen and Paul Karoly. Reprinted by permission.

reference to the hypothetical event described in the vignette. Individuals are asked to indicate the extent to which each thought listed resembles the thought they would have in the same situation. Other researchers have adapted the original CEQ for patients with rheumatoid arthritis (Smith, Christensen, Peck, & Ward, 1994). Although the CEQ is psychometrically sound, I do not use it as an assessment tool. Instead, I prefer to provide a list of the generally accepted categories of cognitive errors, including examples, and use it as a clinical tool when I introduce the concept of automatic thoughts and cognitive errors (see Treatment Module 2).

Assessment of Catastrophizing

In the proliferation of psychosocial pain scales, the measurement of pain catastrophizing has taken a prominent position because of its strong relationship to ratings of the experience of pain, as well as adjustment to chronic pain. Although several measures of pain catastrophizing have been developed (Butler, Damarin, Beaulieu, Schwebel, & Thorn, 1989; Rosenstiel & Keefe, 1983; Sullivan, Bishop, & Pivik, 1995), the Pain Catastrophizing Scale (PCS; Sullivan et al., 1995) has received the most attention in recent research. The PCS has 13 items, which makes the scale quite practical for clinical use. The patient is instructed to reflect on a pain experience and indicate the extent to which she thought about each statement, using a 5-point item response format where 0 indicates "not at all" and 4 represents "all the time." The PCS consists of one general construct, and three empirically derived subscales that are correlated but distinct: Magnification, or exaggeration of the threat value of pain (e.g., "I wonder whether something serious may happen"); Rumination, or focused attention on the pain (e.g., "I can't seem to keep it out of my mind"); and Helplessness, or pessimistic appraisal of the ability to cope (e.g., "There's nothing I can do to feel better"). In the original PCS validation study, the Helplessness and Rumination subscales had satisfactory reliabilities, but the three-item Magnification subscale had less than adequate reliability. Other validation studies have demonstrated adequate internal consistency (reliability) for all three subscales (Osman et al., 2000). The original validation study of the PCS (Sullivan et al., 1995), as well as later studies using community-based samples and outpatient pain clientele, reported sex differences in PCS scores: Women scored higher on the total PCS, as well as on the Rumination and Helplessness subscales. On the other hand, the three-item Magnification subscale has not differentiated men from women (Osman et al., 2000; Sullivan et al., 1995). Although most of the time, PCS results are reported and discussed in terms of the total score, there have been some reports that the specific subscales may vary as a function of duration of pain. For example, the Magnification subscale of the PCS was the best predictor of pain and disability in a sample of patients with whiplash who were approximately 1 year postinjury (Sullivan, Stanish, Sullivan, & Tripp, 2001), whereas the Rumination subscale was the best predictor of severity of disability in patients who had been experiencing pain for approximately 3 years (Sullivan, Stanish, Waite, Sullivan, & Tripp, 1998). Later in the course of chronic low back pain, the Helplessness subscale has been shown to be the best predictor of severity of disability (Viennau, Clark, Lynch, & Sullivan, 1999). Taken together, these studies suggest that the nature of catastrophic cognitions associated with disability may change as the pain condition becomes more chronic.

Because the level of catastrophizing has been shown to be such an important predictor of one's ability to adjust to a chronic pain condition (or to one's ability to tolerate experimental or acute pain, for that matter), I use the PCS as a pretreatment assessment tool, as well as at midtreatment and posttreatment. I also use a patient's responses to the PCS as an educational tool when I am introducing the concept of negative automatic thoughts (Treatment Module 2). Since the treatment program outlined in this book targets dysfunctional thinking, and because pain-related catastrophizing is certainly a crucial aspect of dysfunctional thinking, I consider tracking (and, ideally, changing) the client's catastrophic thought processes to be crucial. An example of how a patient with high levels of pain-related catastrophic thinking might fill out the PCS is included in Figure 4.6.

The PCS, plus a scoring key, is included in Appendix G. In addition, means and standard deviations of PCS scores for patients undergoing evaluation and treatment at a multidisciplinary pain clinic are included (Sullivan et al., 1998).

There has been a great deal of speculation regarding whether the cognitive errors experienced by a patient with pain are tapping something unique to pain, or simply reflect an underlying depressive or anxiety disorder. It is noteworthy that the item content of scales measuring catastrophizing, depression, and anxiety are often very similar, even though they are intended to measure distinct concepts. Not surprisingly, responses on these self-report measures are correlated with each other, suggesting that they are related (Rosenstiel & Keefe, 1983; Sullivan et al., 1995, 1998). Most of the research shows that although there is an association among the conditions of chronic pain, depression, and anxiety, the cognitive errors made by patients with chronic pain are not simply reflections of an anxiety disorder or a de-

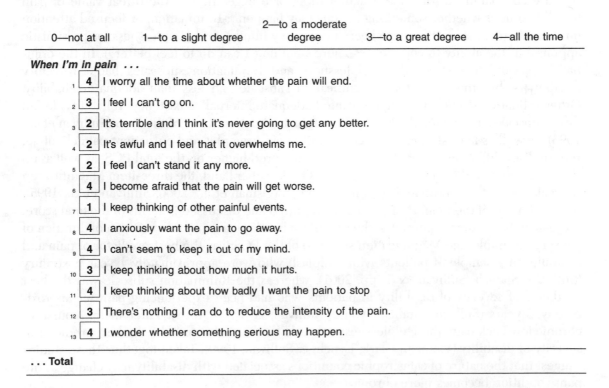

FIGURE 4.6. PCS: Hypothetical endorsements reflecting high Rumination and Helplessness scores, and moderate Magnification score. For the PCS itself, copyright 1995 by Michael J. Sullivan. Reprinted by permission.

pressive disorder (Keefe, Brown, Wallston, & Caldwell, 1989; Sullivan, Thorn, Rogers, & Ward, 2004). The most important conclusion of this research for practitioners is that although many patients with pain may be depressed and anxious, measures of catastrophizing and other cognitive errors predict adjustment to chronic painful states over and above that predicted by depression or anxiety. Thus treating the cognitive errors made by patients with pain is not simply treating their depressive cognitive errors or their anxiety-related cognitive errors. Treating the cognitive errors made by these patients is treating something unique to the pain condition.

Assessment of Other Cognitive Errors

The Inventory of Negative Thoughts in Response to Pain (INTRP; Gil, Williams, Keefe, & Beckham, 1990) was constructed to assess negative thoughts in response to pain flare-ups, and was originally validated on three different populations with chronic pain (i.e., patients with sickle cell disease, rheumatoid arthritis, and mixed chronic pain). In addition to an overall score, three subscale scores reflect a negative sense of self (e.g., "I am worthless"), negative thoughts about interactions with others (e.g., "Other people do not believe I have pain"), and self-blame regarding pain problems (e.g., "I must have done something to bring on this pain") (Gil et al., 1990). The reliability and factor structure obtained in the original study have been supported in later studies (Osman, Bunder, Osman, & Fisher, 1993). Patients with chronic daily pain endorse more frequent negative thoughts during a pain episode than patients having intermittent pain do (Gil et al., 1990). In addition, responding to a pain episode with negative self-statements and negative thoughts about interactions with others is associated with more severe pain and psychological distress during the pain flare-up. The potential value of using the INTRP in addition to the PCS to assess patients' automatic pain-related thoughts is that the INTRP taps into slightly different thought content than the PCS does, particularly as regards patients' perceptions of interactions with others during a pain flare-up. It is not yet known whether the INTRP closely overlaps with measures of depression, or whether it is tapping into a separate construct. However, if you should decide you want to add this to your assessment battery, the instrument can be obtained directly from Gil at *Kgil@email.unc.edu.*

Table 4.4 summarizes this section discussing the assessment of secondary appraisals in patients with pain, and provides a synopsis of the assessment instruments discussed within each category.

ASSESSING COGNITIVE COPING STRATEGIES

Coping involves cognitive or behavioral responses to a stressful situation. Coping, whether adaptive or maladaptive, represents an individual's attempts to resolve pain-related problems, and is strongly influenced by automatic thoughts and beliefs about pain. Given the nature of this book, I focus in this section on the assessment of cognitive coping, rather than on the assessment of cognitive *and* behavioral coping.

As I have mentioned in Chapter 3, there has been some inconsistency when it comes to categorizing cognitive coping strategies; this has made it difficult to evaluate which are strongly related to positive outcome, which are only marginally related to outcome, and which are related to negative outcome.

TABLE 4.4. Assessment of Secondary Pain Appraisals

- *Intermediate beliefs*—Acquired cognitive formulations about the cause and meaning of pain, the way it should be treated, and ability to cope with pain.
  - *Readiness to adopt pain self-management*—Motivation and willingness to adopt various facets of adaptive coping.
    - *MPRCQ* (Nielson et al., 2003) is undergoing validation and revision, but shows promise in terms of assessing patients' readiness to adopt a variety of behaviors shown to be related to positive adaptation to chronic pain.
  - *Beliefs about pain*—Viewpoints regarding the cause of the pain, the nature of the pain experience, and attitudes regarding appropriate and inappropriate response to the pain.
    - *PBPI* (Williams & Thorn, 1989) is reliable, valid, predictive of treatment outcome, and commonly used. Has 16 items with four subscales (Pain as Mystery, Self-Blame, Pain as Permanent, Pain as Constant).
    - *SOPA-R* (Jensen et al., 2000) is reliable, valid, predictive of treatment, and commonly used. Most recent revision has 35 items, with seven subscales (Solicitude, Medication, Disability, Emotion, Medical Cure, Harm, Control).
  - *Beliefs about one's control over pain*—Acquired cognitive understanding regarding one's control over their pain, whether one can execute certain coping responses, and whether particular coping responses will have any impact on one's pain.
    - *SOPA-R* (Jensen et al., 2000) contains a subscale (Control) measuring perceived control over pain and related to self-efficacy. Several other subscales (Medication, Medical Cure, Solicitude) relate to external versus internal LOC.

- *Automatic thoughts*—Cognitive processes that are independent of one's immediate awareness and associated with a specific environmental event or circumstance.
  - *Catastrophizing*—Negatively distorted pain-related cognitions involving magnification of the threat value of pain, rumination about pain, and perceived inability to control pain. Predicts treatment outcome better than many other variables, including pain severity, disease state, age, sex, or depression.
    - *PCS* (Sullivan et al., 1995) is reliable, valid, and robust in its prediction of pain and adaptation to chronic pain. Has 13 items with three subscales (Magnification, Rumination, Helplessness).
  - *Other cognitive errors*—Distorted negative thoughts reflecting a negative sense of self, negative thoughts about interactions with others, and self-blame.
    - *INTRP* (Gil et al., 1990) was constructed to measure cognitions occurring during a pain flare-up, and is associated with poor adaptation to chronic pain. May offer unique information regarding negative perceptions of social interactions.

Cognitive Coping Strategies Inventory—Revised

The original Cognitive Coping Strategies Inventory (CCSI; Butler et al., 1989) was designed to assess cognitive coping strategies used in acute pain situations, although the items are applicable to, and have been used for, populations with chronic pain as well (Boothby, Thorn, Ward, & Overduin, 2004; James, Thorn, & Williams, 1993; Stewart, Harvey, & Evans, 2001). The CCSI items were written to specifically capture and assess various categories of cognitive coping (see Chapter 3), and the instrument was validated on a clinical population of patients with postsurgical pain. In addition to six scales reflecting cognitive coping strategies that were thought to be adaptive, a seventh scale was constructed in an attempt to measure catastrophic thought processes. In the original validation study (Butler et al., 1989), the CCSI subscales were constructed by composing items that fit rationally into each of the scales. Factor analysis of the scales revealed two main components: The first six scales loaded together as one Coping factor, and the seventh scale became the Catastrophizing factor. We found that higher scores on the Coping factor were associated with higher ratings by nurses of patients' ability to tolerate postsurgical pain, and lower pain intensity ratings by the patients themselves. On the other hand, higher scores on the Catastrophizing factor were related to higher self-ratings of postsurgical pain. In a later study, the Coping factor was not significantly related to analgesic use among women undergoing breast surgery, but the Catastrophizing factor predicted greater use of analgesic medications (Jacobsen & Butler, 1996).

One of the criticisms of the original CCSI was that although a factor analysis of the subscales was done, the subscales were not themselves derived through factor analysis, meaning that the subscales might be highly correlated and be subject to poor internal consistency (Stewart et al., 2001). A more recent factor analysis of the items on an abbreviated version of the CCSI resulted in three distinct factors. The first factor was primarily composed of items reflecting the use of distraction techniques (e.g., using imagery, characteristics of the external environment, or cognitions to distract oneself from the pain) This Distraction factor was unrelated to pain tolerance or pain intensity ratings in experimental pain participants, and it was also unrelated to various measures of pain adaptation in a sample of patients with chronic pain (e.g., pain severity, pain interference, perceived life control, mood, or activity ratings). In other words, distraction techniques did not have any association with the way experimental participants dealt with laboratory-induced pain or the way in which patients with chronic pain perceived the pain to affect their lives. The second factor contained the catastrophizing items; as predicted, it was associated with poor tolerance and high pain ratings in experimental participants, and higher pain severity, higher perceived interference, lower sense of life control, and poorer mood in patients with chronic pain.[2] A third factor was primarily composed of items reflecting the use of coping self-statements, attentional focus toward the sensory components of the pain, and emotional distancing, as well as cognitive minimization of the sensory stimulus. This factor was associated with higher tolerance times and lower pain intensity ratings in experimental subjects, but was not significantly associated with pain adaptation in patients with chronic pain (Thorn, Ward, & Clements, 2003).

Recall from Chapter 3 that there is good evidence that positive self-statements are useful cognitive coping strategies, as well as some experimental evidence that focused attention/distancing strategies are helpful in coping with pain. In addition, there appears to be accumulating evidence that distraction strategies are not useful for patients with chronic pain. The CCSI enables the clinician to assess a patient's self-report of these types of cognitive coping strategies and catastrophizing appraisals before treatment, and allows for the assessment of changes in these appraisals and coping strategies after treatment. In particular, it would be useful to determine a patient's baseline levels of catastrophizing and use of distraction strategies before treatment, and to have, as general goals, decreasing catastrophic appraisals and neither increasing nor decreasing distraction strategies. Furthermore, helping patients to increase the other coping strategies (i.e., focusing attention on the sensory qualities of the stim-

---

[2]It is interesting to note that the items on the CCSI Catastrophizing scale, in combination with the PCS items, have been found to result in four factors rather than the three factors originally proposed by Sullivan and colleagues (1995). Thus the CCSI Catastrophizing scale seems to add a unique aspect to the construct of catastrophizing, not previously captured by the PCS. Also, the addition of several CCSI items to the Magnification scale of the PCS increased the internal consistency of that scale (Thorn, Ward, & Clements, 2003).

ulus, redefining the pain sensation, and using positive coping self-statements) would be a useful treatment goal.

The original CCSI has 70 items, each rated by the patient on a 5-point item response format. Since it is quite long for clinical use, clinicians may wish to use an abbreviated version (CCSI-R; Thorn, Ward, & Clements, 2003), which has a total of 32 items but adequately captures the two main coping factors of interest (Distraction and Coping Self-Statements/Cognitive Minimization of Stimulus), as well as the Catastrophizing appraisal factor. An example of how a patient might fill out the CCSI-R (first 10 items) is provided in Figure 4.7. The CCSI-R is included in Appendix H.

Coping Strategies Questionnaire—Revised

The original Coping Strategies Questionnaire (CSQ; Rosenstiel & Keefe, 1983) was constructed specifically for assessing patients with low back pain, and it has been more widely used than any other measure of coping in populations with chronic pain (Jensen, Turner, Romano, & Karoly, 1991). The CSQ, as it was originally constructed, has 48 items (excluding two self-efficacy items) that are rated by the patient on a 6-point item response format. It includes subscales assessing six cognitive coping strategies and two behavioral coping strategies: Diverting Attention, Reinterpreting Pain, Coping Self-Statements, Ignoring Pain, Praying/Hoping, Catastrophizing, Increasing Activity, and Increasing Pain Behaviors. The CSQ also includes two Self-Efficacy items measuring perceived ability to decrease pain and perceived control over pain. In the original validation study, the CSQ subscales were constructed by composing items that fit rationally into each of the scales. Factor analysis of the scales revealed three main components: Cognitive Coping and Suppression (which included items from Reinterpreting Pain, Coping Self-Statements, and Ignoring Pain); Diverting Attention and Praying (which included items from Diverting Attention and Praying/Hoping); and Helplessness (which included items from Catastrophizing, reverse-scored items from

1	2	3	4	5
Never True	Some of the Time True	One-Half of the Time True	Most of the Time True	All of the Time True

1. __3__ I use my imagination to change the situation or place where I am experiencing pain, in order to try and make the pain more bearable.

2. __2__ I think of photographs or paintings that I have seen in the past.

3. __2__ I feel like I just want to get up and run away.

4. __1__ I imagine the pain becoming even more intense and hurtful.

5. __1__ I begin thinking of all the possible bad things that could go wrong in association with the pain.

6. __5__ I "psych" myself up to deal with the pain, perhaps by telling myself that it won't last much longer.

7. __2__ I picture in my "mind's eye" a lush, green forest or other similar peaceful scene.

8. __4__ I try and imagine that for some reason it is important for me to endure the pain.

9. __2__ I tell myself that I don't think I can bear the pain any longer.

10. __2__ I use my imagination to develop pictures which help distract me.

FIGURE 4.7. CCSI-R (first 10 items): Hypothetical endorsements reflecting low Catastrophizing score, moderate Distraction score, and high Coping Self-Statements/Cognitive Minimization of Stimulus score. For the CCSI itself, copyright 1985 by Robert W. Butler. Reprinted by permission.

Increasing Activity, and the two reverse-scored Self-Efficacy items). The items on the Catastrophizing scale of the CSQ are almost identical to those on the Helplessness scale of the PCS (in fact, the original CSQ Catastrophizing items were only slightly adapted and included as part of the PCS items). As was true for the CCSI, the original validation study of the CSQ conducted a factor analysis on the scales rather than the items, and the CSQ has also been criticized for high interscale correlations and low internal consistencies (Stewart et al., 2001). The CSQ has been a subject of a great deal of research, and various attempts to replicate the three factors found in the original study have been unsuccessful. Two studies reported that there were five distinct factors (Swartzman, Gwadry, Shapiro, & Teasell, 1994; Tuttle, Shutty, & DeGood, 1991), whereas later studies have found six factors similar in content to the original rationally derived scales (Riley & Robinson, 1997; Robinson et al., 1997).

The CSQ has since been revised and shortened to 27 items, which makes it more practical to use in a clinical setting (Riley & Robinson, 1997). The CSQ-R has identified six factors based on an item-level factor analysis (Riley & Robinson, 1997). A later study using the CSQ-R identified two factors (Catastrophizing items and Distraction items forming one factor, and all other items forming the second Cognitive Coping factor) (Riley, Robinson, & Geisser, 1999). Three subgroups of patients were identified: the "cognitive copers," who scored high on Cognitive Coping and relatively low on Distraction and Catastrophizing; the "low responders," who scored low on all measures; and the "catastrophizers/distracters," who scored low on Cognitive Coping but high on Catastrophizing and Distraction. An example of how the third type of patient might fill out the CSQ-R (first 10 items) is given in Figure 4.8. The CSQ-R, plus a scoring key, is included in Appendix I.

Table 4.5 summarizes this section discussing assessment of cognitive coping strategies in patients with pain, and provides a synopsis of the assessment instruments discussed within each category.

0	1	2	3	4	5	6
Never do that			Sometimes do that			Always do that

When I feel pain . . .

_1_ 1. I try to feel distant from the pain, almost as if the pain was in somebody else's body.

_1_ 2. I try to think of something pleasant.

_5_ 3. It's terrible and I feel it's never going to get any better.

_2_ 4. I tell myself to be brave and carry on despite the pain.

_1_ 5. I tell myself that I can overcome the pain.

_5_ 6. It's awful and I feel that it overwhelms me.

_4_ 7. I feel my life isn't worth living.

_3_ 8. I pray to God it won't last long.

_1_ 9. I try not to think of it as my body, but rather as something separate from me.

_0_ 10. I don't think about the pain.

FIGURE 4.8. CSQ-R (first 10 items): Hypothetical endorsements reflecting high Distraction and Catastrophizing scores, and low Cognitive Coping score. For the CSQ-R itself, reprinted by permission of Michael E. Robinson and Anne Rosenstiel Gross.

TABLE 4.5. Assessment of Cognitive Coping Strategies

- *CCSI-R* (Thorn, Ward, & Clements, 2003)—32 items assessing cognitive coping strategies and catastrophic pain appraisals. Three factors (Distraction, Coping Self-Statements/Cognitive Minimization of Stimulus, Catastrophizing). Distraction is unrelated to experimental pain or measures of adjustment to chronic pain; Coping Self-Statements/Cognitive Minimization is negatively related to perceived pain; Catastrophizing is positively related to perceived pain and poor adjustment in patients with chronic pain. Catastrophizing factor offers a unique contribution to the original three-domain construct of catastrophizing.

- *CSQ-R* (Riley & Robinson, 1997)—27 items assessing cognitive coping strategies and catastrophic pain appraisals. Six scales (Distraction, Ignoring Pain, Distancing from the Pain, Coping Self-Statements, Praying, and Catastrophizing) and two general factors (Cognitive Coping and Catastrophizing/Distraction). Catastrophizing/Distraction is related to poor indicators of adjustment to chronic pain; Cognitive Coping is related to higher activity levels in patients with chronic pain. Catastrophizing items are very similar in content to PCS Helplessness items.

USING THE ASSESSMENT IN TREATMENT PLANNING

To show you how the instruments described in this chapter can be used in treatment planning, I next present the details of my findings from a sample cognitive assessment. This case example is more specific than what I would typically write for my own use, and certainly more detailed than a summary I would provide to a referring physician. To illustrate how to summarize such findings for a referring health care provider, see Appendix B.

The initial assessment always begins with a clinical interview, as well as liaisons with the appropriate medical or other health care professional(s). Appropriate releases will need to be signed by the patient so that communication with the referring health care provider can be ongoing.

Martha Anne was referred by a rheumatologist in town, following his unsuccessful treatment of her fibromyalgia and chronic fatigue syndrome. A noteworthy aspect of Martha Anne's history was that she had been involved in a life-altering, single-car motor vehicle accident (MVA) 5 years previously. Martha Anne had just purchased the car of her dreams, and almost immediately unintentionally drove it into a culvert filled with rocks and tree trunks. She experienced numerous fractures as well as a concussion, and several surgeries were required to repair her right shoulder, elbow, and wrist. She regained only 50% range of motion in her hand and arm, and reported experiencing daily "aching" pain associated with the injury. Although she had returned to work 6 months following the MVA, she was no longer working by the time she was referred to me. Shortly after the MVA, Martha Anne began to experience increasing generalization of the "aching" sensation to other parts of her body. Four years after the MVA, Martha Anne was diagnosed with fibromyalgia, and shortly before she was referred to me, she had received the additional diagnosis of chronic fatigue syndrome. During the past year, Martha Anne had lost functional capacity in various activities of daily living, and she currently relied on her grown daughter for household management and food preparation. Martha Anne's physician noted that she was taking five different analgesic medications and three psychotropic medications, although they did not seem to make an appreciable difference in her ability to function. In fact, during our clinical interview, Martha Anne noted that she felt the addition of several medications had made things worse in terms of her mood and sleep cycle.

Martha Anne expressed an interest in joining a pain management group. She had been in individual psychotherapy with a local psychologist to deal with a divorce 10 years ago, as well as for supportive therapy subsequent to the MVA. She was therefore receptive to psychotherapeutic interventions.

Following my initial interview, I scheduled Martha Anne for an assessment session, during which I asked her to complete the DAS-24, PAI, PBPI, SOPA-R, PCS, CCSI-R, and CSQ-R. Noteworthy scale scores on the measures, and my interpretations or hypotheses, included the following:

1. *DAS-24*: High Dependency score suggests that Martha Anne may hold distorted beliefs about the importance of others for her happiness. Her dependency needs may promote greater passivity and reliance on others. Assertiveness exercises may be of particular relevance.

2. *PAI*: Exclusive threat/loss appraisals (no challenge appraisals). Threat appraisals suggest that Martha Anne may have a reduced ability to focus her attention away from pain or anticipated pain, as well as a poor capacity for concentration. Loss appraisals may suggest increased passivity and lack of initiative to engage in self-care behaviors. Successfully motivating Martha Anne to engage in treatment may be problematic. High loss appraisals may be partly based on the traumatic MVA, and it will be important to listen for Martha Anne's themes of loss regarding her pain, particularly to determine which components might be associated with unresolved emotions regarding her MVA. Expressive writing exercises may be particularly useful if this is the case.

3. *PBPI*: Low Pain as Mystery score, but high Self-Blame score. Martha Anne seems to have an adequate understanding of her pain, which is a good prognostic sign. Clarify whether this is true for her more recent diagnoses of fibromyalgia and chronic fatigue syndrome. High Self-Blame score is somewhat unusual and often indicative of depression, which may complicate treatment. Listen for themes of self-blame associated with the MVA, which may be related to her high loss appraisals.

4. *SOPA-R*: High Disability, Harm, Emotion, and Solicitude scores, but low Control, Medication, and Medical Cure scores. High disability and harm beliefs will encourage further passivity and avoidance of therapeutic activities. Challenge erroneous beliefs, using cognitive restructuring exercises. High emotion beliefs reflect an awareness that emotions have an impact on physical well-being—a good prognostic sign. High solicitude beliefs may be associated with her high dependency attitudes as indicated on the DAS, and underscore the need to understand Martha Anne's interpersonal relationship factors. Consider giving WHYMPI to obtain responses regarding her perceptions of significant others. Consider conjoint sessions with daughter and Martha Anne. Low medication and medical cure beliefs may be a good prognostic sign, if we can provide other coping strategies to replace reliance on medications. Consider Martha Anne's motivation to reduce her medications, and facilitate desired medication reductions with her physician. Low Control score indicates a poor sense of self-efficacy regarding pain self-management. It will be necessary to proceed slowly, introducing small goals that are likely to produce success experiences.

5. *PCS*: Moderate total catastrophizing score (especially reflected in Rumination and Helplessness subscales), which is likely to be associated with high threat and loss appraisals,

and may compound her passivity and avoidance. Cognitive restructuring aimed at catastrophic automatic thoughts will be particularly important.

6. *CCSI-R*: Low Coping Self-Statements/Cognitive Minimization of Stimulus score and moderate Catastrophizing score. Low positive coping self-statements probably relate to low self-efficacy. Gradual success experiences, coupled with coping self-statement exercises, may increase Martha Anne's sense of her ability to carry out pain self-management tasks. The moderate score on the CCSI-R Catastrophizing factor may indicate a different type of distorted automatic thinking from that reflected by scores on the PCS, and visual inspection of all Catastrophizing items should be undertaken.

7. *CSQ-R*: Low Cognitive Coping score and moderate Catastrophizing score. Martha Anne has few adaptive cognitive coping strategies in her repertoire, and will benefit from coping self-statement training.

CHAPTER SUMMARY

In this chapter, I have provided cognitive assessment tools that can be used as pre- and posttreatment assessments, but also as psychoeducational tools within the treatment regimen itself. The cognitive assessment tools I have provided follow the components of the stress–appraisal–coping model of pain, assessing individual differences (DAS-24), primary appraisals (PAI), secondary appraisals (PBPI, SOPA-R, PCS), and cognitive coping strategies (CCSI-R, CSQ-R). Each of the measures can be incorporated into the corresponding treatment session in order to help illustrate the concept and inform the client of his own individual cognitions, as assessed before the treatment began. It is gratifying for patients (and therapists!) to see how these cognitions change.

The next chapter introduces Part II of the book, which involves the presentation of 10 cognitive therapy treatment modules. The treatment modules follow a similar format across sessions, and session outlines, as well as worksheets, are provided so that you can make copies for your clients and use them as you follow the proposed treatment plan.

PART II

A COGNITIVE TREATMENT PROGRAM FOR CHRONIC PAIN

INTRODUCTION
An Overview of the Treatment Program

In the first three chapters of this book, I have provided the rationale and theoretical model for incorporating a detailed, structured cognitive therapy intervention into a pain management regimen, together with a review of the supporting outcome research. With this conceptual background and Chapter 4's assessment arsenal in hand, you are well prepared to integrate cognitive therapy for pain into your treatment regimen.

Notice that I am suggesting an *integration* of this cognitive program into your treatment approach. Cognitive-behavioral therapy (CBT) already includes well-established and evidence-based behavioral techniques, and I am not advocating discontinuing these interventions. I am suggesting, however, that cognitive interventions—especially when offered early in treatment—are likely to increase clients' receptivity to incorporating various pain self-management skills into their repertoire, as well as decrease their passive reliance on the health care system to "cure" their pain.

Ideally, either during or following the cognitive therapy intervention, clients will begin to engage in a physical therapy-directed exercise program; begin reducing their reliance on analgesic and sedative/hypnotic medication; increase their activities of daily living, including participation in some activities that have previously provided a sense of pleasure, as well as some household management activities; begin to pace their rest–activity cycles so that they neither underengage nor overengage in periods of activity; and begin to utilize some form of relaxation/meditation/self-hypnosis during scheduled periods of rest. These are some examples of pain management behaviors that are frequently part of a multidisciplinary pain management intervention. In essence, then, I am suggesting that using cognitive interventions frees the clients to adopt a wide variety of coping options with established utility.

MODALITY: GROUP VERSUS INDIVIDUAL TREATMENT

Although it is quite reasonable to conduct cognitive therapy in an individual treatment format, I prefer a group therapy format for cognitive therapy and CBT of chronic pain. The research literature supports the efficacy of group treatment for chronic pain (Keefe, Beaupre, & Gil, 2002), and in many ways it is more cost-effective to offer group treatment. Group treatment is also the standard in inpatient pain management clinics (Keefe et al., 2002). At the clinical/process level, I find that group interaction serves an instructional as well as a supportive function. For example, when trying to get the concept of "automatic thoughts" across to clients, I have often found that a patient can more readily identify the automatic thought of a fellow group member than her own. I explain to clients that it is always easier to see a stressful situation objectively when it is not our own; we are not caught up in the emotional relevance of the situation if it is not our stress. Once a client understands the concept behind automatic thoughts by using someone else's real example, she can more easily identify such thinking in her own situation. Clients also learn vicariously from the example of other group members: When one patient identifies a thought pattern and begins to change her thinking, others can benefit from observing the process and tracking the outcome. You will see, throughout the following treatment modules, that I illustrate concepts by working through one or more examples with clients in session. Although you may have time during a session to work through a couple of the clients' examples, the majority of group members during the session are probably participant-observers in the process—learning by working through another group member's example. Group members learn from both types of interactions. In terms of emotional support, group treatment has been documented to be helpful. Patients with chronic pain often feel isolated and misunderstood. Being able to disclose thoughts and feelings to others who have shared similar circumstances gives clients a greater sense that their problems are legitimate. Also, when a patient confronts a fellow patient by pointing out a cognitive error or maladaptive behavior, the confrontation is often easier to accept than when it comes from a nonpatient. For all of these reasons, I advocate group treatment of patients with chronic pain.

Group Size, Composition, and Patient Characteristics

Many logistical questions arise regarding the size and composition of these therapy groups. For example, how big (or small) should the groups be? What kinds of age disparities in group members can be tolerated? What about the gender makeup of the group? What if there are language or cultural disparities among group members? Since this is *cognitive* therapy, how cognitively intact must clients be to benefit from the group? What about issues regarding comorbidity of other disorders (physiological as well as emotional) with chronic pain? And is it better to use single therapists or cotherapists for group treatment?

In response to these questions, I make a distinction between the real and the ideal. Ideally, the group would consist of about five members—large enough to facilitate interaction, but small enough to allow participants their share of "the floor." However, I have run groups with as few as three and as many as nine participants. A group of three did not seem to present problems, but a group of nine was a bit unwieldy. In terms of gender makeup, you will find that more women participate in treatment than men, with the possible exception of work-hardening inpatient pain management programs. Thus you can realistically expect a greater percentage of women in your groups than men. Although age, cultural, and ethnic disparities might lead group members to feel less connected with each other, I have found that chronic pain is a unifying factor that seems to make other potentially divisive issues less important. Although I do not include children in my pain management groups, participants as young as 18 have worked successfully alongside group members in their 60s and 70s.

Regarding single therapist versus cotherapists for groups such as this, you can do either. I have the luxury of having a cotherapist in my groups because I train others to lead these groups. However, the typical "real-world" practice may require a single therapist, and there is nothing inherent in this treatment that would preclude this format.

Comorbidity issues involve physiologically established disease states as well as the disorders presently referred to as "mental disorders." There are many chronic and degenerative diseases that involve pain. Because I accept all pain as real, those patients with identified diseases are not treated as more "entitled" to their pain. However, concomitant disease states necessitate a broader physiological knowledge base on the part of the therapist, as well as frequent consultations with collaborating physicians. In terms of comorbid mental disorders, mood and anxiety disorders are particularly prevalent in patients with chronic pain. Since we already know that cognitive therapy is an evidence-based treatment approach for depression and anxiety, the cognitive intervention program described in this book may have the added benefit of ameliorating the emotional disorders as well.

Who Is Not Suitable for This Kind of Treatment?

Some patients may not be suited to or appropriate for group treatment, given a level of distress or chronic relationship difficulties that would be disruptive to the group process. In addition, individuals with poor reading skills, little formal education, or limited understanding of English may have difficulty with this approach. Certainly, an option for qualified therapists is translation of the treatment into a language easily understood by patients for whom English is a second language. Some patients eschew group treatment because they do not feel comfortable sharing personal issues with other patients. Furthermore, for practical reasons, some individuals cannot modify their personal schedules to fit a group time, and thus need individual accommodation.

Regarding the cognitive status of group members, this should be sufficient to enable participants to benefit from the group. Although I do not include actively psychotic individuals in a group, I have included mildly demented participants. While I cannot say that they received optimal treatment benefits, they were able to incorporate some aspects of the program into their coping repertoire; perhaps more importantly, they were able to connect with the other group members, and the others with them. I would not suggest including potential participants with more than a very mild level of dementia, or ones with other limiting cognitive conditions resulting from, for example, closed head injuries. These individuals are unlikely to be able to understand the concepts being presented, and will probably become confused by the homework and frustrated with the process. It is always better to work with these patients individually, so that you can slow the pace, change the technique, and optimize successful participation in whatever aspects of treatment they *can* engage in.

The bottom line for all of us in real life is that clients ready for group treatment do not present with discrete disorders, in the same age cohort, with similar cultural backgrounds and socioeconomic levels. When you have enough clients to make up a group, start it. The key is to exclude potential group participants who are likely to *interfere* with the group process, or those who would be frustrated and confused by the cognitive and psychoeducational nature of the treatment. Meanwhile, include others, even if you have some questions about their receiving *optimal* treatment benefit.

WHO IS QUALIFIED TO RUN THESE TREATMENT GROUPS?

At least on the surface, any manualized treatment program seems easy to administer: A step-by-step guide is provided, and patient materials are already prepared. The treatment offered in this book, like any other psychotherapeutic intervention, requires basic knowledge and training in the principles of psychotherapy, as well as some understanding of personality and psychopathology. Beyond the *content* of the material to be presented, understanding the *process* of psychotherapy is crucial. "Process" includes, but is not limited to, a client's nonverbal as well as verbal behaviors; the dynamic nature of the relationship between the client and the therapist; and the timing of, as well as the individual tailoring of, interventions based on moment-to-moment developments within the session.

Group treatment is different from individual therapy, in that the therapist attends not only to the content and process of the individual client who is speaking, but also to the interactions among group members. In some ways this complicates the therapist's job, but in other ways it makes for a more exhilarating therapy session. However, administering any group treatment requires knowledge and training regarding group therapy, in addition to the basics of psychotherapy, personality, and psychopathology.

The kinds of training you need for successfully conducting a group like this are not associated with one particular degree; they are certain kinds of didactic and supervised experiential training. If you have not yet gotten these kinds of training, many graduate programs in psychology, social work, counseling, and couple and family therapy, as well as some psychiatric nursing programs, offer the kinds of experiences you need in order to administer this treatment competently. In addition, continuing education workshops can supplement your training, although they do not usually offer the kinds of supervised experiential instruction that are vital to your development as a psychotherapist.

OVERVIEW OF THE TREATMENT

The 10 modules presented in this part of the book provide a step-by-step guide to a cognitive intervention program for pain management. Each module covers a separate treatment session, meant to be presented as a single 90-minute unit. Although each of the treatment modules can be covered in a single session, it is also possible to expand the time used to cover each concept—particularly with individual clients who may be having difficulty grasping the approach, or with groups that have a relatively large number of participants (i.e., five or more). It may also be possible to streamline the treatment into fewer than 10 sessions, although quite frankly, I have had little success with the truncated approach. Although the sessions can be presented more frequently than once per week (e.g., in an inpatient treatment program), I find it ideal to have a week in between sessions in order for each client to have time to practice the material presented and thus incorporate it into his skills repertoire. In my discussion of the treatment, I will use the terms "module" and "session" interchangeably.

Organization of the Treatment Sessions

The 10 treatment sessions include traditional cognitive restructuring modules, as well as modules covering training in coping techniques that are based on a cognitive conceptualization. (See Table II.1 for an overview.) While the initial session is used to acquaint the group members with the cognitive therapy process, it also introduces the stress–pain connection. In addition, Session 1 introduces clients to the concept that our judgments regarding stressful situations, including the stressors associated with chronic pain, influence our choice of coping options. The next three sessions teach clients how to recognize automatic thoughts, how to evaluate them for negative distortions, and how to construct more realistic alternative responses. The modules regarding automatic thoughts are the crux of traditional cognitive restructuring therapy; I spread this topic over three sessions in order to give clients plenty of time to understand the concept and experience success with the cognitive restructuring technique. Sessions 5 and 6 build on the cognitive restructuring process to help clients recognize negatively distorted intermediate beliefs and core beliefs, and to create alternative, more realistic belief systems. Treatment Module 6 focuses specifically on pain-related intermediate and core beliefs, and provides a therapeutic process for examining them, challenging negative distortions, and creating new pain-related belief systems.

Treatment Module 7 teaches clients how to incorporate coping self-statements into their arsenal of cognitive coping techniques. Coping self-statements are somewhat different from the alternative thoughts generated during cognitive restructuring exercises, in that they tend to be somewhat global and to promote self-efficacy and an internal locus of control. Coping self-statements serve as the emotional "cheerleaders" in the cognitive coping arsenal.

Sessions 8–9 present coping techniques based on a cognitive conceptualization, and draw a connection from cognition to affect (expressive writing) and from cognition to behavior (assertiveness training). Treatment Module 8 introduces an expressive writing exercise in order to help clients explore and process their thoughts and emotions regarding their painful condition. Expressive writing encompasses emotions as well as cognitions, and provides an emotional discharge outlet for patients without the risk of overwhelming others. Treatment Module 9 is based on the idea that patients who have a tendency to express catastrophic and other negative thoughts may have a pressing need for support from significant others. Although such expressions of negative thoughts may draw attention and support in the short run, in the long run they have the tendency to elicit negative reactions from others. In Ses-

TABLE II.1. Organization of the Treatment Sessions

- Module/Session 1: The Stress–Pain–Appraisal Connection
- Module/Session 2: Identifying Automatic Thoughts
- Module/Session 3: Evaluating Automatic Thoughts
- Module/Session 4: Challenging Automatic Thoughts and Constructing Alternative Responses
- Module/Session 5: Intermediate and Core Beliefs (General)
- Module/Session 6: Pain-Specific Intermediate and Core Beliefs
- Module/Session 7: Coping Self-Statements
- Module/Session 8: Expressive Writing
- Module/Session 9: Assertive Communication
- Module/Session 10: Final Session

sion 9, I teach clients how to more assertively and more effectively communicate their needs to significant others.

The final treatment module (Session 10) provides a recap of the treatment approaches taught in the cognitive therapy program, and provides some tips for relapse prevention. Helping patients prepare for the inevitable pain flare-ups by providing a different set of thoughts, beliefs, and attitudes to cope with their pain is an important part of generalizing treatment gains beyond therapy.

Rationale for Organization of the Treatment Sessions

When I first began to incorporate cognitive restructuring techniques into my CBT regimen for chronic pain, I devoted one session to negative automatic thinking. But it became obvious that one session devoted to cognitive restructuring was not sufficient, and I decided to experiment with increasing the amount of time devoted to cognitive restructuring in an attempt to allow for a more thorough integration of this process into my CBT regimen. This is one reason why I have chosen to break the typical automatic thoughts worksheet into more discrete components to be presented in sequential sessions, rather than presenting it in its entirety in one session.

Virtually no research has systematically manipulated the number of cognitive restructuring sessions and compared outcomes, and the related available literature is far from conclusive. Based on my clinical observations, for a certain period of time clients struggle with the process of recognizing distorted thoughts, evaluating and challenging those thoughts, and constructing alternative thoughts. However, 3–4 weeks' time seems sufficient to master the concept. In fact, I have observed that clients often experience an "aha!" phenomenon, before which they struggle in confusion and frustration, and after which they seem to have truly grasped the meaning of cognitive restructuring. It is interesting to note that the research literature on cognitive therapy mentions a phenomenon termed "sudden gains," in which there is a rapid gain in positive response over a relatively short treatment period (4–6 weeks) following the introduction of cognitive restructuring techniques (Tan & DeRubeis, 1999). The sudden-gains effect described in the research literature may reflect my clinical observations that clients seem to go from struggling with the concept to rapidly understanding it after working with cognitive restructuring for several sessions.

In developing a deeper appreciation of the process of cognitive restructuring, I came to realize that this technique was not only applicable to automatic thoughts: It was relevant to primary appraisals of pain and associated stressors, as well as to multiple kinds of secondary appraisals—not just automatic thoughts, but also acquired beliefs about the nature of pain and one's ability to control the pain. These acquired pain-related beliefs fit well within the traditional cognitive therapy terminology of intermediate beliefs. And, in the process of developing these ideas, I became aware that a client's acquired belief about himself as a "disabled chronic pain patient" fit well within the traditional cognitive terminology of core beliefs. The cognitive restructuring components of the treatment program began to take on the logical organizational format of a stress–appraisal–coping model, within which the various aspects of primary and secondary appraisals are considered. This explains my organization of the first six treatment modules.

The final three treatment modules (not including the termination session) are based on my interpretation of the cognitive coping literature in pain, as well as the evolving conceptualization of pain-related catastrophic thinking as it translates into emotions as well as behavior. As stated earlier, I do not suggest that we attend only to patients' cognitions, without consideration of their emotions and behavior. Although there are numerous evidence-based behavioral interventions available to you, a cognitive conceptualization of expressive writing and assertion training provides a unique basis from which to view these particular exercises, and their explicit link to catastrophic thinking is explored in detail. Thus these modules become logical supplements to the cognitive restructuring sessions.

Every treatment program needs a final session in which the major points are summarized, misconceptions are clarified, and suggestions for continuing the process begun in treatment are given. If, by the end of the group, clients have come to understand that one of the best therapists for them is themselves, treatment can be viewed as a success. A termination session is also meant to provide a sense of closure for each client, and in group therapy, it further provides a way for members to acknowledge the importance of others' contributions to the group.

A logistical question regards what to do when a group participant misses a session. Since the sessions build upon each other, it is important to attempt to schedule a makeup session prior to the next one if at all possible. What we have done in our clinical research program is to inform clients that if they miss a particular session, they will need to attend a makeup scheduled immediately before the next session. "Prescheduling" the makeups is more practical than attempting to generate a mutually acceptable time after the missed session. Before you know it, the next week's session will be upon you, and the client will not have received the makeup. Also, if the makeup times are prearranged, you can take care of all absentees at the same time, thus holding a "mini-group" if more than one client missed a session.

OVERVIEW OF THE SESSION FORMAT

The sessions follow a specific format, which is presented in Table II.2. With the exception of the initial session, each begins with a presession questionnaire (the "Presession Process Check"; see Appendix J) and an overview of the previous week's session. This is then followed by a fairly extensive review of homework from the prior week. Spending time on the homework emphasizes the essential nature of between-session work and underscores the importance of the collaborative working relationship between client and therapist. Clients must quickly learn that it is not okay for them to have done nothing between sessions.

Troubleshooting Tip: In my experience with clients who do not complete homework assignments during a particular week, a common explanation is that they were in too much pain

---

TABLE II.2. Overview of Standard Session Format

- Presession Process Check
- Review of previous week's session
- Homework review
- Session treatment objectives
- Worksheet
- Homework assignment
- Postsession Process Check

---

or were too sick. When I receive that explanation, I briefly acknowledge their pain or illness without asking them to relay the details of the experience. Although my colleagues and I are empathic to clients' pain and illness conditions, we know that allowing them to dwell on the details of their pain flare-ups does not serve an adaptive function, whereas focusing on concrete pain and stress management strategies does promote positive adaptation to the painful condition. I encourage clients to always do something related to the homework in between sessions, even if they are experiencing a pain or illness flare-up. Often a client has done at least part of the homework, and it is possible to focus on what he has done rather than on whether he has *completed* the homework. The point is to keep the client working on treatment goals in spite of the pain experience.

After the homework review, one or more new concepts are presented in the form of treatment objectives for the session. This presentation takes a psychological–educational approach in the form of a brief and basic "mini-lecture," including pertinent examples. When I am about to present new treatment concepts, I tell clients that I am going to go into my "mini-lecture" part of the session. This prepares them for the more didactic format in this part of the session, which is somewhat different from the interactive makeup of the rest of the session. A simple, straightforward, and personable approach seems to work well when I am presenting the new treatment concepts. Although the treatment outlines help, I encourage my therapists-in-training (and likewise encourage you) not to read from an outline or to use a prepared script, but rather to work toward presenting the concepts in their own words. During this part of the treatment session, you will be providing examples of the concepts you are teaching, and you will also get group members to share relevant examples from their own life situations. Make sure that you acknowledge the clients' participation by restating or rephrasing what they have said, and perhaps weaving it into the context of the concept being discussed. This reinforces the clients for participating, helps the clients to feel that they have been understood, and gives you the opportunity to reword an example (if necessary) to fit the concept being discussed.

A worksheet is usually introduced toward the end of the session. This signals that you are ready for the clients to implement what was just discussed by putting it down on paper. Most of the worksheets are organized in chart form—rows and columns—in order to simplify the process of filling them out. Having a worksheet for each session gives the clients a sense that there is a systematic approach underway, which fits nicely with the cognitive therapy model. Clients will be using the worksheet to complete the homework prior to the next session, so it is important to make sure that they understand what to do with it. You should "walk them through" an example during the session, having them fill in responses as they go, prior to assigning the homework.

Homework, intended for completion prior to the next session, is then assigned. It is key to treatment success. If clients remain passive and continue to expect the treatment to "wash" over them and thereby "cure" them, they will be disappointed. Without nagging clients, the therapist must continually reinforce the fact that practice, via the homework, helps them to consolidate what they have learned in session. Although it seems obvious that these are new skills requiring practice, I have noticed that when I state this directly, it has relevance to clients.

The session ends with a postsession questionnaire (the Postsession Process Check; see Appendix J). This helps determine whether the clients have understood the main point of the session. The first question is simply "List the main point of this week's session." The second question asks clients to list one thing they could do or think differently during the next week as a result of the session. This stimulates their thinking along the lines that they are expected to utilize the session during the next week, and to experiment with changing a relevant thought or behavior. Surprisingly, perhaps, some clients become anxious in filling out the Postsession Process Check, as if they are being evaluated or are taking a test. I clarify that the "test" is for me as the therapist, not for the clients, to see whether I have explained the concepts adequately. The last two questions on the Postsession Process Check give the clients an opportunity to ask questions or express confusion regarding any material presented in session, and to note anything that might have been said that was troubling to the clients. These questionnaires are then collected, and you should go over them immediately following the session. Occasionally, a question or concern merits a follow-up telephone call prior to the next session—the more timely, the better.

For each session, the clients are given a session outline, as well as the worksheet(s) they will be using during the upcoming week. The session outline and worksheet(s) are provided at the back of each module, so that you can copy them for use with your clients. At the beginning of treatment, I give each client a three-ring notebook with the first session outline inserted, and instruct all clients to keep session outlines and worksheets in this notebook. At the beginning of each subsequent treatment week, each client is given the new session outline to include in his notebook. The sheets are prepunched, so that the client can insert them into his notebook immediately upon receiving the week's pages. The notebook also has a built-in folder that clients can use to keep up with various spare note pages that might not be hole-punched. By the end of treatment, each client has a personalized notebook of cognitive therapy for pain management. All of the homework is included in the notebook, so that the client can refer back to the work he has done.

Throughout the 10 modules, I include a number of session transcripts as well as partially filled-in worksheets. The session transcripts are composites made up from the examples of a number of my clients and my students' clients, altered so as to protect identity, and to adequately illustrate the concepts I am trying to get across. The filled-in versions of the worksheets are included to show you how they can be utilized in session and to exemplify the points I am trying to make. The composite group I am using to illustrate my points is made up of eight people: David, Jennifer, Melissa, Tony, Pat, Kristi, Martha Anne, and Kim. You will notice that in the early treatment modules, I focus my examples on two particular group members, David and Jennifer. This helps give a sense of continuity to the treatment sessions, as well as bringing those clients "to life" for you, the reader. However, it is important to understand that in your own "real" groups, you should vary the clients who are working through their examples in session. I try to use examples that get at some of the complexities that evolve in cognitive therapy for patients with pain. Nonetheless, I have created the illustrations to have the desired outcome by the end of each example. Don't expect real life to go quite that smoothly—it doesn't in my groups!

THERAPEUTIC CHALLENGES

As I have stated earlier, patients with pain are often resistant to referral to a psychotherapist for pain management. Within the context of multidisciplinary pain management programs, both inpatient and outpatient psychotherapeutic approaches have become more acceptable to patients because they are part of the standard of care within these programs, and every patient (ostensibly) gets the same thing. Individuals referred by physicians or other health care providers to private practitioners, though, may feel that they are being singled out, and may resent the implication that their pain is not "real." Patients are often referred for psychotherapy if they seem unusually distressed when seeing their health care providers, if they make an unusual number of office or emergency department visits, or if they make inordinate requests for pain medication. In addition, patients may be referred for psychotherapy when other health care providers have run out of diagnostic or intervention options, and nothing has worked to eliminate the pain (or at least make it manageable for the patients).

As I have stated in the Preface, I see the greatest therapeutic challenge regarding pain management to be the barrier posed by our culture's promotion of the patient as a passive recipient of diagnosis, treatment, and cure. A passive stance is the antithesis of what our clients need; they must work actively to adopt new thoughts and belief systems regarding chronic pain in order to implement appropriate restorative behaviors. This is why establishing a truly collaborative relationship with a client who has chronic pain is so critically important. And, as you well know, these patients are not used to collaborative treatment, and thus part of the therapeutic endeavor needs to involve shaping them into that process. The homework is the key to collaboration. If the clients are attempting homework, they are collaborating; if they are not doing the homework, something is wrong. Below, I present some ideas to consider when it is apparent that a client is not engaged in collaborative treatment.

Therapeutic Alliance

Ideally, if you have given careful consideration to conceptualizing the patient and each patient's pain via a cognitive model, you really understand and empathize with how the patient may have gotten where she is. When we empathize with clients, we are less judgmental, less punitive, and more on the clients' side than against them. Nonetheless, some patients, including patients with pain, are difficult to like. Particularly when patients display high levels of negative emotion and "neediness," we may feel overwhelmed by them and tend to back away from their seemingly insurmountable problems. I tell my students that they must find a way to like their clients, because if they don't, they will be withdrawing from rather than approaching the clients (whether the students are aware of this tendency or not). Liking one's clients can sometimes be a therapeutic challenge, but I believe it is a necessity rather than just a beneficial "extra." Developing a liking for an "unlikeable" client may mean implementing a flexible approach to a manualized agenda and getting to know the person behind the problem before attempting to tackle the problem. Allowing the client to see you as a human being in addition to a knowledgeable health care professional also helps build a therapeutic alliance. Both getting to know the person within the client, and allowing him to know you, can be accomplished without violating necessary and important boundaries between therapist and patient.

Client Goals

Although we as therapists clearly have goals for the clients we work with, we also need to be aware of the goals clients have for themselves. Some of their goals, though realistic, workable, and attainable, would not necessarily be the focus of our treatment unless we knew they were important to the clients. One simple question for assessing goals is to ask each patient, "How would you like to be different by the end of therapy?" (J. S. Beck, personal communication, June 2002). On a related note, although it is important for clients to have goals, we want them to be realistically tailored for each individual. Patients with pain often hold the goal of total eradication of their pain. This is more often than not impossible for patients who have endured long-term chronic pain, and letting go of this goal may feel like a tragic loss to such patients. On the other hand, helping them to adopt other, more attainable goals—and, in doing so, helping them to regain functioning—has been repeatedly shown to be highly satisfying to clients with intractable pain.

Clients' "Buy-In" to the Stress–Appraisal–Coping Model of Pain

If a client does not come to the point where she believes in the importance of thoughts and feelings regarding the experience of pain, the cognitive interventions will not work. Bear in mind that "buy-in" to a stress-and-coping model is meant to be a gradual process, rather than an immediate endorsement of a totally foreign concept. Beginning with the premise that the client's pain is indeed real and stress-related, you are setting the stage for helping the client understand the impact of her thoughts and feelings on pain, and on how she copes with pain. Yet there are clients who remain jaded and resolute in their assertion that real pain is not "in my head." It is as if they fear that accepting the importance of thoughts and feelings delegitimizes their pain, and therefore they must struggle to hold onto a belief that serves them ill. Occasionally, I will make some headway with this kind of resistance by asking the clients to consider whether their beliefs are in some ways serving them (as explained in Treatment Module 6). Also consider that even if buy-in is not complete, there may be some long-term changes in the clients' thinking at a point beyond the termination of therapy, simply because they were exposed to a new point of view.

CHAPTER SUMMARY

Now that you are acquainted with the logistics of the group treatment approach and the general session format, it is time to consider each session in turn. The following 10 modules provide the details of each session of the cognitive treatment program for chronic pain.

THE STRESS–PAIN–APPRAISAL CONNECTION

The first session is used to establish a collaborative working relationship with each client. To do so, therapists must provide a sound rationale for treatment and discuss treatment goals. This phase of treatment is a typical first session in most cognitive therapy as well as cognitive-behavioral therapy (CBT) approaches, yet it continues throughout the therapeutic endeavor. The session begins by introducing the format and overall goals of treatment, as well as helping the clients understand the concept of shared responsibility for treatment and issues of confidentiality; it ends with working on the first treatment concept, the stress–pain–appraisal connection. Therapist Handout 1.1, found at the back of this module, provides an outline of Session 1 to be used by the therapist. Client Handout 1.1 is also found at the back of this module and can be copied and given to clients as a session outline at the beginning of the session.

SESSION 1 TREATMENT OBJECTIVES

- Welcome clients and introduce the treatment.
- Introduce the stress–pain connection.
- Introduce the stress–appraisal connection.

SESSION OBJECTIVE: WELCOME CLIENTS AND INTRODUCE THE TREATMENT

Rationale, Overall Goals, and Format

In describing the treatment rationale to patients, I begin by highlighting that pain is a physical reality, and that it is also stress-related. It is important to emphasize that in using this treatment approach, we do *not* assume that the pain is "all in the head," "psychogenic," or in any way "not real." Patients with pain who have been referred to mental health practitioners have already heard these messages, either quite explicitly or by implication. Following a firm assertion that experienced pain is a reality, I point out that all pain is processed by the brain—the same organ that sorts through thoughts and feelings, stores and retrieves memories, responds to stress, and translates all incoming information into meaning. A basic understanding of how the brain does this allows us to tap into the way the brain processes pain, and use it to our benefit. Following this brief introduction, I then move to the main concepts behind this treatment approach:

1. Pain is real, *and* pain is stress-related.
2. Pain triggers stress.
3. Stress makes pain worse.
4. Stress can be made better or worse by how one thinks about pain.
5. Learning about stress, and how to manage stress, can reduce one's pain.

We will build on these concepts throughout the treatment program.

I describe the treatment format as an educational–psychological process. Group discussion is focused on clients' experiences with stress and pain, and patients learn about their thoughts, emotions, and behaviors before and during pain flare-ups. Describing the treatment approach as a "class" often helps to reduce resistance to psychological intervention. It is very important to explain that weekly homework assignments are given, that an integral part of treatment is the work done outside the therapy session, and that discussion of each homework assignment occurs during the next treatment session. I also explain to clients that although they are not given "tests" the way they would be in a standard classroom experience, they will be asked to note at the beginning and end of each session what they learned from the session and from their homework in between sessions.

As a general introduction to the goals of the group, you can describe (or list on a flipchart) the following:

1. To learn about the connection between stress and pain.
2. To reduce the frequency and seriousness of pain flare-ups, by learning to think differently about stressful situations.
3. To learn what is most helpful and least helpful in coping with pain and managing stress.
4. To learn the best ways of getting social and emotional support.
5. To learn promising coping techniques that may help during a painful episode.

Shared Responsibility for Treatment

A primary emphasis of treatment is on building positive rapport and creating a collaborative working relationship with each client. A positive relationship with a client has been repeatedly shown to be a nonspecific factor associated with psychotherapeutic treatment gain, regardless of the treatment model adopted (Turk & Holzman, 1986)—and, of course, this relationship has to be considered from the moment the therapist speaks with each client about possible treatment. Building positive rapport encompasses a wide range of therapist behaviors demonstrating caring about and acceptance of clients, empathy regarding their situation, and active listening skills. I teach my students that although therapists have a different background and knowledge base than clients do, we are not in any way "above" our clients, and we must resist the temptation to lean on our intellects when it becomes unclear what to do next. Building positive rapport involves approaching all clients with a respectful attitude and inviting them to explore with us a different way of managing their pain. Building positive rapport sets the stage for an active working alliance with each client.

Establishing a working alliance may be one of the most important aspects of a therapist's work. Shared responsibility for treatment is bedrock for cognitive therapy, and you need to help every client adopt the mindset of active collaboration. This is a foreign concept to most clients—especially for patients with pain, who are typically entrenched in a biomedical system, where patients are often the passive recipients of diagnoses, treatments, and "cures." One way to approach this is to emphasize the "flip side" of responsibility, which is empowerment. The skills clients learn in this treatment program are practical tools that they can use on their own to control their pain and their lives.

In cognitive treatment, the therapist has specific knowledge, teaches the use of helpful tools, and provides ongoing consultation and feedback. But it is the client who does the great majority of the work. Much of this work is done between therapy sessions and after formal therapy has ended. Bear in mind that many patients dealing with chronic pain begin treatment with a high level of dependency; a poor sense of self-efficacy; an external locus of control; distorted appraisals, automatic thoughts, and beliefs about pain; and a passive, avoidant, helpless behavioral stance. Thus starting clients on the journey of pain self-management requires the therapist to set small, sequential, and manageable goals toward changes in cognitions—goals whose accomplishment will lead to a gradual willingness to try new ways of coping. Of course, changing the way one thinks is a new way of coping in and of itself.

Confidentiality

All psychotherapy, regardless of format, involves a discussion of issues of client confidentiality and potential limits to confidentiality. In raising the issue of confidentiality, I first outline my legal and ethical responsibilities to group members. The responsibilities and limits of confidentiality differ somewhat across states, and so you should follow the rules and regulations set forth by your state. Common therapist responsibilities include not disclosing any personal or identifying information regarding a client to another source or person unless the client presents a danger to self or others. In other words, your clients need to know that unless they give you explicit permission, you will not disclose personal information to family members or other health care providers.

Group treatment formats necessitate discussion of additional confidentiality issues: the responsibilities of group members toward one another. I emphasize the importance of never revealing the name of another group member, but also explain that revealing details of another's personal experiences may inadvertently lead someone outside the group to be able to identify a group participant. For this reason, I ask group members to limit any discussion outside the group to their own personal experiences and no one else's. I ask all members for their word on this matter, and give them a written copy of the confidentiality policy as part of the session outline.

SESSION OBJECTIVE: INTRODUCE THE STRESS–PAIN CONNECTION

In this phase of the first session, the connection between stress and pain is introduced, with particular attention to cognitive interpretation (appraisal) of potentially stressful events. Although the term *"primary* appraisal" is not used with clients, this part of the treatment session incorporates Lazarus and Folkman's (1984) concept of primary appraisals into the treatment protocol—specifically, the judgment that an event is benign/positive or stressful (i.e., taxing one's ability to cope). In order to introduce the stress–pain connection, you will need to present a "mini-lecture" defining the term and discussing the stress response. You can use the material below in an almost script-like fashion. However, as you become more comfortable with the information, use your own words and your own style to present these ideas to your groups.

> The physical pain you experience is real, and this real pain produces a stress reaction. Stress reactions make pain worse. What is stress? "Stress" is defined as a biological, emotional, and cognitive (that is, mental) reaction to an event that you think you might not be able to cope with. Let's look at the three parts of a stress reaction.
>
> *Biological.* Stress reactions are biological. Your body automatically prepares for either "fight or flight." The fight-or-flight response evolved in early humans and is quite useful in life-or-death situations—encountering a saber-toothed tiger, for example, or a robber with a gun.
>
> The biological response to stress includes an increase in blood pressure, heart rate, and respiration, and a decrease in digestive processes. Certain hormones that help these biological processes are released into the bloodstream. There is a reduction in blood flow to organs and an increase in blood flow to large body muscles—those used for fight or flight. These biological responses evolved to produce short-term responses, but many present-day stressors are quite different. They are ongoing rather than short-lived. Yet the body responds in the same way, as if every stressor were a saber-toothed tiger. On a long-term basis, these biological changes produce wear and tear on the body and reduce the ability of the immune system to function.
>
> *Emotional.* In addition to biological responses, stress also sets off emotional reactions. Many patients with pain tell us that they react to the stress of chronic pain with nervousness, sadness, depression, anger, embarrassment, and shame, to name some of the more common emotions.
>
> *Cognitive.* Stress also sets off cognitive, or mental, reactions. "Cognitions" are thoughts, images, or beliefs. For example, cognitions include what we tell ourselves about the stress, what we tell ourselves about our ability to cope, and what we think about ourselves. These thoughts, by themselves, can be negative, overwhelming, and stressful. The way we think—our cognitions—can trigger stress reactions by themselves.
>
> Chronic pain is a major ongoing stressor. It can and does produce the biological, emotional, and cognitive stress responses just described. But non-pain-related stressors can also worsen pain. Anything that triggers stress can produce physical changes in blood flow, hormonal changes, and immune response suppression, as well as changes in our emotions, thoughts, and behaviors.

Exercise: Listing Stressors

Following this introduction to the stress–pain connection, you should provide blank sheets of paper to clients and ask them to list situations that they find stressful and/or that trigger pain flare-ups. Explain that they don't have to go into great detail in this list; just noting each situation in general is sufficient.

Troubleshooting Tip: For some patients, succinct identification of a stressful situation is difficult. When asked to identify the situation, they may provide unnecessary context to introduce the situation, and follow this by giving a "blow-by-blow" description of the details involved. When a client begins a lengthy discourse, it may be because he feels a need to convince the therapist or group members that he was justified in his reaction to a particular situation, and it may indicate that he has a strong need for emotional support regarding the event. For some clients, the group therapy experience may be the first forum in which they have felt really listened to, and they may not want to give up the floor! While recognizing that these are legitimate needs, the therapist can help shape the client's verbal description of the situation in such a way that he does not take up inordinate group time and does not miss the point of the exercise. If it becomes necessary to interrupt the client, the therapist, with great sensitivity, can offer a synopsis of the stressful situation that he might "jot down" on his paper.

SESSION OBJECTIVE: INTRODUCE THE STRESS–APPRAISAL CONNECTION

Once you have obtained at least one example of a stressor from each client, you can move on to introduce the concept of "appraisal" or interpretation of stress, whereby situations are judged as harmless or stressful. A situation judged to be stressful is further appraised as a challenge (the perception that the ability to cope is not outweighed by the potential danger of the situation), a threat (the perception that the danger posed by the situation outweighs the individual's ability to cope), or a loss (the perception that damage has occurred as a result of the situation). Depending upon one's interpretation of a circumstance, one will think about it differently, feel different emotions about it, and behave differently.

It's helpful to start by coming back to the basic definition of stress given earlier: "Stress is a three-part reaction you have to an environmental event that you think you might not be able to cope with."

> Let's go back to our definition of stress. What's important in setting off the stress reaction isn't so much the actual situation, but how we interpret or "appraise" the situation. We are constantly sorting out which events need our attention, which can be ignored, and which should be avoided. These judgments are cognitive processes (what we call "appraisals"). Can we relax about it? It's not stressful if you decide you can relax. When we judge a situation as stressful, we make some other interpretations. There are three basic ways that people appraise or interpret a stressful situation: as a challenge, as a threat, or as a loss.
>
> *Challenge.* People who interpret the stressful situation as a challenge think that their ability to cope is enough to see them through.
>
> *Threat.* People who see stress as a threat think that their coping ability will be overwhelmed by the situation.
>
> *Loss.* People who see stress as a loss think that they've already been damaged by the situation.
>
> Depending on how we interpret stress—as a challenge, a threat, or a loss—we will feel different emotions, think different thoughts, and behave in different ways.
>
> Let's look at an example: A young couple wishing to have children is unable to conceive after 6 months. The situation is stressful for them, but they could interpret the stressful situation in three different ways. They may think of this as a challenge ("Let's learn all we can about optimizing our chances to conceive, and then give it our best shot"), a threat ("This may mean we will not be able to have children"), or a loss ("Our in-

ability to conceive a child has robbed us of a critical part of our life"). Would the couple feel, think, and behave the same or differently, depending on how they interpreted the situation?

Once group members are provided with the example above, they are encouraged to discuss how each of these ways of appraisal (challenge, threat, loss) would affect the couple's thinking, feeling, and subsequent behavior. Most participants are able to give some general examples of how the type of appraisal would influence the partners' emotions, their coping attempts, and things they might tell themselves or each other about the situation. Even more specifically, I guide clients to reflect upon how each type of appraisal might focus the couple's attention and concentration toward one dimension of their lives, to the exclusion of other components. For example, if the couple judges their difficulty in conceiving as a threat, they are likely to be much more vigilant to any potential physical changes in either partner (e.g., changes signifying stage in fertility cycle, changes associated with sexual functioning in the male). They may begin charting the female's ovulation cycles and reading about causes for infertility. They may be less likely to interact with friends who do not share their present difficulty. The couple is likely to magnify the potential importance of small physical changes because they are so intensely focused on these, and *any* perceived physical changes—big or small—may be met with fearful anticipation and anxiety. If the couple judges their potential infertility as a loss, they are likely to tell themselves that there is not much they can do about it; they are likely to feel grief and sadness, and may even become depressed. They are likely to feel helpless, leave it up to their fertility specialist to attempt to solve, and not engage in many self-directed coping activities. On the other hand, if the couple views their delay in procreation as a challenge, they are likely to focus on the aspects of the situation they do have control over, engage actively and enthusiastically in those potential problem-solving activities, and use more empowering self-statements—and thus they are likely to feel energized and hopeful!

Note that the initial example used is not a pain-related example. I choose a non-pain-related illustration first, in order to initially minimize the emotional identification with the example that the clients might otherwise have. Subsequent case illustrations become increasingly relevant to the clients' personal situation.

Exercise: How Do You Appraise Your Stressors?

Following discussion of the case example above, you should direct group members back to their own initial examples of identified stressors, and guide them through the process of how they appraise each stressor: as a threat, a loss, or a challenge. Following their identification of the appraisal type, help them discuss how their own appraisal of the stressor might affect their focus of attention, their thoughts, their feelings, and their subsequent behavior. Note that in general, when stressors are appraised as "threats," doing so causes a narrowing of the focus of attention toward the stressors, making it harder to direct attention elsewhere. Focused attention toward pain or potential pain may have the effect of increasing anxiety and fear, and promotes avoidance. Also, when we appraise our stressors as "losses," it unduly focuses our thoughts toward what we *cannot* do; these thoughts increase our feelings of grief and sadness, and decrease our motivation to try things that might be useful in managing the pain situation.

Discussion of Clients' PAI Responses

At this point in the session, it is useful to hand clients their responses to the Pain Appraisal Inventory (PAI; see Chapter 4) to illustrate how they had initially appraised their pain-related stressors. Recall from Chapter 4 that the PAI covers two broad categories of appraisals: threat/loss and challenge. The point of using the PAI here is not to make clients expert at categorizing stressors, but to serve as a discussion aid. For most clients, appraising their pain as a challenge is not typical, whereas appraising their pain as a threat or a loss is commonplace. Once you have helped them go over their responses and discuss the types of appraisals they seem to use, you can next introduce the Stress–Pain Connection Worksheet.

WORKSHEET: STRESS–PAIN CONNECTION WORKSHEET

The Stress–Pain Connection Worksheet (see Client Handout 1.2 at the end of this module) is next introduced as a tool for charting stressful situations; the appraisal category assigned to each stressor; and the impact of the situation/appraisal on thoughts, feelings, and behavior. In session, clients are directed to transfer an example they had written down on their blank sheet of paper during the Listing Stressors exercise (see above) to the Stress–Pain Connection Worksheet, and then to use the worksheet to write down the appraisals and thoughts associated with the stressor. You will find that one particular stressful situation can have more than one appraisal component to it. When more than one appraisal category is identified for a single stressor, help the client consider each component separately, in terms of how each appraisal might influence his thoughts and feelings in a different way. Clients are also directed to the "Any specific thoughts . . . ?" column of the worksheet. By asking whether clients are aware of any specific thoughts associated with the stressful situation, you are beginning to emphasize the importance of the thought category. If you are already familiar with cognitive therapy, you will recognize that this worksheet provides the context for introducing the idea of automatic thoughts, to be covered in the next session. I find that introducing the concept of different types of stress appraisals helps clients to begin identifying associated automatic thoughts. Although I focus here on the appraisal category and the impact it has on the clients' thoughts, emotions, and behavior, I have laid the groundwork for the next session as well.

An example of a partially completed Stress–Pain Connection Worksheet from a client (David) is included in Figure Mod. 1.1 as an illustration. David is a 42-year-old married father of three children, ages 17, 14, and 12. David's wife works as a secretary at a nearby university, and he is a production worker at the local tire manufacturing plant. David has had low back pain for 7 years, and he has undergone three surgeries. The first surgery (a laminectomy) was undertaken to treat a herniated disc in his lumbar spine. The second surgery was to remove a bone spur, and the third surgery was to remove scar tissue resulting from his first two surgeries.

Note that in this particular example, David identified going to the doctor about his pain as a threat, and he made a connection between that appraisal (threat) and an emotional response (dread). He was also able to identify an image associated with the stressful situation (i.e., seeing himself in the hospital, awaiting yet another surgery). Without being fully aware of it, David has made an association in his mind between an increase in pain and going to the

Stressful situation	Appraisal category (threat, loss, challenge)	Impact on emotions, thoughts, behavior	Any specific thoughts associated with stressful situation? (can also be an image)	Comments/ other notes to self
Going back to my doctor because my pain has gotten worse.	Threat	Dread	Image of me in the hospital, waiting for another surgery.	

FIGURE MOD. 1.1. David's in-session Stress–Pain Connection Worksheet.

doctor, which means surgery. This link and others like it are critically important associations, and they will be addressed in the next several sessions.

HOMEWORK ASSIGNMENT

As homework, clients are directed to continue adding to their list of stressful situations and/or situations that may trigger pain flare-ups. They are asked to use the Stress–Pain Connection Worksheet to identify how each stressor was appraised and how their appraisal might affect their emotions, thoughts, and behaviors. They are asked to pay particular attention to any specific thoughts or images associated with each stressful situation, and to write them down in the column provided for these on the worksheet. I emphasize that this homework is central to the process of the treatment, and that we will be discussing group members' findings, by way of the worksheet, during the next session.

POSTSESSION PROCESS CHECK

Even if the treatment is delivered properly, if a client does not understand the main point of the session, he is unlikely to incorporate it into his pain management repertoire. As I have indicated in the introduction to Part II, I find it useful to include a very brief questionnaire at the end of each session asking clients first to list the main point of the session, and then to list one thing they could do or think differently during the following week based on this week's session. Even though clients will have an explicit homework assignment each week, this exercise cues them to be thinking about how they can utilize the session content. I also give clients an opportunity to write questions or concerns they might have following the session. A copy of the Postsession Process Check is included in Appendix J.

  Troubleshooting Tip: Sometimes toward the end of a session, time is short, and a patient may defer a question regarding some point he did not understand. Also, it is possible that something happens during the session that a client finds troubling, upsetting, or distasteful. We don't want clients to sit on these issues for a week, stewing over them. Worse yet, we don't want them to discontinue treatment over something that could have been addressed between sessions. For example, a few weeks ago, one of my students was giving an illustration and used the word "hell" in his example. A client noted in her feedback sheet that she was offended by his profanity. After the student and I discussed why it was a good idea to avoid profanity in treatment sessions, he was able to address this with her over the phone prior to the next treatment session.

THERAPIST HANDOUT 1.1

Session 1 Outline for Therapists: The Stress–Pain–Appraisal Connection

SESSION OBJECTIVES

- Welcome clients and introduce the treatment.
- Introduce the stress–pain connection.
- Introduce the stress–appraisal connection.

NEEDED MATERIALS, HANDOUTS, AND WORKSHEETS

- Session 1 Outline for Therapists (this handout)
- Three-ring notebook for client Session Summaries and client worksheets
- Session 1 Summary for Clients (Client Handout 1.1)
- Stress–Pain Connection Worksheet (Client Handout 1.2)
- Results from each client's Pain Appraisal Inventory (PAI), completed during assessment (Appendix D)
- Postsession Process Check (Appendix J)

SESSION OBJECTIVE: WELCOME CLIENTS AND INTRODUCE THE TREATMENT

Treatment Rationale

- Pain is real, *and* pain is stress-related.
- Pain triggers stress.
- Stress makes pain worse.
- Stress can be made better or worse by how one thinks about pain.
- Learning about stress and how to manage it can reduce pain.

Overall Treatment Program Goals for Group Members

- To learn about the connection between stress and pain.
- To reduce the frequency of pain flare-ups by learning to think differently about stressful situations.
- To learn what is most and least helpful in coping with stress and pain.
- To learn promising coping techniques that help during a pain episode.

Format: Psychological–Educational Group—A Class

- Tell clients: "We'll give you information about stress and pain."
- "We'll discuss how it applies to your experiences with stress and pain."
- "We'll teach stress management skills you can use."
- "There will be weekly homework assignments for practicing the skills."

(continued)

From *Cognitive Therapy for Chronic Pain* by Beverly E. Thorn. Copyright 2004 by The Guilford Press. Permission to photocopy this handout is granted to purchasers of this book for personal use only (see copyright page for details).

Shared Responsibility for Treatment Success

What's Expected from the Leaders?

- "We will teach you skills and help you problem-solve."
- "We will work with you in your treatment."

What's Expected from Group Members?

- *Regular attendance*: "You are important contributors to this group. Without your regular attendance, the group is likely to be negatively affected."
- *Active participation*: "Our treatment requires you to take an active role in changing the way you respond to pain and other stressors."
- *Between-session activities*: "Practice the skills learned in between sessions."
- *Reporting back*: "Share with the group your successes with what you have begun to practice, as well as places you get stuck."

Confidentiality

Therapists' Responsibility

Therapists do not reveal personally identifying information to anyone outside the group.

- *Exceptions*: Therapists are legally required to report any cases where a client presents a clear threat of imminent harm to self (e.g., potential suicide), imminent harm to others (e.g., potential homicide), or suspected child abuse or elder abuse.

Clients' Responsibility

Tell clients: "Feel free to discuss what you learn with others outside the group. *But* protect the privacy of group members! It is *not okay* to use group members' names or other identifying information outside the group."

SESSION OBJECTIVE: INTRODUCE THE STRESS–PAIN CONNECTION

Introducing the Stress–Pain Connection

- Pain produces stress.
- Stress increases pain.
- Managing stress reduces pain.

What Is the Stress Response?

- The stress response is a three-part reaction to something (an event, emotion, physical feeling) that people think they cannot cope with. These are the three parts of the reaction:
  - *Biological*: Increased blood pressure, muscle tension, stress hormones; lowered immune response.
  - *Emotional*: Anxiety, sadness, anger, embarrassment, shame, depression.
  - *Cognitive*: Thoughts and images about the event and about the self.

(continued)

- Anything that triggers the three-part stress response is a "stressor."
- Pain is a stressor: Chronic pain itself can be a major ongoing stressor, and can lead to the stress response (see above).
- Physical changes, emotions, thoughts, and behaviors can all be (non-pain) stressors that can trigger pain flare-ups.

Exercise: Listing Stressors

- Give out paper. Ask clients to jot down a list of situations (pain-related and non-pain-related) that each considers "stressful."
- Get at least one example of a stressor from each client. Then ask clients to put the sheet aside for a little while and move on.

SESSION OBJECTIVE: INTRODUCE THE STRESS–APPRAISAL CONNECTION

Introducing the Stress–Appraisal Connection

- Review definition of "stressful"—"anything you think you may not be able to cope with."
- How we judge or "appraise" a situation and then react is more important than the actual situation.
- Stressors are judged as threats, losses, or challenges.

Example

A young couple wishing to have children, but unable to conceive for 6 months, may think of this situation as:

- *A challenge*: "Let's learn all we can about optimizing our chances to conceive, and then give it our best shot."
- *A threat*: "This may mean we will not be able to have children."
- *A loss*: "Our inability to conceive a child has robbed us of a critical part of our life."

Discussion

- Using the example above, have clients discuss how each different appraisal category would affect the couple's emotions, thoughts, and behaviors.
- Review clients' answers to the PAI to see how they said they judge typical pain-related stressors.

WORKSHEET: STRESS–PAIN CONNECTION WORKSHEET

- Give out copies of the Stress–Pain Connection Worksheet.
- Ask clients to transfer their initial list of stressors onto the worksheet.
- Ask: "How do you appraise *your* stressors? (Threat, loss, or challenge?)"
- "Do you have any thoughts or images associated with the stressor?"

(continued)

HOMEWORK ASSIGNMENT

- Tell clients: "Using the Stress–Pain Connection Worksheet, continue adding to your list of pain-related and pain-unrelated situations that are stressful for you and/or you identify as eliciting pain. Try doing this each day."
- "Beside each stressor, write down the category of how you appraise that situation (threat, challenge, loss, other)."
- "Note how the stressor (and your appraisal of the stressor) might have an impact on your focus of attention, emotions, thoughts, and behaviors."
- "Are you aware of any specific thoughts you have about the stressful situation? If so, write these down. (Hint: These could be images as well as thoughts.)"
- "Bring your homework to the next session, and be prepared to discuss what you have learned."

POSTSESSION PROCESS CHECK

- Hand out Postsession Process Check and have clients fill it in before they leave.

Session 1 Summary for Clients: The Stress–Pain–Appraisal Connection

GOALS FOR THIS TREATMENT PROGRAM

- To learn about the connection between stress and pain.
- To reduce the frequency of your pain flare-ups by learning to think differently about stressful situations.
- To learn what is most and least helpful in coping with stress and pain.
- To learn and use promising coping techniques that help during a pain episode.

WHAT YOU CAN EXPECT FROM THE LEADERS

- We will teach you skills and help you problem-solve.
- We will collaborate with you in your treatment.
- *Confidentiality*: As therapists, we do not reveal personally identifying information to anyone outside the group. But there are important exceptions: We are legally required to report any cases where a client presents a clear threat of imminent harm to self (e.g., potential suicide), imminent harm to others (e.g., potential homicide), or suspected child abuse or elder abuse.

WHAT THE LEADERS EXPECT FROM GROUP MEMBERS

- *Regular attendance*: You are important contributors to this group. Without your regular attendance, the group is likely to be less helpful for everyone.
- *Active participation*: Our treatment requires you to take an active role in changing the way you think about, and act in response to, pain and other stressors.
- *Between-session activities*: Practice the skills learned in between sessions.
- *Reporting back*: Share with the group what you have learned that has helped, as well as places you get stuck.
- *Confidentiality*: Feel free to discuss what you learn with others outside the group. *But* protect the privacy of group members! It is *not okay* to use group members' names or other identifying information outside the group.

THE STRESS–PAIN CONNECTION

- Pain produces stress. Stress increases pain. Managing stress reduces pain.
- What is the stress response?
  - The stress response is a three-part reaction to something (an event, emotion, physical feeling) that you think you cannot cope with. These are the three parts of the reaction:
    - *Biological*: Increased blood pressure, muscle tension, stress hormones; lowered immune response.
    - *Emotional*: Anxiety, sadness, anger, embarrassment, shame, depression.
    - *Cognitive*: Thoughts and images about the event and about yourself.

(continued)

From *Cognitive Therapy for Chronic Pain* by Beverly E. Thorn. Copyright 2004 by The Guilford Press. Permission to photocopy this handout is granted to purchasers of this book for personal use only (see copyright page for details).

- Anything that triggers the three-part stress response is a "stressor."
- Pain is a stressor: Chronic pain itself can be a major ongoing stressor, and can lead to the stress response (see above).
- Physical changes, emotions, thoughts, and behaviors can all be (non-pain) stressors that can trigger pain flare-ups.

THE STRESS–APPRAISAL CONNECTION

- Any situation can be "stressful" if you think you may not be able to cope with it.
- If you think you can relax, it's not a stressful situation.
- How we judge (that is, "appraise") a situation *and* our coping ability is more important than the actual situation.
- Stressful situations can be appraised (that is, judged) as threats, losses, or challenges. For example, a young couple wishing to have children, but unable to conceive for 6 months, may think of this situation as:
  - A *challenge*: "Let's learn all we can about optimizing our chances to conceive, and then give it our best shot."
  - A *threat*: "This may mean we will not be able to have children;"
  - A *loss*: "Our inability to conceive a child has robbed us of a critical part of our life."

SUMMARY OF KEY POINTS

- The stress response is biological, emotional, and cognitive (mental/thoughts).
- Chronic pain is a stressor.
- Any stressor (pain or non-pain) can trigger pain flare-ups.
- The way we judge stress can shape what we think, feel, and do about the stress.

HOMEWORK ASSIGNMENT

- Using the Stress–Pain Connection Worksheet, continue adding to your list of pain-related and pain-unrelated situations that are stressful for you and/or you identify as eliciting pain. Try doing this each day.
- Beside each stressor, write down how you appraise that situation (threat, challenge, loss, other).
- Note how the stressor (and your appraisal of the stressor) might have an impact on your focus of attention, emotions, thoughts, and behaviors.
- Are you aware of any specific thoughts you have about the stressful situation? If so, write these down. (Hint: These could be images as well as thoughts.)
- Bring your homework to the next session, and be prepared to discuss what you have learned.

CLIENT HANDOUT 1.2

Stress–Pain Connection Worksheet

Stressful situation	Appraisal category (threat, loss, challenge)	Impact on emotions, thoughts, behavior	Any specific thoughts associated with stressful situation? (can also be an image)	Comments/other notes to self

From *Cognitive Therapy for Chronic Pain* by Beverly E. Thorn. Copyright 2004 by The Guilford Press. Permission to photocopy this handout is granted to purchasers of this book for personal use only (see copyright page for details).

IDENTIFYING AUTOMATIC THOUGHTS

The second treatment session introduces the concept of automatic thoughts and teaches clients how to begin identifying such thoughts as they occur in response to environmental events. Session 2 also teaches clients the link between shifts in emotion or in one's sense of physical well-being and the occurrence of automatic thoughts. Therapist Handout 2.1, found at the back of this module, provides an outline of Session 2 to be used by the therapist. Client Handout 2.1, also at the back of the module, can be copied and used as a session outline to be given to clients at the beginning of the session.

SESSION 2 TREATMENT OBJECTIVES

- Introduce the stress–appraisal–coping model of pain.
- Identify automatic thoughts or images.

PRESESSION PROCESS CHECK

Each session begins with a presession process check, very similar to the postsession check given at the end of the session. Copies of the Pre- and Postsession Process Check measures are included in Appendix J. The first few times you give clients these measures, you will need to reiterate that these questions are not meant to be a quiz or test; rather, they are meant for you as a therapist to make sure that everyone has understood the material presented in the session, and to clarify any questions or concerns that might have come up.

REVIEW OF PREVIOUS WEEK'S SESSION

The session proceeds with a brief review of the previous week's session. The main points I want clients to have gotten from Session 1 are the following:

1. The stress response is a biological, emotional, and cognitive response (with a reminder that cognitions are thoughts).
2. Chronic pain is itself a stressor, and non-pain-related stressors can trigger pain flare-ups.
3. The manner in which we judge stress (i.e., stress appraisals of threat, loss, or challenge) can shape what we think, feel, and do about our stress.

You will notice in the client outline for Session 2 (Client Handout 2.1) that the second bulleted list contains the main points from the previous session. During the session review, clients are given the opportunity to ask follow-up questions and express any concerns they might have. If you noticed questions or concerns from clients' responses to the Postsession Process Check following Session 1, or from the Presession Process Check they have just filled out, now is the time to address them.

HOMEWORK REVIEW

Homework review is the next step in every session, and serves as a means for clients to share what they have been working on with the rest of the group members. Recall that as homework following Session 1, group members were asked to continue adding to the Stress–Pain Connection Worksheet by noting stressful situations that seemed to have an impact on their thoughts, emotions, or physical functioning (see Client Handout 1.2). Once clients are informed about the stress response, they are usually quick to acknowledge the connection between stress and shifts in physical sensations. Often they can readily give examples of how stressful situations trigger pain episodes or make painful conditions worse. You may notice from their Stress–Pain Connection Worksheets that they have also been able to identify thoughts associated with stressful situations, in addition to identifying the type of appraisal they used to categorize the stressor.

Between Sessions 1 and 2, our client David did more work using his Stress–Pain Connection Worksheet. (Figure Mod. 2.1 illustrates the worksheet that he brought into the session, and a brief session transcript illustrating how to go over the homework is included below.

THERAPIST: David, I see you added a few things to your Stress–Pain Connection Worksheet during this past week. Is it okay if we go over these now in the group?

DAVID: Sure. The first line was what I did in here before I left.

THERAPIST: I remember that. You were able to identify a stressful situation—going back to your physician because the pain had gotten worse. Most important, you were able to recognize that you judged that situation to be in the "threat" category of appraisal. You also identified an image of yourself as being in the hospital waiting for another surgery. We'll work with that image later in the session, okay? In the meantime, let's move on to your next example.

Stressful situation	Appraisal category (threat, loss, challenge)	Impact on emotions, thoughts, behavior	Any specific thoughts associated with stressful situation? (can also be an image)	Comments/ other notes to self
Going back to my doctor because my pain has gotten worse.	Threat	Dread	Image of me in the hospital, waiting for another surgery.	
The doctors can't do anything to help, anyway.	??	Mad at the world. Why try?		
Had a fight with my kids.	Loss	Left the house in a huff.	They don't respect me any more.	

FIGURE MOD 2.1. David's Session 1 homework Stress–Pain Connection Worksheet.

DAVID: Okay. I listed that the doctors can't do anything to help anyway, which always gets me so mad, I just feel like giving up!

THERAPIST: Those are good examples of emotional responses to thinking that the doctors can't do anything to help. You felt mad at the world, and you felt like not trying to help yourself any more. Let me clarify something, though: Thinking that the doctors can't do anything to help—is that a stressful situation?

DAVID: Hell, yeah, it's stressful! Sometimes I just cancel the appointment I have, or don't even show up, because it's no use anyway!

THERAPIST: So there's something else to list in that third column, under "Impact on emotions, thoughts, behavior"—a behavior in response to the thought "The doctors can't do anything to help, anyway."—You cancel your appointment or don't show up. Go ahead and put that down there as a behavior under column 3.

DAVID: Okay.

ANOTHER GROUP MEMBER: I don't think David's thought that the doctors can't do anything is the stressor. I think it's another response to having to go to the doctor in the first place.

THERAPIST: I think you're right, Kristi. It seems to me that the stressful situation is going to the physician. David appraised that stressor as a threat, and had an image of himself lying in the hospital waiting for surgery. I wonder also, David, if you judge that situation to be a loss, which then makes you mad and makes you feel like canceling the appointment.

DAVID: Well, it seems to be a waste of time—so it's a loss of my time and energy, that's for sure.

THERAPIST: So here's my suggestion for altering your worksheet. Go ahead and cross out "The doctors can't do anything to help, anyway" under the "Stressful situation" column, and put it instead in the "Any specific thoughts . . . ?" column. Then go ahead and add under the "Appraisal category" column the category "Loss." I think you might appraise the stressor of going back to your physician as both a threat and a loss. Those appraisals

Stressful situation	Appraisal category (threat, loss, challenge)	Impact on emotions, thoughts, behavior	Any specific thoughts associated with stressful situation? (can also be an image)	Comments/ other notes to self
Going back to my doctor because my pain has gotten worse.	Threat <u>And</u> loss	Dread Mad at the world. Why try? Cancel my appointment.	Image of me in the hospital, waiting for another surgery. The doctors can't do anything to help, anyway.	
~~The doctors can't do anything to help, anyway.~~	??			
Had a fight with my kids.	Loss	Left the house in a huff.	They don't respect me any more.	

FIGURE MOD. 2.2. David's Session 1 homework Stress–Pain Connection Worksheet, after in-session review.

seem to have different effects on your emotions, behaviors, and thoughts. Now let's take a look at the worksheet.

Figure Mod. 2.2 illustrates David's homework worksheet after the in-session review. The session transcript continues:

DAVID: Geez, this is complicated. I see what you mean, but it looks like I get a "D" on homework!

THERAPIST: Not at all, David! If you work with your homework, you get an "A" every time. And the more cross-outs and add-ins, the better! This *is* complicated stuff—it really points out how complex and powerful our thoughts really are! It's not important to get all the categories "right." What's important is that you work with identifying thoughts and feelings in response to stressful situations, and that you begin to notice how your appraisals and other thoughts affect how you feel and what you do. Let's talk some more now about why thoughts are so important. Take a look at your outline for Session 2, and let's move on to the next part of the session.

SESSION OBJECTIVE: INTRODUCE THE STRESS–APPRAISAL–COPING MODEL OF PAIN

It is now time to drive home the assertion that clients' thoughts have an influence on everything they do (or don't do) to deal with pain and pain-related stressors. In order to underscore the importance of thoughts, you will provide a brief overview of the current theories of pain, including a formal introduction of the stress–appraisal–coping model of pain. In actuality, the material you presented in Session 1 (on the stress–pain connection and the stress–appraisal connection) has provided an experiential introduction to the stress–appraisal–coping model of pain. Introducing the entire model in Session 1 might have been overwhelming to the clients, so this is saved for Session 2. In Session 2, you provide a more complete introduction to the model, by way of a mini-lecture.

> Last week, you learned that pain is stress-related—the stress–pain connection. You also learned that our interpretation, or appraisal, of a situation makes a difference in how we feel, think, and behave in reaction to that situation—the stress–appraisal connection. The ideas that we discussed last week are actually part of a larger theory of pain, called the "stress–appraisal–coping model of pain." In order to understand that model, it helps to give you a bit of the history behind other theories of pain.
>
> For over 300 years, biomedical theories of pain stated that the amount of pain someone feels is directly related to the amount of tissue damage that has occurred: More tissue damage equals more pain. However, we have learned from recent research that physical damage to the body *does not* explain how much pain someone will experience. Newer theories of pain have been developed in order to better explain how much pain someone might experience, and how well someone will adjust to chronic painful conditions. These newer theories of pain emphasize that the brain has tremendous influence on the way pain signals are processed, and therefore the brain influences our perception of pain. Since the brain processes our thoughts and emotions, it makes sense that thoughts and feelings could also have an influence on the experience of pain. And there is mounting research evidence that thoughts and feelings have a direct physical impact on the way the brain processes pain. In other words, *our thoughts and feelings can rewire the part of the brain that perceives pain.* Thoughts and feelings can make things much worse, or much better, in terms of coping with pain.
>
> Let's take the example of patients with terminal cancer to illustrate the point I am trying to make here. No one assumes that the pain a patient with cancer may experience is "all in his head." But the cancer itself (the tissue damage associated with the cancer) does not tell us how much pain that patient will experience, and it doesn't tell us how distressing it will be for the patient. There are many examples of patients with the same type of cancer, the same size tumor, and the same life expectancy, where one patient will be suffering terribly and be bedridden while another patient will be getting along without any major disruption in her life. How can this be? While we certainly don't have all the answers, we do know that physical damage to the body is *not* what determines the amount of pain we experience, and that physical damage doesn't determine whether the pain is "real."
>
> The stress–appraisal–coping model of pain—the model we use in this treatment program—states that to a great extent, people's thoughts about pain and pain-related stressors determine how they will adjust to chronic painful conditions.
>
> The idea behind the stress–appraisal–coping model of pain is simple, but important: Our thoughts focus our attention on certain things, our thoughts influence our emotions, our thoughts influence our behavior, and our thoughts influence our physical well-being. Our thoughts give rise to *other* thoughts, and *those* thoughts also have an impact on our emotions, behavior, and physical functioning.
>
> Thoughts come in a variety of categories. We've already discussed one of the categories of thoughts—the category called "appraisals." When we label a stressful situation as "threatening," we are *thinking* "THREAT!" and our bodies go on high alert: We focus our available attention on the situation; we feel apprehensive, anxious, or frightened; and we try to escape or avoid the situation if we can (or fight it if we can't). In the stress–appraisal–coping model of pain, there are other kinds of thoughts that are equally important to consider. These kinds of thoughts include categories with the labels "automatic thoughts," "beliefs," and "coping thoughts."

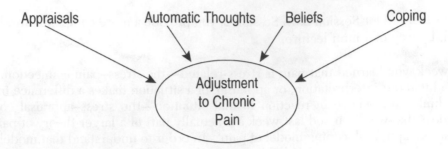

FIGURE MOD. 2.3. The stress–appraisal–coping model of pain.

[At this point in the session, I provide clients with a simple illustration of the stress–appraisal–coping model of pain, depicting appraisals, automatic thoughts, beliefs, and coping. You can redraw Figure Mod. 2.3 on a flipchart during your mini-lecture, or you can enlarge this one and tack it up on the wall.]

The model shows appraisals influencing adjustment, and we talked about appraisals last week. Over here is the category "automatic thoughts." Automatic thoughts are thoughts that come up in response to situations before we're even fully aware of them. Automatic thoughts, just like our appraisals of a stressful situation, have a direct impact on our mood, our physical well-being, and our behavior. Another broad category of thoughts is the "beliefs" category, and this category represents more firmly held ideas about the pain problem, the self, and the world around us. In this treatment program, we will be covering each of these thought categories in detail, and we will show you how each category of thoughts has an important influence over how you cope and adjust to chronic pain. We will also show you how certain kinds of coping can be used to help deal with pain flare-ups when they occur.

It is certainly not necessary for a client to understand all of these ideas right now; they are only presented in this mini-lecture by way of introduction. As a reminder, Session 1 has introduced the idea of appraisals as thoughts judging a potentially stressful situation as a threat, a loss, or a challenge. The next part of this session gets more specific about another important category of thoughts—those we call "automatic thoughts."

SESSION OBJECTIVE: IDENTIFY AUTOMATIC THOUGHTS OR IMAGES

As we talked about in our first session, some thought processes help us sort out cues in our surroundings that need our attention, those that can be ignored, and those that should be avoided. These thought processes (which we call "appraisals") are like thermometers measuring our complicated surroundings. When we judge a situation as stressful, we also decide how easy or hard it will be for us to "cope" with it. So we make a second interpretation. Are we up for making the effort? Can we do it? Can we handle the stress? These interpretations are called "automatic thoughts." Automatic thoughts, just like our appraisals of a stressful situation, have a direct impact on our mood, our physical well-being, and our behavior.

We are most interested in negative, distorted automatic thoughts, because such thoughts have a harmful effect on the way we cope and adjust to pain. Negative automatic thoughts are typically associated with appraising pain, or pain-related stressors, as a threat or loss. [Provide a diagram of the appraisal–automatic thoughts–pain connection—see Figure Mod. 2.4—using a flipchart.] Negative automatic thoughts are also associated with a tendency to focus on pain or pain-related cues. Focusing on pain or pain-related cues results in an accentuated perception of pain, an inability to direct thoughts away from the pain, and beliefs that one is helpless when it comes to having any control over one's condition. Research has repeatedly shown that the tendency toward negative, distorted automatic thoughts is associated with greater pain, greater distress, more medication used, more loss of function, and more disability. Since such automatic thoughts can occur without our awareness, the first step in changing them is to become aware of them. Let's look at an example.

To help illustrate the concept of automatic thoughts, I provide a simple case example for group discussion. I have provided one below, but you can make up your own if you prefer; if you are working with a specific pain clientele that has unusual characteristics, you can devise an example tailored to your particular population. The example below offers some background regarding the client, a description of the stressful situation, and an easy-to-recognize automatic thought.

Nancy is a 54-year-old woman who has lived in a rural area for the past 30 years. She has been diagnosed with fibromyalgia, chronic fatigue, and mixed migraine–muscle tension headaches. Nancy's husband works at a local automobile assembly plant. Nancy's daughter and two children have recently moved back into her home following the daughter's divorce. Nancy is suddenly faced with increasing responsibilities for child care, food preparation, and homemaking. Her self-expectations are to help her daughter through this difficult time by making it "easy" for her, thus taking the load on herself. However, Nancy is unable to set limits or attend to her own needs. A few months after her daughter moves in, Nancy experiences a severe pain flare-up, during which she tells herself, "I just can't handle my life."

At this point in the session, it is only necessary to get group members to recognize the stressful situation (increased responsibilities in the home resulting from Nancy's daughter and grandchildren moving in) and the automatic thought ("I just can't handle my life"). You should help group members discuss how such an automatic thought might affect Nancy's emotions, her behavior, her other thoughts, and even her physical well-being.

Since people are often not even aware of the automatic thoughts they have, these thoughts are sometimes difficult to identify. For this reason, it is useful to offer examples of types of negatively distorted thoughts in order to facilitate the discussion. A list of the categories of cognitive errors—patterned after those noted by Burns (1980) and Beck (1995), with examples—is found in Client Handout 2.2 at the end of this module, and can be copied and

Stress appraisal as threat or loss	→	Attention focused on pain and pain-related issues	→	Negative, distorted automatic thoughts	→	Magnify the perception of pain
					→	Contribute to inability to distract self
					→	Lead to sense of helplessness

FIGURE MOD. 2.4. Diagram of appraisal–automatic thoughts–pain connection.

distributed to your clients. The point here is not to make the clients experts in categorization. The point is to stimulate the clients' thinking so that they can begin to recognize automatic thoughts, particularly the negative ones. Once you have gone over the categories in the handout, ask the group members whether they recognize a certain category as characteristic of them, and if so, to share a specific example with the group. Once again, when clients are offering specific examples from their own life situations, it is important for the therapist to acknowledge each example by restating or paraphrasing it. This helps each client feel heard and understood.

Discussion of Clients' PCS Responses

Another useful tool for this session is to bring in the group members' initial responses to the Pain Catastrophizing Scale (PCS; see Chapter 4). The PCS taps specific kinds of negative pain-related cognitions, and using it in this part of the session can enhance the discussion, because it provides an illustration to clients consisting of what they actually reported their thoughts to be in response to pain. Since these are not yes or no responses, but responses made on a scale of 0–5, helping each client look at how strongly she endorsed a particular type of thought can also be enlightening.

WORKSHEET: AUTOMATIC THOUGHTS WORKSHEET–1 (ATW-1)

The next step in Session 2 is to introduce the worksheet clients will be using during the coming week's homework. Worksheets helping clients identify automatic thoughts have been used widely in cognitive therapy, and the ones used in this book are similar to those used in Beck (1995), Burns (1980), and Caudill (2002), among others. To begin with, clients are asked to go back to their homework assignment from the previous week (the Stress–Pain Connection Worksheet), and to pick a specific thought or image associated with a stressful situation that they wrote down on their worksheet. They are asked to record the situation and the thought or image on the Automatic Thoughts Worksheet–1 (ATW-1; see Client Handout 2.3 at the back of this module). If they have not come up with a thought or image associated with the stressful situation, they leave that column blank for the moment. They are then asked to think back to a specific situation during which they noticed a change in their emotions and/or a shift in their physical comfort level. Those practitioners already familiar with cognitive therapy principles will recognize the technique of having clients identify a shift in emotions with an automatic thought. For patients with chronic pain, it may be quite useful to have them note physical changes as well as emotional changes associated with stressful situations. Often an initial increase in muscle tension can trigger a pain flare-up, particularly if the situation is allowed to progress. Explain to the group that changes in emotion or physical changes in response to a stressful situation often occur right after an automatic thought. We are often aware of the emotional or physical change, but not aware (without training) of the automatic thought. Thinking back to the emotional change or physical shift related to the situation is a useful tool to get at the automatic thought. Once the clients have identified a situation and a change in emotions or physical shift, ask them, "What thought or image might have gone through your mind right around the time of the shift in emotions or your physical sense of well-being?" I use recent examples from my own life by way of illustration, such as the one below:

Situation: It is a school day, and my 9-year-old son has to be at school in 15 minutes. I discover he has math homework, which he has not even begun.

Emotional and/or physical shift: Angry, anxious, increase in neck tension.

Thought or image: "I can't let down my guard for even one night! If I do, he will fail!"

Clients are guided through the process of completing one row on the ATW-1. It is quite common at this point for clients to be confused about what an automatic thought or image might be. You may need to ask leading questions and suggest possible automatic thoughts related to the situation in order to help the clients with the initial exercise. Also, some clients have more than one automatic thought related to a stressful situation. In fact, there are many automatic thoughts occurring all the time. The way to decide which automatic thought to focus on and identify is to establish which one "grabs" a client the most. One way to do this is to say to clients, "How much do you believe that thought? On a scale of 0–100%, if you believe a particular thought about 20%, it is not worth writing down or working with. If, on the other hand, you believe a thought 70–100%, it is an important component of your reaction to the situation." In the example provided above, at the time that I had the automatic thought "I can't let down my guard for even one night! If I do, he will fail!", I believed it 90%. You can bet the thought contributed to my neck tension and my feelings of anxiety and anger!

HOMEWORK ASSIGNMENT

As homework, clients are asked to continue working with the ATW-1. They are asked to use the ATW-1 to identify situations during the week, to recognize changes in their emotions and/or shifts in their physical state, and to attempt to distinguish thoughts or images associated with the emotional/physical shifts. Specifically, they are instructed to be aware of shifts in their emotions and/or physical well-being, and to ask themselves immediately, "What just went through my mind?" They are reminded that an automatic thought can also take the form of an image. Be sure to remind group members that they can (and probably will) have more than one automatic thought in response to a situation, and to write down all that seem relevant. They should also rate how much they believe each automatic thought on a scale of 0% ("not at all") to 100%. Once again, emphasize that this homework is central to the process of the treatment, and that we will be discussing group members' findings by way of the worksheet during the next session.

POSTSESSION PROCESS CHECK

The very last part of the session involves having group members fill out the Postsession Process Check. Remind them that this is not a "test" for them; rather, it helps you as the therapist figure out whether you got the main points across during the session. It also provides the clients with an opportunity to give you feedback, ask questions, or express concerns.

Session 2 Outline for Therapists: Identifying Automatic Thoughts

SESSION OBJECTIVES

- Introduce the stress–appraisal–coping model of pain.
- Identify automatic thoughts or images.

NEEDED MATERIALS, HANDOUTS, AND WORKSHEETS

- Flipchart and markers
- Session 2 Outline for Therapists (this handout)
- Session 2 Summary for Clients (Client Handout 2.1)
- Presession Process Check (Appendix J)
- Results for each client's Pain Catastrophizing Scale (PCS), completed during assessment (Appendix G)
- Examples of Negative (Distorted) Thinking (Client Handout 2.2)
- Automatic Thoughts Worksheet–1 (ATW-1) (Client Handout 2.3)
- Postsession Process Check (Appendix J)

PRESESSION PROCESS CHECK

- Hand out Presession Process Check and have clients fill it in.

REVIEW OF PREVIOUS WEEK'S SESSION

- Stress is a biological, emotional, and cognitive response.
- Chronic pain is a stressor, and non-pain-related stressors can trigger pain flare-ups.
- Appraisal of stress (as threat, loss, or challenge) shapes what we think, feel, and do about it.

HOMEWORK REVIEW

- Review Stress–Pain Connection Worksheet with clients.
- Ask several clients: "Pick one stressful situation from your Stress–Pain Connection Worksheet, and share what you wrote with the group."
- "What did you learn about the importance of the appraisal category?"
- "What did you learn about specific thoughts associated with the stressful situation?"

(continued)

From *Cognitive Therapy for Chronic Pain* by Beverly E. Thorn. Copyright 2004 by The Guilford Press. Permission to photocopy this handout is granted to purchasers of this book for personal use only (see copyright page for details).

SESSION OBJECTIVE:
INTRODUCE THE STRESS–APPRAISAL–COPING MODEL OF PAIN

- Early theories of pain (tissue damage equals pain) have been proven incorrect.
- Newer theories of pain suggest that the centers for thoughts and feelings in the brain can influence how the brain processes pain signals—and hence the experience of pain.
- The stress–appraisal–coping model of pain, emphasizes the importance of thoughts:
  - Our thoughts influence our emotions, our behavior, and our physical functioning, and also give rise to other thoughts.
  - These *other* thoughts influence our emotions, behavior, and physical functioning (and so on).
  - Provide illustration of stress–appraisal–coping model of pain, using flipchart.
  - Thought categories in the stress–appraisal–coping model of pain include these:
    - Appraisals
    - Automatic thoughts
    - Beliefs
    - Coping
- Often thoughts in response to pain or stress are automatic. That is, we are not even consciously aware of the thoughts.

SESSION OBJECTIVE: IDENTIFY AUTOMATIC THOUGHTS OR IMAGES

- Stress appraisals are the "thermometers" checking our environment.
- Automatic thoughts are related to stress appraisals.
- Automatic thoughts shape whether, and which, coping attempts will be made.
- Provide diagram of appraisal–automatic thoughts–pain connection, using flipchart.
- Negative, distorted automatic thoughts are related to stress appraisals of threat and loss.
- Such automatic thoughts are harmful for these reasons:
  - They tend to focus our attention on pain or pain-related cues.
  - They result in magnification or accentuation of the perception of pain.
  - They contribute to an inability to direct thoughts away from the pain.
  - They lead to beliefs that one is helpless to exert any control over one's condition.

Example

Nancy is a 54-year-old mother and wife with fibromyalgia, chronic fatigue, and headaches. Her recently divorced daughter and grandchildren have moved into her home. Nancy has increased responsibilities, doesn't set limits, and experiences a severe pain flare-up. She tells herself, "I just can't handle my life."

Discussion

- Using the example above, have clients determine what Nancy's automatic thought is.
- Give out Examples of Negative, Distorted Thinking (Client Handout 2.3). Ask clients:
  - "Is a certain type of negative automatic thought characteristic of you?"
  - "Can you give an example?"
- Review clients' answers to the PCS to see how they said they think in response to pain.

(continued)

WORKSHEET: AUTOMATIC THOUGHTS WORKSHEET–1 (ATW-1)

- Give out copies of the Automatic Thoughts Worksheet–1 (ATW-1).
- Tell clients: "Go back to your homework with the Stress–Pain Connection Worksheet."
- "Pick a specific stressful situation that you wrote down on your worksheet."
- "Were you able to identify a specific thought or image associated with a stressful situation?"
- "Transfer your notation of this situation and thought/image to the ATW-1."
  - "On a scale of 0–100%, how much did you (or do you) believe that thought?"
  - "Note the specific shift in emotions and/or physical shift associated with the stressful situation."

HOMEWORK ASSIGNMENT

- Tell clients: "Using the ATW-1, continue identifying automatic thoughts. Try doing this each day."
  - "When you notice a change in your emotions or a physical change, note that down. Note the time, date, and situation."
  - "What automatic thoughts or images were present immediately prior to, during, or after the event? Note all that seem relevant."
  - "Rate how strongly you believe each of the automatic thoughts/images."
- "Bring your homework to the next session, and be prepared to discuss what you have learned."

POSTSESSION PROCESS CHECK

- Hand out Postsession Process Check (Appendix J) and have clients fill it in before they leave.

Session 2 Summary for Clients: Identifying Automatic Thoughts

THE GOALS OF THIS SESSION

- To introduce you to the stress–appraisal–coping model of pain.
- To help you identify negative automatic thoughts or images.

REVIEW OF PREVIOUS WEEK'S SESSION

- Stress is a biological, emotional, and cognitive (thoughts) response.
- Chronic pain is itself a stressor.
- Non-pain-related stressors also trigger pain.
- Your appraisal of stress (threat, loss, challenge) shapes how you think and feel, and what you do about it.

HOMEWORK REVIEW

- Pick one stressful situation from your Stress–Pain Connection Worksheet, and share what you wrote with the group.
- What did you learn about the importance of the appraisal category?
- What did you learn about specific thoughts associated with the stressful situation?

INTRODUCTION TO THE STRESS–APPRAISAL–COPING MODEL OF PAIN

- Early theories of pain (tissue damage equals pain) are incorrect.
- Newer theories of pain emphasize the importance of the brain as a pain filter.
- The centers for thoughts and feelings in the brain influence how the brain processes pain signals, and influence the experience of pain.
- The stress–appraisal–coping model of pain emphasizes the importance of thoughts:
  - Our thoughts influence our emotions, our behavior, and our physical functioning.
  - Thought categories in the stress–appraisal–coping model of pain include these:
    - Appraisals (the topic of last week's session)
    - Automatic thoughts (the topic of this week's session)
    - Beliefs
    - Coping
  - Often thoughts in response to pain or stress are automatic. That is, we are not even consciously aware of the thoughts.

(continued)

From *Cognitive Therapy for Chronic Pain* by Beverly E. Thorn. Copyright 2004 by The Guilford Press. Permission to photocopy this handout is granted to purchasers of this book for personal use only (see copyright page for details).

IDENTIFYING AUTOMATIC THOUGHTS OR IMAGES

- Automatic thoughts are related to stress appraisals.
- Negative, distorted automatic thoughts are related to stress appraisals of threat and loss.
- Such automatic thoughts are harmful for these reasons:
  - They focus our attention on pain or pain-related cues.
  - They result in magnification or accentuation of the perception of pain.
  - They contribute to an inability to direct thoughts away from the pain.
  - They lead to beliefs that you are helpless to exert any control over your condition.
- There are different kinds of negative thoughts, and certain types may be characteristic of your kind of thinking.
- Learning to identify negative, distorted automatic thoughts is the first step to changing them.

SUMMARY OF KEY POINTS

- The brain controls how we experience pain. The centers for thoughts and emotions in the brain influence our perception of pain.
- The stress–appraisal–coping model of pain emphasizes thoughts, and each category of thoughts (appraisals, automatic thoughts, beliefs, coping) influences your adjustment to pain.
- Automatic thoughts are those that arise in response to situations, and you may not even be consciously aware of their presence.
- Negative, distorted automatic thoughts are harmful, and the first step to changing them is becoming aware of them.

HOMEWORK ASSIGNMENT

- Using the Automatic Thoughts Worksheet–1 (ATW-1), continue identifying automatic thoughts. Try doing this each day.
- When you notice a change in your emotions or a physical change, note that down. Note the time, date, and situation.
- What automatic thoughts or images were present immediately before, during, or after the event? Note all that seem relevant.
- Rate how strongly you believe each of the automatic thoughts/images.
- Bring your homework to the next session, and be prepared to discuss what you have learned.

Examples of Negative, Distorted Thinking

Category	Definition	Example
All-or-nothing thinking	Viewing a situation as two distinct categories rather than on a continuum—"black-versus-white" thinking.	"I can't work any more, so nothing I can do is worthwhile."
Fortunetelling	Predicting the future negatively without considering other possible outcomes.	"Oh, man, here comes a migraine aura. I'll wind up in the emergency room for sure!"
Disqualifying the positive	Telling oneself that positive experiences don't count.	"I was able to cook dinner last night, but one night out of 20 doesn't mean much."
Emotional reasoning	Assuming that because one feels or believes something so strongly, it must be true.	"I can just feel my bones grinding together when I move. I don't care what the physical therapist says; it can't be good for me to do those exercises."
Labeling	Attaching a global, extreme, negative label to oneself or others.	"All doctors are uncaring jerks!"
Magnification/minimization	Magnifying the negative or minimizing the positive.	"My pain is totally unbearable!"
Mental filter	Paying undue attention to a single negative detail instead of seeing the whole picture.	"My fibromyalgia means that I am less than a whole person."
Mind reading	Believing that one knows what others are thinking.	"My husband thinks that I am exaggerating how bad I feel."
Overgeneralization	Making global negative conclusions that go well beyond the current situation.	"I can't do the work I was trained for any more, so I won't be able to go back to work at all."
"Should" statements	Holding fixed ideas about how the world "should," "ought to," or "must" be.	"A competent doctor would be able to get rid of my pain."
Personalization	Seeing oneself as the cause of negative external events for which one is not necessarily responsible.	"This pain is a punishment from God for something I did wrong."

From *Cognitive Therapy for Chronic Pain* by Beverly E. Thorn. Copyright 2004 by The Guilford Press. Permission to photocopy this handout is granted to purchasers of this book for personal use only (see copyright page for details).

Automatic Thoughts Worksheet–1 (ATW-1)

Date/time	Stressful situation	Shift in emotion and/or physical change	Automatic thought or image* (How much do you believe it? 0–100%)	Comments/notes

*Automatic thoughts often occur immediately before a shift in emotion (e.g., anxiety) or physical sensation (e.g., neck tension).

From *Cognitive Therapy for Chronic Pain* by Beverly E. Thorn. Copyright 2004 by The Guilford Press. Permission to photocopy this handout is granted to purchasers of this book for personal use only (see copyright page for details).

EVALUATING AUTOMATIC THOUGHTS

The third treatment session shows clients how to evaluate automatic thoughts. Therapist Handout 3.1, found at the back of this module, provides an outline of Session 3 to be used by the therapist. Client Handout 3.1, also at the back of the module, can be copied and used as a session outline to be given to clients at the beginning of the session.

SESSION 3 TREATMENT OBJECTIVE
• Evaluate automatic thoughts.

PRESESSION PROCESS CHECK AND REVIEW OF PREVIOUS WEEK'S SESSION

The session begins by having group members fill out the Presession Process Check and reviewing the previous week's session and homework. During Session 2, the specifics of the stress–appraisal–coping model of pain were introduced. This model states that our thoughts influence our feelings, behavior, other thoughts, and physical well-being. The role of automatic thoughts in the stress–appraisal–coping model was highlighted—particularly because negative, distorted automatic thoughts can magnify our perception of pain, contribute to our inability to distract ourselves from the pain, and lead to a sense of helplessness. The other treatment objective for Session 2 was to help clients begin identifying automatic thoughts, by giving them examples of negatively distorted thoughts, going over their Pain Catastrophizing Scale (PCS) responses, and teaching them to recognize the connection between shifts in emotion and/or changes in their sense of physical well-being and automatic thoughts. In reviewing Session 2, remind clients that since we are often not aware of automatic thoughts as they occur, shifts in emotions or our sense of physical well-being can cue us to ask, "What just

115

went through my mind?" Identifying automatic thoughts is an important step in taking more control over how the brain responds to stressful situations, including pain.

HOMEWORK REVIEW

The Automatic Thoughts Worksheet–1 (ATW-1; see Client Handout 2.4) was used to help clients identify automatic thoughts, particularly negative automatic thoughts. At this point in the session, obtain some examples from clients regarding homework with the ATW-1. It should again be noted that this is a new skill for clients, and they should not expect to become experts on the first go-round. Rather, it should be emphasized that this work takes practice and repetition to become good at identifying automatic thoughts.

The following transcript is from a session during which a client was asked to report on her homework using the ATW-1. Jennifer is a 46-year-old working mother with a supportive husband and family. She has had mixed migraine and muscle tension headaches for over 30 years. She works full time at a local bank. Although she is not the head teller, coworkers seem to look to her for guidance.

THERAPIST: Jennifer, can you share with the group one of the automatic thoughts you identified during your homework? If you would, give us a brief synopsis of the situation, the shift in emotion or physical well-being that cued you to the automatic thought, and then the automatic thought.

JENNIFER: Well, since we got on our new computer networking system, our machines have consistently gone down one or two times per week. It never fails that when our screens go blank, regardless of whether I have a line of customers out the door, the other clerks will look at me and call, "Jennifer, what do I do?" It makes me so angry, because they have lived with this system flaw as long as I have. Why do they ask me? They know as much as I do! But it never fails—they turn to me and begin calling to me, like a flock of sheep looking for a leader. I feel the muscles in my neck tensing up, and my hands tighten, and I can just feel the headache starting.

THERAPIST: Wonderful example! So the situation involved being interrupted by your coworkers, and you noticed a shift in your emotions (anger), and a physical shift as well (neck tension, hands tightening). In fact, you said you could just *feel* the headache starting. So what do you think your automatic thought was?

JENNIFER: "I'm so mad!"

THERAPIST: Well that certainly was your emotional response to the situation, wasn't it? So the emotion you became aware of in response to being interrupted by your coworkers was anger. And the shift in your physical being in response to the situation was increased tension in your neck and hands. Chances are there was an automatic thought that occurred in response to the situation, right before you experienced anger and an increase in muscle tension.

JENNIFER: Well, I just hate to turn people down. It makes me feel guilty. But I really can't do two things at once any more than anyone else can. Maybe my automatic thought was "Why do you people put me in the position of having to do two things at once?", which then made me mad. As a matter of fact, I often feel like I'm not in control of my own time, and it always makes me really mad and tense.

THERAPIST: That is very insightful. It sounds like you have two related automatic thoughts there: "Coworkers put me in the position of having to do two things at once," and "I'm not in control of my own time at work." Does one of those grab you more than the other?

JENNIFER: Well, for the exact situation, it would be about my coworkers making me do two things at once, but the reason it bothers me so much is that it is the story of my life! I'm just not in control of my own time! So the second grabs me more than the first.[1]

THERAPIST: How much do you believe the thought "I'm not in control of my own time at work" on a scale of 0%, being "not at all," to 100%, being "totally"?

JENNIFER: Oh, at least 90%! On some level, I realize that no one can *make* me do anything I refuse to do—so it's not really that people force me to do things I don't want to do—but it still grabs me emotionally.

THERAPIST: We'll deal with testing the reality of that automatic thought in a little while, but for now, I think you've really hit on an important automatic thought in response to interruptions by coworkers. You're saying that the thought was a real grabber, which means it's an important automatic thought to put on your list. Let's go back to the worksheet for a minute. What you noticed first were anger and an increase in muscle tension in response to the situation. As you looked back on it, you were able to discover an important automatic thought. Does this make sense to you?

JENNIFER: Yes, now that you helped me figure it out. But I felt totally lost before you saved me.

THERAPIST: Well, actually, I didn't save you. I helped you decode the clues. You provided the most important input, and you did the hard work of dissecting the stressful situation as part of your homework, and sharing it with the group.

ANOTHER GROUP MEMBER: It seemed so easy to figure out the gist of Jennifer's automatic thought, but when it came to figuring out mine, I had that same lost feeling that Jennifer did.

THERAPIST: Well, especially at first, it is much easier to "think" about someone else's situation and help them, because you are not emotionally caught up in the situation yourself. That's one of the benefits of the group. We help each other. But still, the majority of the work is done by each individual, as you continue to do these homework exercises and work with the concepts on a daily basis. So, just for practice, let's take a look at your thought worksheet that you completed during the week. Of course, you see three important columns on the thought record. The first two columns are "Date/time" and "Stressful situation." The third column is "Shift in emotion and/or physical change." The fourth column is "Automatic thought or image." So, Jennifer, I see you filled in the "Stressful situation" column exactly right—"Coworkers hassling me." Under "Shift in emotion and/or physical change," you put "Headache," and under "Automatic thought or image," you put "I'm so mad!" Based on our discussion, how would you go about changing this somewhat?

---

[1]Note that both of these are automatic thoughts, and one is very specific to the described situation, while the other is more global. I took the more global thought, and narrowed it to the work situation so that it would be easier to work with. Although I could also have steered Jennifer to work with the very specific thought, the thought that coworkers want her to be able to do two things at once is probably less distorted than the thought that she is not in control of her own time at work. Therefore, I chose to guide Jennifer toward working on the thought most likely to be distorted.

JENNIFER: Well, I guess I'd put "anger" down for the emotion, and "muscle tension" down for the physical shift. The headache came later.

THERAPIST: Very important point—which goes back to our session last week, where we introduced the connection between stress response and pain. Maybe the stress of the situation led to the anger and muscle tension, which then led to the headache. How about for the automatic thought?

JENNIFER: Well, I put "I'm so mad" before, but now I'd put either "My coworkers make me do two things at once," or "I'm not in control of my own time at work." The second thought grabs me more.

THERAPIST: Excellent. I think you are correct in identifying both as automatic thoughts, and selecting the most important one to work on.

JENNIFER: And I had those thoughts without even being aware of them! That's kind of creepy.

THERAPIST: It's kind of creepy when you realize you're having all these automatic thoughts and didn't even know it. It's very powerful, however, when you learn how to recognize the automatic thoughts and bring them under your control. That's what we're going to tackle next.

Remember that we spend so much time on the homework from Session 2, rather than getting into new material, because the homework is the integral "meat" of the session and provides the opportunity for consolidation of the material. The example above illustrates how even motivated clients need careful tutoring following the initial try at identifying automatic thoughts. Going over their work carefully helps them to understand the concept and increases the likelihood that they will continue to work with the identified treatment goals. Jennifer's ATW-1, as modified following the in-session review, is included as Figure Mod. 3.1 to illustrate the process of identifying and refining the automatic thoughts.

Another common occurrence when clients are first learning to identify automatic thoughts is that they are often surprised to find they have so *many* automatic thoughts. Determining which automatic thought to work on is often a challenge for these clients. Another example—David's ATW-1, as illustrated in Figure Mod. 3.2—illustrates this.

Date/time	Stressful situation	Shift in emotion and/or physical change	Automatic thought or image (How much do you believe it? 0–100%)	Comments/notes
9/26/02, 10:30 A.M.	Coworkers hassling me.	~~Headache~~ Hands tense up. Neck tenses up. Angry. Headache starts.	~~I'm so mad!~~ My coworkers make me do two things at once. I'm not in control of my own time at work. (90%)	Note: Headache came after anger, tension. Note: Anger was the emotion, not the thought.

FIGURE MOD. 3.1. Jennifer's Session 2 homework Automatic Thoughts Worksheet–1 (ATW-1), after in-session review.

Date/time	Stressful situation	Shift in emotion and/or physical change	Automatic thought or image (How much do you believe it? 0–100%)	Comments/notes
9/2/02, 9:00 A.M.	Spending more time standing at work than usual.	Back pain began increasing. Getting irritable.	I'm getting so tired of having this pain. (100%). I'm so disappointed, because I'm trying so hard but it's not working. (80%) The pain is just eating me up! (90%) I can't afford to miss work. (100%) It's going to get worse if I don't go home and go to bed. (90%) It's gonna be a horrible day with me here. (80%)	

FIGURE MOD. 3.2. David's Session 2 homework Automatic Thoughts Worksheet–1 (ATW-1).

Troubleshooting Tip: Since thoughts are usually related to each other, clients *can* (and do) tend to work on multiple automatic thoughts at the same time. But it is probably easier for them to grasp the concept initially if they work on one automatic thought at a time. At this point in treatment, I usually guide clients to choose the automatic thought that seems to have the most emotional pull for them, and work on examining that one thought in particular. In the case illustrated in Figure Mod. 3.2, David believed two of the automatic thoughts 100%. The thought that had the most emotional pull for him, however, was "The pain is just eating me up!", which he believed 90%. I encouraged him to focus on and examine this thought.

SESSION OBJECTIVE: EVALUATE AUTOMATIC THOUGHTS

The treatment objective for Session 3 is to help clients learn to evaluate automatic thoughts to determine whether they are accurate.

Troubleshooting Tip: Clients do not like to hear that their thoughts may contain distortions, and they object to calling these thoughts "maladaptive." When I first began offering these groups, I used thought worksheets entitled "Dysfunctional Thought Records." My initial groups objected to my labels, and in the process helped me to realize that terms such as "distorted," "dysfunctional," and "maladaptive" are emotionally loaded for clients, as well as denigrating. Hence I have chosen to use the label "Automatic Thoughts Worksheet." Nonetheless, some automatic thoughts *are* distorted and *do* damage the clients' ability to cope with chronic painful conditions. Thus learning to critically evaluate them is an important component of treatment. It is the therapist's job to treat the issue with great sensitivity, and to be mindful of terminology in doing so—as in the following mini-lecture.

Now that you have a sense of how to identify negative automatic thoughts, it's time to figure out whether or not they are true. First, let me emphasize that *some* thoughts in response to pain or stress are precisely accurate. *Many* thoughts in response to pain or stress are at least partly based on fact—in other words, many thoughts are at least partly true. Often, though, thoughts in response to pain or stress become partly distorted in the negative direction. As we talked about last week, automatic thoughts with a negative distortion have a powerful, damaging influence on our emotions, behavior, and physical functioning. So it becomes very important to learn how to evaluate the accuracy of automatic thoughts, so that we can come up with more realistic and less damaging thoughts. We'll talk about coming up with alternative thoughts next week, but for now, let's use our next worksheet to learn now to evaluate the ones we have.

WORKSHEET: AUTOMATIC THOUGHTS WORKSHEET–2 (ATW-2)

Following this introduction to the concept of evaluating automatic thoughts, you should present the Automatic Thoughts Worksheet–2 (ATW-2; see Client Handout 3.2). Using the ATW-2, clients are guided through a process of Socratic questioning to help them determine for themselves whether the thought is completely true, partially true, or not at all true. As you can see from the ATW-2, this process mainly involves first listing all of the factual evidence that the thought is true, and then listing the evidence that the thought is not true. Taking Jennifer's example from above, we would begin by listing the situation and the automatic thought—in this case, coworker interruptions, and "I'm not in control of my own time at work." Next, we would ask Jennifer to assign a weight to how much she believes that automatic thought on a scale of 0–100%. Note from the homework discussion above that Jennifer had already begun to question the validity of the thought by noting that in reality, people can't "make me" do two things at once. If the client has already begun to evaluate the automatic thought, this is a good place to facilitate the process by having her list the evidence she has come up with. In Jennifer's case, she would be encouraged to list, in the "Evidence that the thought/image is not true" column, "Coworkers can't make me do two things at once."

Troubleshooting Tip: Because clients have chosen to work with an automatic thought that has real emotional valence for them (i.e., they believe the thought 70–100%), it is important not to jump too quickly into the "evidence against" side of things. As the therapist, you need to make sure that the evidence supporting the automatic thought is considered as well as honored. If clients believe that you do not disparage the evidence supporting the thought, and that in doing so you validate the rationale for having the thought in the first place, they will be less likely to resist attempts to evaluate the evidence refuting the thought.

In Jennifer's case, her coworkers *were* behaving as if they are helpless, and implying that they could not function without her input. It is also a fact that at work, one is not totally in control of one's time. Part of an explicit or implicit work contract involves taking direction from supervisors and, in Jennifer's case, serving customers. Another "fact" that Jennifer ultimately listed as evidence supporting the automatic thought was that she had taken several network computing classes that her coworkers had not taken, and thus she did know more than they did. She reasoned that if she did know more about the computer snafu, then she should stop what she was doing and help her coworkers.[2]

Following the generation of a list of facts supporting the automatic thought, clients should be guided to generate a list of facts that refute the automatic thought. Jennifer started with her initial fact that "Coworkers can't make me do two things at once." Jennifer then

---

[2]This "should" statement, by the way, is an intermediate belief that should be mentally noted by the therapist. Intermediate thoughts are tackled at a later point, when the client has gained success in recognizing, challenging, and reconstructing automatic thoughts. If the therapist has already made note of intermediate and core beliefs as they appear, it will be easier to help the client identify and work with them when the time is right. In Jennifer's case, an intermediate belief seems to be "If I know more than someone else, I *should* put my own needs aside and help them out."

Date/time	Stressful situation	Emotional/ physical shift	Automatic thought or image (How much do you believe it? 0–100%)	Evidence that the thought is true	Evidence that the thought is not true	Re-rate belief (0–100%)
9/26/02, 10:30 A.M.	Coworkers interrupt me.	Hands tense up. Neck tenses up. Angry. Headache starts.	I'm not in control of my own time at work. (90%)	My coworkers do act helpless. No one is in total control of her time at work. I do know more than they do, so I should help them out.	Coworkers can't make me do two things at once. I can set limits with coworkers. I can say yes or no to coworkers. I can control when I help coworkers out.	20%

FIGURE MOD. 3.3. Jennifer's in-session Automatic Thoughts Worksheet–2 (ATW-2).

noted that she was responsible for setting limits with coworkers and others, and that she could determine when to say yes and when to say no. She also noted that although she was not in control of *all* her activities at work, she was certainly in control over when, and whether, she deferred her own work in order to help a coworker.

An illustration of Jennifer's ATW-2 is provided as Figure Mod. 3.3.

HOMEWORK ASSIGNMENT

As homework, ask clients to continue working with the ATW-2. You should instruct them to use the ATW-2 to identify automatic thoughts or images that occur as situations arise during the week. Just the way they did with the ATW-1, they should identify changes in their emotions and/or shifts in their physical state, and identify the thoughts or images associated with the emotional/physical shifts. In the ATW-2, though, they go a step further and evaluate each automatic thought by generating a list of facts supporting the thought and a list of facts refuting the thought. After they have generated these lists of facts, they should re-rate the strength of their belief in the original automatic thought. This sets the stage for helping the clients to construct alternative thoughts, which will be a treatment goal in Session 4. Be sure to tell clients that the stressful situations they list do not have to be major, extremely upsetting events. Even minor stressors probably elicit automatic thoughts that can be examined via this exercise. When clients get good at the skill of examining automatic thoughts in "minor" situations, they will be able to utilize this valuable technique in more significant stressful situations with greater ease.

POSTSESSION PROCESS CHECK

Remember to administer the Postsession Process Check at the end of each treatment session. If you have a chance, glance at the responses to make sure that there is not a question you need to address before dismissing the group. To illustrate the relevance of my point, see Figure Mod. 3.4, which is Kristi's completed Postsession Process Check form.

1. List the main point of this week's session.
   • *Evaluate and challenge untrue automatic thoughts.*
   • *Come up with more realistic and positive alternative thoughts.*

2. List one thing you can do or think differently during the next week as a result of this week's session.
   • *I'm already doing this. As soon as I recognize a bad thought, I tell myself that it's not true and come up with another one. I can do more of this.*

3. Was there anything said during this week's session that confused or troubled you?
   • *The homework steps aren't really relevant because it's already happening automatically.*

4. Do you have any questions from this week's session?

FIGURE MOD. 3.4. Kristi's Postsession Process Check after Session 3.

Since Kristi was about to leave the session assuming that the steps of working through the homework assignment weren't really relevant to her (and thus she would be unlikely to do the homework), I decided to delay dismissing the group for a few minutes so that I could clarify the issue she raised. The session transcript is included below.

THERAPIST: Before you all go, I'm noticing on one of the Postsession Process Check forms that there is a question that might be applicable to several of you. It has do with what happens if as soon as you recognize your unrealistic automatic thought, you almost automatically replace it with a more realistic alternative, but you haven't gone through all the steps.

KRISTI: That was mine. This isn't really relevant to me, because ever since you taught us how to recognize automatic thoughts last week, my mind just sort of automatically challenges it as "not realistic" and comes up with a replacement thought. I didn't even know about all these steps to go through to do that.

THERAPIST: Actually, our minds are probably doing that all the time anyway, without our awareness. A thought pops in, we evaluate it, and maybe we change it, without even being fully aware of it. But there are thoughts, especially the negative ones, that may pop in and get stuck. Either way, the point is to help you become consciously aware of the process so that it is under your control.

KRISTI: It's like I just needed a little reminder of what I was doing wrong, and it seems to be taken care of.

THERAPIST: As an experiment, I'm wondering if you'd be willing to try something slightly different this next week, Kristi.

KRISTI: Oh, oh! I should have kept my big mouth shut!

THERAPIST: Not at all! This is the way we all learn from each other. Here's my suggestion: When you find that you've had a negatively distorted automatic thought, and that as soon as you recognize it you almost immediately replace it with a more realistic alternative, write them both down. Then go backward with the exercise to see if you can figure out what the situation was that triggered the thought, what the emotional or physical shift was, and what the evidence was supporting and refuting the automatic thought. Chances are, even if it happened very quickly, you'll be able to go back and reconstruct some of the pieces.

KRISTI: I can give that a try.

THERAPIST: Good! That way, you'll be able to put the process under your conscious control, rather than just letting your mind sweep whichever way it cares to go. Okay? See you all next week.

Session 3 Outline for Therapists: Evaluating Automatic Thoughts

SESSION OBJECTIVE

- Evaluate automatic thoughts.

NEEDED MATERIALS, HANDOUTS, AND WORKSHEETS

- Session 3 Outline for Therapists (this handout)
- Session 3 Summary for Clients (Client Handout 3.1)
- Presession Process Check (Appendix J)
- Automatic Thoughts Worksheet–2 (ATW-2) (Client Handout 3.2)
- Postsession Process Check (Appendix J)

PRESESSION PROCESS CHECK

- Hand out Presession Process Check and have clients fill it in.

REVIEW OF PREVIOUS WEEK'S SESSION

- The stress–appraisal–coping model of pain: Thoughts influence feelings, behavior, other thoughts, and physical well-being.
- Automatic thoughts are thoughts or images that can occur without our full awareness of them.
- Negative, distorted automatic thoughts are harmful for these reasons:
  - They focus our attention on the pain and pain-related stressors.
  - They magnify the perception of pain.
  - They contribute to an inability to direct thoughts away from the pain.
  - They lead to a sense of helplessness.
- Identifying automatic thoughts: These thoughts or images usually occur right before shifts in emotions or physical well-being.

HOMEWORK REVIEW

- Ask several clients: "Pick one automatic thought from your Automatic Thoughts Worksheet–1 (ATW-1), and share what you wrote with the group."
- "Were you able to identify the effect of the automatic thought on your emotions, behavior, other thoughts, or physical well-being?"
- "What did you learn about identifying automatic thoughts?"
- "What problems did you encounter in identifying automatic thoughts?"

(continued)

From *Cognitive Therapy for Chronic Pain* by Beverly E. Thorn. Copyright 2004 by The Guilford Press. Permission to photocopy this handout is granted to purchasers of this book for personal use only (see copyright page for details).

SESSION OBJECTIVE: EVALUATE AUTOMATIC THOUGHTS

- *Some* thoughts in response to pain or stress are completely factual.
- *Most* thoughts in response to pain or stress are at least partly based on fact.
- *Often*, however, thoughts in response to pain or stress are somewhat distorted.
- Negative thought distortions have the most (negative) influence on our emotions, behavior, and physical functioning.
- Evaluating automatic thoughts can help reduce negative distortions, and this can have a positive influence on the ability to cope.

WORKSHEET: AUTOMATIC THOUGHTS WORKSHEET–2 (ATW-2)

- Give out copies of the Automatic Thoughts Worksheet–2 (ATW-2).
- Tell clients: "Go back to your ATW-1 and choose an automatic thought to evaluate."
- "Choose the automatic thought that grabs you the most (usually, the thoughts that you believe the most on a scale of 0–100%)."
- "Transfer that automatic thought onto your ATW-2."
- "Next, list *all* the evidence that the automatic thought is true or factual. You should be able to list more than one thing that makes the thought true."
- "Next, list *all* the evidence that the automatic thought is not true. You should be able to list more than one thing that makes the thought false."
- "Remember that most automatic thoughts have some truth to them, but that they also often contain some negative distortion of the facts."
- "Remember: Negative, distorted automatic thoughts are the most damaging."

HOMEWORK ASSIGNMENT

- Tell clients: "Using the ATW-2, note all important automatic thoughts that you become aware of (those that you believe 70–100%). Try doing this each day."
- "Rate how strongly you believe your automatic thought."
- "Just like you did in the ATW-1, note any shift in emotions or physical functioning, as well as the situation, time, and date."
- "Construct a list of factual evidence supporting that automatic thought, as well as a list of factual evidence that does not support that automatic thought."
- "After generating your lists of facts supporting and refuting your automatic thought, re-rate it for how much you believe the automatic thought now."
- "Bring your homework to the next session, and be prepared to discuss what you have learned."

POSTSESSION PROCESS CHECK

- Have clients fill out Postsession Process Check before they leave. Glance at responses and trouble-shoot if necessary.

Session 3 Summary for Clients: Evaluating Automatic Thoughts

THE GOAL OF THIS SESSION

- To evaluate automatic thoughts.

REVIEW OF PREVIOUS WEEK'S SESSION

- Thoughts influence feelings, behavior, other thoughts, and physical well-being (the stress–appraisal–coping model of pain).
- Automatic thoughts are thoughts or images that can occur in response to pain or pain-related stressors without your full awareness of them.
- Negative, distorted automatic thoughts are harmful for these reasons:
  - They focus your attention on the pain and pain-related stressors.
  - They magnify the perception of pain.
  - The contribute to an inability to direct thoughts away from the pain.
  - They lead to a sense of helplessness.
- Automatic thoughts usually occur right before shifts in emotions or physical well-being.

HOMEWORK REVIEW

- Pick one automatic thought from your Automatic Thoughts Worksheet–1 (ATW-1), and share what you wrote with the group.
- Were you able to identify the effect of the automatic thought on your emotions, behavior, other thoughts, or physical well-being?
- What did you learn about identifying automatic thoughts?
- What problems did you encounter in identifying automatic thoughts?

EVALUATING AUTOMATIC THOUGHTS

- *Some* thoughts in response to pain or stress are completely factual.
- *Most* thoughts in response to pain or stress are at least partly based on fact.
- *Often*, however, thoughts in response to pain or stress are somewhat distorted.
- Negative thought distortions have the most (negative) influence on your emotions, behavior, and physical functioning.
- Evaluating automatic thoughts can help reduce negative distortions, which has a positive influence on your ability to cope.
- Using the Automatic Thoughts Worksheet–2 (ATW-2) can help you work through the process of evaluating automatic thoughts.

(continued)

From *Cognitive Therapy for Chronic Pain* by Beverly E. Thorn. Copyright 2004 by The Guilford Press. Permission to photocopy this handout is granted to purchasers of this book for personal use only (see copyright page for details).

SUMMARY OF KEY POINTS

- Automatic thoughts, usually outside your immediate awareness, must be recognized before they can be changed.
- Negative, distorted automatic thoughts are harmful to your adjustment.
- Once you have learned to recognize automatic thoughts, you can use a system to evaluate what part of them is true and what part is distorted.
- Most thoughts are partially true and partially distorted.
- The ATW-2 guides you through the process of evaluating automatic thoughts.

HOMEWORK ASSIGNMENT

- Using the ATW-2, note all important automatic thoughts that you become aware of (those that you believe 70–100%). Try doing this each day.
- Rate how strongly you believe each automatic thought.
- Just as you did on the ATW-1, note any shift in emotions or physical functioning, as well as the situation, time, and date.
- Construct a list of factual evidence supporting that automatic thought, as well as a list of factual evidence that does not support that automatic thought.
- After generating your lists of facts supporting and refuting your automatic thought, re-rate it for how much you believe the automatic thought now.
- Bring your homework to the next session, and be prepared to discuss what you have learned.

Automatic Thoughts Worksheet–2 (ATW-2)

Date/time	Stressful situation	Emotional/physical shift	Automatic thought or image (How much do you believe it? 0–100%)	Evidence* that the thought is true	Evidence* that the thought is not true	Re-rate belief (0–100%)

*What are the *facts* regarding this automatic thought or image? Automatic thoughts are almost always partly true, but they often contain some negative distortions of the facts.

From *Cognitive Therapy for Chronic Pain* by Beverly E. Thorn. Copyright 2004 by The Guilford Press. Permission to photocopy this handout is granted to purchasers of this book for personal use only (see copyright page for details).

CHALLENGING AUTOMATIC THOUGHTS AND CONSTRUCTING ALTERNATIVE RESPONSES

The fourth treatment session teaches clients how to challenge negative, distorted automatic thoughts and construct alternative, more realistic responses. Therapist Handout 4.1, found at the back of this module, provides an outline of Session 4 to be used by the therapist. Client Handout 4.1, also at the back of the module, can be copied and used as a session outline to be given to clients at the beginning of the session.

SESSION 4 TREATMENT OBJECTIVES

- Challenge negative, distorted automatic thoughts.
- Construct realistic alternative responses.

PRESESSION PROCESS CHECK AND REVIEW OF PREVIOUS WEEK'S SESSION

After having group members fill out the Presession Process Check, conduct the review of the previous week's session. For Session 3, the treatment goal was to learn to evaluate automatic thoughts for their accuracy. Remind the group that although most automatic thoughts in response to pain and associated stressors are at least partly factual, there is often some distortion involved in these thoughts, usually in the negative direction. The Automatic Thoughts Worksheet–2 (ATW-2) was used to help clients begin to examine the authenticity of their automatic thoughts and to identify possible distortions. The therapeutic rationale for identifying negative distortions should be reemphasized; that is, such automatic thoughts have a powerful influence over our subsequent thoughts and feelings, and over what we do as a result.

Troubleshooting Tip: Clients will often come up with some negative automatic thoughts that they believe to be completely true—and, in fact, they may be. Not every negative automatic thought is distorted, and when such a thought is a statement of fact, you should not work to try to make it seem distorted. Consider, however, that this *true* negative automatic thought may in turn generate other, *distorted* automatic thoughts. You can sometimes help clients look behind the true thought and examine subsequent thoughts for negative distortions. An example of this technique, taken following examination of the Presession Process Check forms, is included in the session transcript below.

THERAPIST: Now that we've briefly reviewed our last session, I want to give an opportunity for group members to ask questions. I also see that some questions were listed on several of this week's Presession Process Check sheets. One group member has listed a question about automatic thoughts that, upon examination, seem to be true, although they are very negative. What are you supposed to do with *true* negative thoughts?

KRISTI: That was *my* question. I was at a family gathering this weekend, and my sister-in-law started bad-mouthing my religion again. My thought was "She is disagreeable, and I don't like to be around her." I examined the facts, and that thought is true! (*Group members laugh.*)

THERAPIST: Since you've talked about your sister-in-law before, we know this isn't an isolated instance. It sounds like you had an automatic thought that, while negative, is true. The question you're asking though, is "What do I do with automatic thoughts that are negative but true?"

KRISTI: Yes. I certainly found myself tensing up and feeling put down. I didn't want to be there, and I know it made my pain worse thinking these things.

THERAPIST: Sometimes negative thoughts that are true can mobilize us to do something about a disagreeable situation. In this case, are there things that you can do to change the situation or minimize your sister-in-law's impact on you?

KRISTI: Well, I could refuse to go to the family outings, but that would hurt my husband, and then I would have another stress on my hands. Unless I want to make a family stink, I guess I just have to put up with her.

ANOTHER GROUP MEMBER: I think what you just said is the part that's not true. You don't have to put up with that!

KRISTI: Well, I do if I want to keep peace in the family!

THERAPIST: It sounds like there are other automatic thoughts that come up when you think about your options for changing the situation with your sister-in-law. One theme behind those thoughts—"Unless I want to make a family stink, I just have to put up with her"— is that it makes you sound pretty helpless to change anything.

KRISTI: That's how I feel. I feel stuck in a bad situation.

THERAPIST: So in this case, your original thought—"She is disagreeable, and I don't want to be around her"—is true and might motivate you to change the situation. But then you have other thoughts that keep you stuck, like "I have to put up with it." Sounds like you need to list the other thoughts and examine them for their truthfulness. Would you be willing to do this as part of your homework during this week?

HOMEWORK REVIEW

As a homework check, you should once again obtain an example from clients regarding their work with the ATW-2, particularly the columns examining the evidence supporting and refuting the automatic thought. By way of example, I have included David's ATW-2 from his homework (see Figure Mod. 4.1). Later in this module, further work with this homework sheet in session is described.

SESSION OBJECTIVE: CHALLENGE NEGATIVE, DISTORTED AUTOMATIC THOUGHTS

Once a client's list of facts supporting and refuting the automatic thought is complete, he needs to be able to determine where the distortion is in the original automatic thought in order to construct an alternative, more realistic thought. At this point in the session, it helps to explain more about how thoughts can be distorted, and to provide examples.

> Now that you've been able to create a list of facts that support and don't support your original automatic thought, it's time to decide whether there is any negative distortion in the thought. There are lots of different ways an automatic thought can be distorted. The distortion may be in the "always" or "never" part of the thought—for instance, "I will *never* be able to play ball with my kids again." Or the distortion could be in the level of intensity attributed to the pain, or in the threat value of the pain—for example, "This pain is *intolerable*. I *cannot survive* this pain." Another example of a distortion can be in forecasting the outcome of an event before it has happened—for example, "Oh, oh, there's a twinge in my back. Today *is* going to be a bad day." Let's go back to our list of examples of

Date/time	Stressful situation	Emotional/ physical shift	Automatic thought or image (How much do you believe it? 0–100%)	Evidence that the thought is true	Evidence that the thought is not true	Re-rate belief (0–100%)
9/2/02, 9:00 A.M.	Spending more time standing at work than usual.	Back pain began increasing. Getting irritable.	The pain is just eating me up! (90%)	I'm on a lot of medicine. The medicine isn't working. I am missing a lot of work. I have had to be hospitalized five times. I've had to have three back surgeries. The MRI still shows problems with my discs.	I was able to stay at work on Thursday, and it wasn't unbearable. I did get up and go to work on Friday. I was able to use positive self-talk to get up and go to work, and to stay at work. I feel better being distracted at work than sitting around feeling useless at home.	

FIGURE MOD. 4.1. David's Session 3 homework Automatic Thoughts Worksheet–2 (ATW-2).

negative thinking from Session 2 and look them over again [provide copies of Client Handout 2.3, if necessary.] There are as many examples of types of distortions as categories of cognitive errors, and this list should give you a sense of the variety of distortions that can occur in an automatic thought. Does anybody have any other examples, now that they've seen this list again?

Another important point about distortions in thinking is that our negative, distorted automatic thoughts are often quite widespread and global. When I say to myself, "I just can't stand it," am I talking specifically about the pain sensation I feel at that moment, or am I creating a widespread and global thought about my pain condition and all of its associated stressors? By the way, it is natural and understandable to tend to have global, sweeping automatic thoughts during a pain flare-up or during times of associated stress. But when you learn how to identify globally distorted thoughts and make them more specific, this has the effect of decreasing the part of your life you feel you have no control over, and expanding the part you *can* take control over.

In order to help clients recognize where the distortion is in the automatic thought they are examining, direct them back to their homework with the ATW-2. Now that they have heard your "mini-lecture" about types of distortions, and having listed both the facts supporting *and those refuting* the thought, they should be able to specify where the distortion is. David, for example, was able to identify that his automatic thought "The pain is just eating me up!" was overgeneralized and exaggerated. Note also that the image his automatic thought offers is quite grim! Automatic thoughts can sometimes take the form of images, without even any well-formed associated cognitions, and still have a profound negative impact on the client.

SESSION OBJECTIVE: CONSTRUCT REALISTIC ALTERNATIVE RESPONSES

Once a client has learned to evaluate an automatic thought realistically (i.e., generated a list of facts supporting and refuting the automatic thought, and identified the source of the distortion), she should be ready to construct an alternative, more realistic thought.

WORKSHEET: AUTOMATIC THOUGHTS WORKSHEET–3 (ATW-3)

The Automatic Thoughts Worksheet–3 (ATW-3; see Client Handout 4.2) is used as a tool for helping the client construct an alternative thought as a rejoinder to the compelling, but negative and distorted, automatic thought. Have the group members pick one automatic thought from their ATW-2 homework sheet (one that has a strong emotional pull for them) and transfer it to the ATW-3. Next, walk them through the process of constructing an alternative thought. First, make sure that they have generated adequate lists of facts supporting and facts refuting the automatic thought on the ATW-2. If necessary, help the clients to expand on the list of facts refuting the distorted part of their original automatic thought. Once you feel that they have a sufficiently developed list of refuting facts, ask the clients whether there is an alternative response that might be worth adopting in place of the original automatic thought. You might wish to have clients ask themselves, "What would I tell a friend in a similar situation?", as suggested by Beck (1995). If the clients have sufficiently grasped (and worked with) the preceding two sessions' concepts, they should have little trouble constructing an alternative thought, and probably will begin to do so as they construct a list of facts refuting the automatic thought.

Once an alternative response has been constructed, it is important for the clients to assess whether this has resulted in a change in their thinking. One way to evaluate this is to have the clients ask themselves how much they *now* believe the original automatic thought. It is likely that the clients will still believe the original thought somewhat, but there should be a substantial decline in the percentage assigned to that belief.

Troubleshooting Tip: Following the construction of an alternative thought, if there is little change—that is, if a client still believes the thought to a high degree, or if there continues to be distortion in the alternative thought—more work needs to be done. It is possible that there are layers of negatively distorted automatic thoughts imbedded underneath the original thought, and/or that the client did not spend enough time constructing his list of facts supporting and refuting the automatic thought. Also, if the client continues to have difficulty generating an alternative response to the original automatic thought, it is possible that he is actually struggling with an intermediate or core belief, rather than an automatic thought. Underlying beliefs will sometimes be expressed as automatic thoughts. If this occurs early in the therapeutic process and you recognize the thought as a belief, go ahead and identify it for the client as an underlying belief that gives rise to automatic thoughts, and then help the client formulate an associated automatic thought. Remember that intermediate and core beliefs are more ingrained, and thus more difficult to challenge. Clients need success experiences with recognizing and challenging automatic thoughts before they tackle more deeply held beliefs, and you must therefore be able to redirect them to another automatic thought when necessary. We will discuss intermediate and core beliefs in the next two treatment modules. Meanwhile, let's go to David's ATW-3 (Figure Mod. 4.2) and see what happened when he constructed an alternative response.

After David generated his lists of "facts" supporting and refuting his automatic thought that the pain was "just eating me up," he initially decided that his alternative response was "The pain is chipping away at me." When I asked him how much he *now* believed the thought that the pain was "just eating me up," he replied that although he still believed it "this much," he had previously believed it "**THIS MUCH!!!**" He also acknowledged feeling that the thought had somewhat less of an emotional hold on him (from 90% to 60%).

Date/time	Stressful situation	Emotional/physical/other change	Automatic thought or image (How much do you believe it? 0–100%)	Alternative thought (Use questions below to review the evidence and compose alternative)	Results 1. How much do you *now* believe original thought? 2. Emotional/behavioral/physical response to alternative thought
9/2/02, 9:00 A.M.	Spending more time standing at work than usual.	Back pain began increasing. Getting irritable.	The pain is just eating me up! (90%)	The pain is chipping away at me.	1. 60%. 2. Less of an emotional hold on me, but still a hell of a way to live.

FIGURE MOD. 4.2. David's initial in-session Automatic Thoughts Worksheet–3 (ATW-3)

Note that although there was an appreciable change in the degree to which David believed the original thought, he still believed it to a pretty high degree. In addition, his alternative thought, "The pain is chipping away at me," is hardly what I would hope for in the kind of alternative response that would increase a client's sense of control over the painful situation. In David's case, he still believed the original automatic thought 60%, and his alternative thought still contained a distorted image, even though the pain was now chipping away instead of eating away at him. I made the decision to go back to his lists of facts supporting and refuting his original automatic thought, in order to determine whether embedded automatic thoughts were interfering with his ability to adopt a more realistic alternative thought. A brief session excerpt follows:

THERAPIST: David, let's take a closer look at your original thought and your alternative thought. Although you went from believing the original thought 90% to believing it 60%, that's still pretty significant. It still has an impact on you. And if you look at your alternative thought, it's similar in theme, although not identical.

DAVID: It's a better thought, I guess, but still a hell of a way to have to live.

THERAPIST: Let's take a look at the alternative thought you came up with, which is "The pain is chipping away at me." Would you go back to your list of facts supporting your original thought and take a minute to read them over to us?

DAVID: Okay, then: "I'm on a lot of medicine."—You know I am; you even said so yourself. "The medicine isn't working."—You got me to admit that the first time I came in here! "I am missing a lot of work."—I'm lucky I haven't lost my job already! Then there's all of this physical evidence: "I've had three surgeries, five hospitalizations, and even so, the MRI shows I have continuing damage to my discs!" These are all facts![1]

THERAPIST: I agree, David. These are all facts, and as facts, they lent support to your original thought that the pain was eating you alive. *But* you were also able to identify some facts that did not support that automatic thought, and in doing so, you were able to believe that thought less—it has less of an emotional hold on you. I'm wondering about something, though. Let's go back again to your list of facts supporting your original thought. Does anything on that list also support your alternative thought, "The pain is chipping away at me"?

DAVID: Well, yeah, especially the MRI. If the MRI shows that new damage is occurring, even

---

[1]*Troubleshooting Tip:* Note that this single response offered a great deal of grist for the therapeutic mill. First, I noticed that David was showing some irritation or even anger at me: "You got me to admit that . . . " Second, there were apparently some unspoken automatic thoughts behind the comment "I am lucky I haven't lost my job already!" You may have already noticed that on his ATW-2, David's list of four facts refuting his original automatic thought all had an association with going to work or staying at work, supporting the hypothesis that work-related thoughts would be important to explore more fully at some point. Third, David asserted that the MRI shows "continuing damage" to his discs, implying that he perceived an ongoing deterioration of his spine. This assumption of degenerating damage might be directly related to David's alternative response that "The pain is chipping away at me." One challenging aspect of therapy is to recognize that there are multiple possible intervention choice points as they are occurring within each session, and to select the option that may provide the most gain. A cognitive therapist does not ignore the importance of interpersonal process, and acknowledging, honoring, and working with a client's irritation or anger can be an appropriate intervention within cognitive therapy, especially when it is well timed. In this case, I made a mental (and, later, written) note to be on the lookout for continuing issues of irritation or anger directed toward me, and also to pursue a more in-depth exploration of automatic thoughts related to potential job loss. At this juncture, though, I chose to pursue thoughts that might be directly tied to David's new, but not greatly improved, alternative thought: "The pain is chipping away at me."

though I've had three surgeries to correct the old damage, it seems like a losing battle to me.[2]

THERAPIST: You know, MRIs, CAT scans, and X-rays are great technologies for helping physicians see what's going on inside the body. The problem is that they don't tell us much about who will or will not experience continuing pain. To give you an example, there was a really important research study comparing the MRIs of patients *with* back pain to the MRIs of people *without* back pain. It turns out that very few of the people *without* any back pain complaints had "clean" MRIs. The majority of the people, even if they did not have any back pain, showed abnormalities on their MRIs [M. C. Jensen et al., 1994]. So, while this kind of physical evidence may be of some use, it doesn't tell us who are going to be troubled by their backs and who are not.

DAVID: So why the hell does everybody rely on them so much?

THERAPIST: Well, it's the best tool there is for now, and it can tell physicians about certain conditions that require immediate correction because the spinal nerves themselves are being damaged. But it's not a good tool for predicting who has pain, or how much pain you'll have. Let's experiment here with listing another automatic thought down on your worksheet—one that holds importance for the way you think about your pain. How about listing "My MRI shows continuing damage to my spine" under the "Automatic thought or image" column?

DAVID: All right, then. Actually, now that we're talking about it, my thought has been "The MRI shows my spine disintegrating." I realize that may be an overstatement of the situation.

THERAPIST: How would you feel about listing this as a fact *not* supporting that thought: "MRIs do not tell us how much pain someone will have"?

DAVID: It kind of takes some of the importance away from the MRI.

ANOTHER GROUP MEMBER: How about "The MRI is not a crystal ball"? (*David laughs.*)

THERAPIST: That's a good one, Pat, and it captures the spirit of what we're talking about here. MRI results tell us some things, but they don't tell us how much pain someone is going to have, or whether they'll be incapacitated by discomfort, and they don't give us a "death sentence" about the future. Okay, David, if we now know that the MRI results aren't as crucial in determining the future of your condition, what does that do to your automatic thought that "The pain is chipping away at me"?

DAVID: Well, come to think of it, that MRI stuff has always raised a picture in my mind of my spine just grinding down, further and further—like my spine was chipping away, bit by bit, and there was nothing that could be done. That's how I saw that MRI!

THERAPIST: Does thinking about the MRI differently now have any effect on your thoughts?

DAVID: Yeah, it has less power over me. Like the MRI isn't that important—it doesn't mean that much.

THERAPIST: That's good to hear, and now I understand much better where your thoughts

---

[2]***Troubleshooting Tip:*** Note that this thought could be characterized as an automatic thought or as a belief. I decided to go ahead and treat it as an automatic thought for the moment, to see whether I could make any headway on helping David move toward a more adaptive alternative thought.

were coming from. Can you think of another alternative thought based on what we've just talked about?

DAVID: How about "The MRI doesn't control how much pain I feel"? If that's true, then maybe there is more that I can do about my situation.

THERAPIST: I really believe that's true, David. And I think you are really getting the idea of just how powerful our thoughts or images can be. Our own thoughts can do us powerful damage, or they can do us powerful good. Would you be willing to work with these thoughts and images some more during the next week?

DAVID: Yeah, definitely. I can see there's more to be done with this list.

Figure Mod. 4.3 illustrates David's ATW-3 after his work on it in session.

As a result of believing the original automatic thought *less* (and perhaps believing the alternative response *more*), the client should experience a change in his emotions, sense of physical well-being, and subsequent thought processes. This change is the second part of the "Results" in the last column of the ATW-3. Once the client has constructed an alternative thought and rated how much he now believes the original automatic thought, the therapist should ask him to list any effects the new thought has on his emotions, other thoughts, and physical well-being. In David's case, he reported feeling more hopeful, thinking maybe he had more control than he thought, and physically feeling himself "sitting up a little taller."

Date/time	Stressful situation	Emotional/ physical/other change	Automatic thought or image (How much do you believe it? 0–100%)	Alternative thought (Use questions below to review the evidence and compose alternative)	Results 1. How much do you *now* believe original thought? 2. Emotional/behavioral/ physical response to alternative thought
9/2/02, 9:00 A.M.	Spending more time standing at work than usual.	Back pain began increasing. Getting irritable.	Original: The pain is just eating me up! (90%)	The pain is chipping away at me.	1. 60% 2. Less of an emotional hold on me, but still a hell of a way to live.
			Second: The pain is chipping away at me. (100%) Third: The MRI shows my spine disintegrating. (80%)	The MRI doesn't control the amount of pain I will have. (The MRI is not a crystal ball!)	1. Original thought: 20%. Second thought: 35%. Third thought: 5% (almost completely gone!). 2. Emotion: Less hopeless. Thought: Maybe there's more I can do for myself. Physical: Sitting up straighter.

FIGURE MOD. 4.3. David's revised in-session Automatic Thoughts Worksheet–3 (ATW-3).

HOMEWORK ASSIGNMENT

For homework, instruct group members to continue working with the ATW-3. They should continue working on the "unfinished" automatic thoughts they began working on in session, and they should construct, and work on, new automatic thoughts as they arise during the week. Remind clients that although they will continue to identify automatic thoughts by noticing shifts in emotions or shifts in their physical state, they now also evaluate, challenge, and reconstruct the original automatic thoughts into more realistic alternatives.

POSTSESSION PROCESS CHECK

Hand out the Postsession Process Check, and ask clients to fill it out before they leave.

Session 4 Outline for Therapists: Challenging Automatic Thoughts and Constructing Alternative Responses

SESSION OBJECTIVES

- Challenge negative, distorted automatic thoughts.
- Construct realistic alternative responses.

NEEDED MATERIALS, HANDOUTS, AND WORKSHEETS

- Session 4 Outline for Therapists (this handout)
- Session 4 Summary for Clients (Client Handout 4.1)
- Presession Process Check (Appendix J)
- Extra copies of Examples of Negative, Distorted Thinking (Client Handout 2.3)
- Automatic Thoughts Worksheet–3 (ATW-3) (Client Handout 4.2)
- Postsession Process Check (Appendix J)

PRESESSION PROCESS CHECK

- Hand out Presession Process Check and have clients fill it in.

REVIEW OF PREVIOUS WEEK'S SESSION

- *Some* thoughts in response to pain or stress are exactly factual.
- *Most* thoughts in response to pain or stress are at least partly factual.
- *Often*, however, thoughts in response to pain or stress are somewhat distorted.
- Negative, distorted thoughts have the most (negative) influence on our emotions, behavior, and physical functioning.

HOMEWORK REVIEW

- Ask several clients: "Pick one automatic thought from your Automatic Thoughts Worksheet–2 (ATW-2), and share what you wrote with the group."
- "Were you able to generate a list of facts supporting the automatic thought and a list of facts not supporting the automatic thought?"
- "After generating the lists of facts, how much did you believe the automatic thought?"

SESSION OBJECTIVE:
CHALLENGE NEGATIVE, DISTORTED AUTOMATIC THOUGHTS

- To challenge a negative, distorted automatic thought, the way to start is by identifying the source of the distortion.

(continued)

From *Cognitive Therapy for Chronic Pain* by Beverly E. Thorn. Copyright 2004 by The Guilford Press. Permission to photocopy this handout is granted to purchasers of this book for personal use only (see copyright page for details).

- Have clients go back to the list of examples of negative, distorted thoughts from Session 2 (Client Handout 2.3), and see whether any of these categories are characteristic of your negative automatic thoughts."
  - Tell clients: "Notice whether your negative automatic thought is very specific or very global (we tend to have sweeping, generalized, automatic thoughts when in pain or stress)."
  - "Evaluating the source of the distortion in your automatic thought can help you to formulate alternative, more realistic thoughts."
  - "Believing *less* in the original automatic thought has a positive influence on your ability to cope with pain."

SESSION OBJECTIVE: CONSTRUCT REALISTIC ALTERNATIVE THOUGHTS

- Say to clients: "First, look back at your responses on the ATW-2 and pick an automatic thought that was important to you."
- "Did you generate a list of facts supporting the automatic thought and a list refuting the automatic thought?"

WORKSHEET: AUTOMATIC THOUGHTS WORKSHEET–3 (ATW-3)

- Give out copies of the Automatic Thoughts Worksheet–3 (ATW-3).
- Tell clients: "Transfer your ATW-2 thought to the ATW-3."
- "Is there an alternative, more realistic thought that you could use to replace the original automatic thought?"
- "It may help to ask yourself this: If one of your friends had a similar automatic thought, or was in a similar situation, what would you tell your friend?"
- "On a scale of 0–100%, how much do you now believe the original automatic thought?"
- "Believing the original automatic thought *less*, and believing the alternative thought *more*, has a positive influence on your ability to cope with pain."

HOMEWORK ASSIGNMENT

- Tell clients: "Using the ATW–3, complete any unfinished work with the automatic thought you began working on during this week's session."
- "During the week, note any important new automatic thoughts that you become aware of, and rate how strongly you believe those automatic thoughts. Try to do this each day."
- "Evaluate each automatic thought, using facts supporting and facts refuting the thought."
- "Use the questions at the bottom of the worksheet to help you construct an alternative thought, and write it down."
- "Re-rate how much you believe the original automatic thought."
- "What is the result of constructing the alternative thought? That is, what is the influence on your thoughts, feelings, and physical well-being?"
- "Bring your homework to the next session, and be ready to discuss what you have learned with other group members."

POSTSESSION PROCESS CHECK

- Have clients fill out Postsession Process Check before they leave. Glance at responses and troubleshoot if necessary.

Session 4 Summary for Clients: Challenging Automatic Thoughts and Constructing Alternative Responses

THE GOALS OF THIS SESSION

- To challenge negative, distorted automatic thoughts.
- To construct realistic alternative responses.

REVIEW OF PREVIOUS WEEK'S SESSION

- *Some* thoughts in response to pain or stress are exactly factual.
- *Most* thoughts in response to pain or stress are at least partly factual.
- *Often*, however, thoughts in response to pain or stress are somewhat distorted.
- Negative, distorted thoughts have the most (negative) influence on your emotions, behavior, and physical functioning.

HOMEWORK REVIEW

- Pick one automatic thought from your Automatic Thoughts Worksheet (ATW-2), and share what you wrote with the group.
- Were you able to generate a list of facts supporting the automatic thought and a list of facts not supporting the automatic thought?
- After generating the lists of facts, how much did you believe the automatic thought?

CHALLENGING NEGATIVE, DISTORTED AUTOMATIC THOUGHTS

- To challenge a negative automatic thought, start by identifying the part that is distorted. (It helps to go back to the list of examples of negative thoughts—Client Handout 2.3.)
- Notice whether your negative automatic thought is very specific or very global (we tend to have sweeping, generalized, automatic thoughts when in pain or stress).
- Evaluating the part that is distorted in your automatic thought can help you to formulate alternative, more realistic thoughts.
- Believing *less* in the original automatic thought has a positive influence on your ability to cope with pain.

CONSTRUCTING REALISTIC ALTERNATIVE RESPONSES

- First, look back at your responses on the ATW-2 and pick an automatic thought that was important to you.
- Did you generate a list of facts supporting the automatic thought and a list refuting the automatic thought?

(continued)

From *Cognitive Therapy for Chronic Pain* by Beverly E. Thorn. Copyright 2004 by The Guilford Press. Permission to photocopy this handout is granted to purchasers of this book for personal use only (see copyright page for details).

- Transfer your ATW-2 thought to the Automatic Thoughts Worksheet–3 (ATW-3).
- Is there an alternative, more realistic thought that you could use to replace the original automatic thought?
- It may help to ask yourself this: If one of your friends had a similar automatic thought, or was in a similar situation, what would you tell your friend?
- On a scale of 0–100%, how much do you now believe the original automatic thought?
- Believing the original automatic thought *less*, and believing the alternative thought *more*, has a positive influence on your ability to cope with pain.

SUMMARY OF KEY POINTS

- Although almost all thoughts are partly true, they often contain some negative distortion.
- Identifying facts supporting and refuting the original automatic thought can help clarify the thought.
- Identifying the distorted part of the thought can help you create a more realistic alternative response.
- Creating a more realistic alternative response should help you believe the original thought less, and the alternative thought more.
- Creating a realistic alternative response from a negatively distorted thought should have a positive impact on your thoughts, your emotions, and your behavior.

HOMEWORK ASSIGNMENT

- Using the ATW-3, complete any unfinished work with the automatic thought you began working on during this week's session.
- During the week, note any important new automatic thoughts that you become aware of, and rate how strongly you believe those automatic thoughts. Try to do this each day.
- Evaluate each automatic thought, using facts supporting and facts refuting the thought.
- Use the questions at the bottom of the worksheet to help you construct an alternative thought, and write it down.
- Re-rate how much you believe the original automatic thought
- What is the result of constructing the alternative thought? That is, what is the influence on your thoughts, feelings, and physical well-being?
- Bring your homework to the next session, and be ready to discuss what you have learned with other group members.

CLIENT HANDOUT 4.2

Automatic Thoughts Worksheet–3 (ATW-3)

Date/time	Stressful situation	Emotional/physical other change	Automatic thought or image (How much do you believe it? 0–100%)	Alternative thought (Use questions below* to review the evidence and compose alternative)	Results 1. How much do you *now* believe original thought? 2. Emotional/behavioral/physical response to alternative thought

*Questions from ATW-2: What is the evidence that the thought is true? What is the evidence that the thought is *not* true?

From *Cognitive Therapy for Chronic Pain* by Beverly E. Thorn. Copyright 2004 by The Guilford Press. Permission to photocopy this handout is granted to purchasers of this book for personal use only (see copyright page for details).

INTERMEDIATE AND CORE BELIEFS (GENERAL)

The fifth treatment session introduces the concept of intermediate and core beliefs. Therapist Handout 5.1, found at the back of this module, provides an outline of Session 5 to be used by the therapist. Client Handout 5.1, also at the back of the module, can be copied and used as a session outline to be given to clients at the beginning of the session.

- Identify general underlying belief systems.
- Challenge negative, distorted beliefs and construct new beliefs.

PRESESSION PROCESS CHECK AND REVIEW OF PREVIOUS WEEK'S SESSION

After having clients fill out the Presession Process Check, as always, review the previous week's session. For Session 4, the treatment goals were to challenge negative, distorted automatic thoughts and to construct alternative, adaptive, and more realistic responses to the original automatic thoughts. The Automatic Thoughts Worksheet–3 (ATW-3) was used to guide clients in constructing alternative responses, and to examine the "results" of the alternative responses on their emotions, their sense of physical well-being, and their subsequent thoughts. Clients were also asked to re-rate the amount they believed in each original automatic thought after constructing the alternative response.

Remind group members that making sure to list all the facts supporting and refuting an automatic thought helps them to identify the distortion in the thought and makes challenging the thought easier. It also may help to ask, "What would I tell a friend in this situation?" when constructing an alternative thought.

HOMEWORK REVIEW

As a homework check, you should once again obtain an example from group members regarding their work with the ATW-3, focusing particularly on the column with the alternative response and the "Results" column. Ideally, clients will have followed up with work begun in the previous session and progressed further with challenging new automatic thoughts and creating alternative responses. Obviously, though, this is the time to deal with areas where group members are stuck, as well as to deal with success experiences.

During our homework check for this session, Jennifer came in with the following:

JENNIFER: The other day a coworker walked up to me, right as I was waiting on another customer, and I actually set limits! I actually turned her away! I was polite, but I said, "I am in the middle of doing this, and I can't do two things at once. You'll have to go ask the supervisor." It felt great to do that! But I noticed my hands were shaking after she left.

THERAPIST: Did you actually have an automatic thought that you were able to challenge and reconstruct into an alternative thought in this situation?

JENNIFER: Yes, well, it all happened so fast that it almost seemed like my alternative response was pretty automatic, too! I went back later and thought about it, and put it down on my sheet—sort of reconstructed it. It was like this: BAM, she came up to me; BAM, I had my initial knee-jerk reaction of telling myself I had to stop what I was doing; and BAM, I had my alternative response. I can't say that I deliberately went through all the steps until later.

THERAPIST: I think that the fact that you've been practicing this technique paid off big-time for you. Once you get good at a new skill, you don't have to be quite so deliberate in all the steps. But, Jennifer, I *am* glad you went back and retraced your steps to see what happened in your thinking process.

ANOTHER CLIENT: It's like we're retraining our minds to stop the knee-jerk reactions as they're happening, and substitute a better thought. I've recognized that, too. It happens fast!

THERAPIST: I'm glad others are finding this to be the case, too. If this method is still a step-by-step process for some of you, that's okay, too. The more you practice it, the better you'll get at it, and the less effort it will take. So, Jennifer, was it worth it to examine and challenge those automatic thoughts you'd been having?

JENNIFER: Oh, yes! Even though my hands were shaking, I wasn't the kind of tense I've been before. And I wasn't mad! And amazingly, I didn't get a headache that day!

The part of Jennifer's homework (ATW-3) related to the situation described above is included in Figure Mod. 5.1.

By this point in treatment, clients should recognize the connection among challenging a negatively distorted automatic thought, constructing an alternative response, and ultimately reducing the amount they believe the original automatic thought. We also want them to understand that believing the original thought less, and the alternative thought more, influences their emotions, their subsequent thoughts, and even their sense of physical well-being. When a client begins to realize that her thoughts can actually have an impact on how her body feels, and that she has some control over her thoughts, she is at a turning point in cognitive therapy:

Date/time	Stressful situation	Emotional/ physical/other change	Automatic thought or image (How much do you believe it? 0–100%)	Alternative thought (Use questions below to review the evidence and compose alternative)	Results 1. How much do you *now* believe original thought? 2. Emotional/ behavioral/physical response to alternative thought
10/20/02, 11:00 A.M.	Coworker <u>tried</u> to interrupt me.		I have to stop what I'm doing and see what she wants. (Immediate: 70%)	I should <u>not</u> stop what I'm doing! I can <u>and will</u> set limits with her.	1. 0%!! 2. I set limits with her. My hands were shaking. I still felt <u>great!</u> I didn't get a headache that day!

FIGURE MOD. 5.1. Jennifer's Session 4 homework Automatic Thoughts Worksheet–3 (ATW-3).

She now has an internal tool for exerting control over her physical well-being. This tool is not dependent on drugs, and not dependent on physicians or other health care professionals. The power, and the responsibility, lie within her.

SESSION OBJECTIVE: IDENTIFY GENERAL UNDERLYING BELIEF SYSTEMS

One of the treatment goals for session 5 is to learn to identify underlying belief systems. Recall from Chapter 2 that core beliefs and intermediate beliefs are less situation-specific than automatic thoughts, and that these underlying belief systems are said to provide the thematic content of automatic thoughts. Intermediate beliefs are generally held attitudes, assumptions, and rules (Beck, 1995), and they are assumed to stem from core beliefs. Intermediate beliefs often express themselves in terms of a "should," a "must," or an "ought to." Core beliefs (sometimes referred to as "cognitive schemas") are considered to reflect one's most central beliefs about the self and the world. People hold both realistic and distorted intermediate and core beliefs, so we certainly aren't out to change them all—only the negatively distorted ones. It's important to emphasize that negative beliefs are not everyday thoughts; when things are going well, people tend to have positive belief systems. However, environmental stressors are likely triggers for negatively distorted beliefs. Certainly, the stress associated with a chronic pain disorder is sufficient to activate negative belief systems.

In addition to having general underlying belief systems, patients with pain hold entire sets of underlying beliefs, attitudes, and assumptions that are specific to their pain condition. It is also crucial to help the clients consider and change these pain-specific belief systems, if they are negatively distorted. Pain-specific belief systems will be tackled in the next treatment session (Treatment Module 6). The aim in the present session is to help the clients identify more general beliefs because they are relevant, and because understanding the general concept of belief systems helps them more easily understand pain-related beliefs.

Troubleshooting Tip: Be forewarned that identifying underlying beliefs, particularly negative core beliefs, tends to be more distressing for clients than identifying automatic thoughts. This makes sense when one considers that underlying beliefs are not specific to particular situations, and that they tend to be more firmly held than automatic thoughts. Nonetheless, I have encountered groups where one or more clients insist that they do not hold negative beliefs about themselves, and they can't quite understand others' doing so. In cases like this, I assure clients that we are not assuming that they all go around "branded" by fixed, negative core beliefs that guide their every move. However, especially during stressful and unpleasant times, it is quite natural and normal to have negative belief systems triggered. These beliefs then provide a theme for negative automatic thoughts, guiding which, if any, coping responses are attempted.

In preparation for introducing the concept of intermediate and core beliefs, it is useful to go back through the clients' homework records from previous sessions. Ideally, you will be making notes along the course of treatment that will help you generate hypotheses about clients' intermediate and core beliefs in preparation for this session. Often clients give clues about their distorted beliefs with the language they use, or the images that come to mind when they are describing their automatic thoughts. (I illustrate this later in the session, where I use an example from Jennifer's previous work on automatic thoughts.) Another way to identify clients' distorted underlying belief systems is to look for common themes across automatic thoughts.

Troubleshooting Tip: As I have mentioned earlier, a client sometimes mistakes an underlying belief for an automatic thought and brings it into an earlier session, when he is not yet ready to work on underlying beliefs. If so, inform the client that what he has proposed as an automatic thought is probably a more deeply held belief (which will be examined in a later session), and help the client come up with an associated automatic thought that he can work on for the moment. Then file the client's underlying belief away in your notes so that you can bring it up and work on it in the appropriate session.

In basic cognitive therapy texts (e.g., Beck, 1995), it has been suggested that negatively distorted core beliefs tend to take on themes of either helplessness or unlovability, and that it helps to determine whether core beliefs are on the helplessness side or on the unlovability side. Core beliefs associated with these two themes are listed in Figure Mod. 5.2.

> We've spent the last three sessions learning about how to recognize and change automatic thoughts. You've probably noticed that some of your automatic thoughts have common "themes" to them. For example, the subject matter of your automatic thoughts might include some notion of not being in control of certain aspects of your life. Some automatic thoughts are "frequent flyers"; that is, the same automatic thoughts seem to keep coming up in response to similar situations. We call these kinds of automatic thoughts

Helplessness:

- Can't do, can't cope, ineffective
- Needy, weak, need protection
- Inferior in comparison to others (don't achieve as well, not as effective, etc.)

Unlovability:

- Rejected, abandoned
- Different, defective, not good enough to be loved
- Bad, worthless, toxic, evil

FIGURE MOD. 5.2. Core beliefs associated with the themes of helplessness and unlovability.

"*key* automatic thoughts," and they stem from underlying belief systems. Everyone has belief systems—they are the way we make sense of the world. Belief systems can be divided into two types: "intermediate beliefs" and "core beliefs." Intermediate beliefs are the "rules" we hold for ourselves and for others. When we tell ourselves that something *should* be a certain way, or that we *must* do such-and-such, those are intermediate beliefs. Core beliefs are the very deeply held notions we have about ourselves and about the world around us. Core beliefs are our basic notions about the general goodness (or badness) of people, and about our own self-worth and capability. When things are going fine in our lives, we usually operate under positive belief systems about ourselves and the world around us. But in times of stress, belief systems are more likely to become distorted in the negative direction. Negative core beliefs often have themes of helplessness ("I'm weak, needy, ineffective, inferior to others") or unlovability ("I'm defective, unworthy, worthless, bad, toxic, or evil"). It's important to examine our own belief systems, because they can be negatively distorted just they way automatic thoughts can be negatively distorted. Belief systems are trickier to change than automatic thoughts, because they are more general and deeply held. That's why it's so important that you've had success with recognizing and changing automatic thoughts before we tackle underlying beliefs. In this session, we'll learn how to recognize and challenge negatively distorted intermediate and core beliefs.

Discussion of Clients' DAS-24 Responses

In order to help clients understand the idea of underlying beliefs, it is useful to go over their responses to the Dysfunctional Attitude Scale–24 (DAS-24), one of the assessment questionnaires that clients filled out prior to the beginning of the group sessions. Recall that the DAS-24 is a questionnaire aimed at measuring people's general attitudes and beliefs, particularly *negative* attitudes and beliefs (see Chapter 4). You should hand out the clients' original DAS-24 responses to them, so that they can see what kinds of responses they made to these items. Again, these items assess general negative attitudes and beliefs. The higher the "score" on the item, the more negative a belief the client holds. In addition, since there are three scales on the DAS-24 (Dependency, Achievement, and Self-Control), clients can also see whether their belief systems tend toward one theme or another. It is fine to give clients the scoring key, so that they can tally up the relative weight they are giving to the various themes (although I do not give them the comparative mean scores that I have provided in Appendix C for this measure, along with the scoring key). However, don't encourage clients to get too caught up in their scores on these measures. The point is to use their responses to stimulate their thinking, get the point across, and generate discussion.

Troubleshooting Tip: At times, clients will want to point out and discuss particular items on the DAS-24 that they found confusing or objectionable. I assure clients that not every item on all of the questionnaires they were asked to fill out will be relevant to them in particular. I explain to the clients that the items on the questionnaires are written in such a way as to tap a wide array of individual differences, and therefore there has to be a wide variety of questions. If a question is not relevant to them, they can always skip it. Also, at times clients will want to justify why they believe so strongly in a particular item that is being labeled a "dysfunctional attitude." Rather than get into a struggle with the clients by trying to convince them that holding general, negative, distorted attitudes is "dysfunctional," I simply state that the exercise is meant to provide examples and food for thought, rather than to challenge clients on general beliefs they might hold.

WORKSHEET: IDENTIFYING BELIEFS WORKSHEET

As its name indicates, the Identifying Beliefs Worksheet (Client Handout 5.2) is used to help clients identify their underlying beliefs. There are a number of ways to help clients get at their core and intermediate beliefs. One helpful method, detailed by Burns (1980), is called the "downward-arrow" technique. First, have clients identify a problem situation, and then help them identify a key automatic thought. Again, key automatic thoughts are ones that seem to come up again and again. Once a key automatic thought is identified, help the clients try to get at the meaning behind the automatic thought. To get at intermediate beliefs, you can ask, "If that automatic thought were true, what does it mean to you?" The meaning behind the automatic thought is considered to be the intermediate belief. After identifying an intermediate belief, then ask, "If that automatic thought were true, what does it mean *about* you?" The meaning about the self, based on the automatic thought, is considered the core belief. In the abstract, these concepts are pretty meaningless, so working through an example is always essential.

To pick up on one of Jennifer's automatic thoughts from Treatment Session 3 ("I'm not in control of my own time at work"), recall that she described a situation of coworkers' looking to her for guidance. In describing the situation, Jennifer said, "Why do they ask me? They know as much as I do! But it never fails—they turn to me and begin calling to me, like a flock of sheep looking for a leader. I feel the muscles in my neck tensing up, and my hands tighten, and I can just feel the headache starting." An important statement made by Jennifer at the time was "I just hate to turn people down. It makes me feel guilty." Jennifer's comment that she felt guilty when she turned people down suggested to me that a dysfunctional belief might be the basis for her automatic thought in that situation. Also, her visual image of a flock of sheep looking for a leader gave me an idea for helping her get at the deeper belief system underlying the automatic thought. Although I would not have brought this material into the earlier session, where Jennifer was just learning to identify automatic thoughts, I did choose to bring this information back into this later session as a means of helping the group understand the concept of underlying beliefs. (See the session transcript below.)

THERAPIST: To illustrate how we go about identifying the belief systems underlying certain automatic thoughts, I wonder if we could go back to your example at the office, Jennifer. Do you remember the one I mean, where your automatic thought was "I'm not in control of my own time at work"?

JENNIFER: Yes, I certainly do. I've been working on variations of that ever since!

THERAPIST: Well, some automatic thoughts seem to crop up again and again, almost like "frequent flyers." These can be useful ones to examine to see if underlying belief systems are triggering those thoughts. Shall we give it a try?

JENNIFER: Yes, *please!* I'd like to figure this one out.

THERAPIST: Okay. First, let's begin with the question, what does it mean to have the thought "I'm not in control of my own time at work"?

JENNIFER: It means that I get mad! It's like an emotional trigger for me that also makes me tense up like crazy, and before I know it, I have a killer headache.

THERAPIST: Those were the exact reactions you described before, and it sounds like you are continuing to have them to some extent with other related automatic thoughts. Let's try this: If the thought "I'm not in control of my own time at work" is true, what does that thought mean to you?

JENNIFER: Mad and tense, mad and tense. I just can't get beyond that!

THERAPIST: Let's dig a little deeper. Another clue to our automatic thoughts and belief systems is the mental picture that a situation creates. Can you remember the mental picture you described when you were telling us about your coworkers hassling you?

JENNIFER: Uh, no, not really. I don't think I had a mental picture. I'm not sure what you mean.

THERAPIST: (*to other group members*) Can anyone help Jennifer out? When she was first describing the situation with her coworkers, does anyone remember the very vivid image she described for us?

TWO GROUP MEMBERS: (*in unison*) Sheep!

THERAPIST: Yes! Excellent! Jennifer, you described a flock of sheep searching for a leader. I had a vivid image of little lambs surrounding you and bleating at you all at once! (*Group members laugh, as does Jennifer.*)

JENNIFER: But I don't want to be their leader. I've got my own stuff to do. But I feel like I just *can't* turn anyone away!

THERAPIST: "I just can't turn anyone away." (*pause*) Is that what the thought "I'm not in control of my own time" means to you?

JENNIFER: Oh, yes. It's like I just throw a mental switch, and if anyone asks, I have to drop everything and help—even if it messes me up!

THERAPIST: Do you suppose that could be an underlying belief that makes the automatic thought so emotionally meaningful to you?

JENNIFER: Oh, of course, I'm sure it is! I tell myself that these people need me—that they can't get along without me—when in reality, if I'm not there, I suppose they muddle through somehow. (*Everyone laughs.*)

ANOTHER GROUP MEMBER: Oh, I feel that way too—about my family. The problem is . . . I've become their doormat! It's not a great way to live, Jennifer. You should change that particular belief.

THERAPIST: So this belief may be relevant to some folks in addition to Jennifer, which makes her work on this even more important. Jennifer, when you were first telling us about that situation, you said, "I just hate to turn people down. It makes me feel guilty." On a scale of 0–100%, how much would you say you believe the, quote, "rule" that "I just can't turn anyone away"?

JENNIFER: Oh, probably at least 80%. If they ask, I should help them, particularly if I know more than they do or if I'm better off than they are.

THERAPIST: Do you see how that is a rule you've constructed for yourself, which may or may not be true?

JENNIFER: Yes, and it most likely comes from my family background. We were always taught that if we *could* help, we *should* help.

THERAPIST: Although that might be an unselfish and charitable standard to live by, can you see how it could get you into hot water at times? Are there times when it is inappropriate to help?

ANOTHER GROUP MEMBER: Jennifer talks about being really mad a lot. No wonder she's mad if her family taught her that she always has to drop everything to help someone else out.

A DIFFERENT GROUP MEMBER: But she's holding onto that rule just like I do, and now instead of my family telling me it's my duty, I tell myself it's my duty!

JENNIFER: And when I put other's needs above my own, and it results in such a headache that I have to go ahead and leave work, that's certainly a sign that I'm doing something wrong. That seems pretty dumb, come to think of it.

ANOTHER GROUP MEMBER: Hey, you turned one of your coworkers away last week, and that made you feel pretty good!

JENNIFER: That was one time out of about a thousand! I still feel dumb.

THERAPIST: There's no need to feel dumb here. These are common traps many of us fall into. Just look around the room and see how many of your fellow group members are nodding their heads! What makes you all different from other people is that you are beginning to learn connections between your thoughts, your feelings, and your physical well-being that you have never made before. And, more importantly, you are starting to learn how to question distorted or unrealistic thoughts and construct more realistic and useful thoughts. With underlying beliefs, we can learn to do the same thing. Let me summarize so far: You had the thought "I'm not in control of my own time" in response to the work situation where coworkers are interrupting you and asking for help at an inconvenient time. I asked you what that thought meant to you, and you responded with "I just can't turn anyone away." That's an underlying rule you have for yourself, apparently. That rule puts you in a bind when saying "yes" to others means that you are not taking care of yourself. Now there's one more question I want you to consider: If the thought "I'm not in control of my own time" is true, what does the thought mean *about* you? This is different from the question of what the thought means *to* you.

JENNIFER: It means I'm not in control of my own time. Other people are, so I might as well just give up!

THERAPIST: Hang on. If it's true that you're not in control of your own time—that you should always put others' needs ahead of your own and never turn anyone away—what does it mean *about* you as a person?

ANOTHER GROUP MEMBER: It means that her needs aren't worth very much. I mean, I don't believe that about you, Jennifer, but I think you do.

JENNIFER: Well, yes! I do believe that my needs aren't worth very much—that I'm not worth much!

THERAPIST: And how much do you believe that on a scale of 0–100%?

JENNIFER: Oh, it varies, depending on what's going on. But when I'm feeling depressed, or when the pain is particularly bad and wearing, I feel that between 90% and 100%.

ANOTHER GROUP MEMBER: But you shouldn't believe that about yourself, Jennifer. It's just not true!

THERAPIST: These beliefs we call "core beliefs" are really tricky, because they *feel* more true to us than automatic thoughts or intermediate beliefs. They are harder to challenge, but it's quite possible to challenge them, especially after you've had success with challenging automatic thoughts. For the moment, Jennifer, would you be willing to consider that this belief you sometimes have so strongly about yourself is not a fact, but an idea—and that as an idea, it can be tested, just like the way we did it with automatic thoughts?

JENNIFER: (*warily*) I suppose, but this seems like a biggy—a tough one to challenge.

THERAPIST: Which is exactly why we want to help you work on what we call "core beliefs"— those deeply held belief systems that help shape our automatic thoughts, particularly the negative ones. So, for now, let's put down on your paper your automatic thought "I'm not in control of my own time at work." You said that the thought means "If I can help, I should help," which is your intermediate belief. And finally, you said that what this means about you is, quote, "I'm not worth much," which is your core belief.

Jennifer's Identifying Beliefs Worksheet from the exercise above is provided in Figure Mod. 5.3.

SESSION OBJECTIVE:
CHALLENGE NEGATIVE, DISTORTED BELIEFS AND CONSTRUCT NEW BELIEFS

In order to help clients challenge distorted belief systems, we use a similar process to the one used for challenging automatic thoughts; that is, we get them to list the facts supporting and refuting each underlying belief. For beliefs, we also ask the clients to consider any potential advantages or disadvantages there might be for holding onto a particular belief. Clients can often readily pick up on the disadvantages to holding onto a belief, but have more difficulty understanding that there are sometimes advantages to holding onto dysfunctional beliefs.

Situation: Coworkers keep interrupting me.

Automatic Thought: I'm not in control of my own time at work.

Intermediate Belief: If I can help, I should help.

Core Belief: I'm not worth much,

FIGURE MOD. 5.3. Jennifer's in-session Identifying Beliefs Worksheet.

WORKSHEET: CHANGING BELIEFS WORKSHEET

The Changing Beliefs Worksheet (Client Handout 5.3), which is similar to the Automatic Thoughts Worksheets, is used to examine the facts as well as the advantages and disadvantages of holding beliefs. (The idea of there being both disadvantages and advantages to holding onto beliefs is quite important when it comes to pain-specific beliefs, and I will save a detailed example illustrating this point for the next treatment module.) An example, Jennifer's in-session Changing Beliefs Worksheet, is included as Figure Mod. 5.4.

After helping group members list the facts supporting and refuting their intermediate and core beliefs, and after helping them identify some disadvantages and advantages to holding the belief, ask them to consider whether an alternative belief could be adopted and tested. Rather than helping them take on an unrealistically positive belief in place of the unrealistically negative belief, it may be more useful to help them experiment with a belief that is *relatively* more positive than the original belief.

Bear in mind that clients may need to experiment with a new belief in order to test out whether it has potential merit. To help them do this, you should suggest a behavioral test of-

Automatic thought (How much do you believe it? 0–100%)	Intermediate belief (How much do you believe it? 0–100%)	Evidence for/against Advantages/ disadvantages	Core belief (How much do you believe it? 0–100%)	Evidence for/against Advantages/ disadvantages	Alternative belief (use questions below to review the evidence and compose alternative)
I'm not in control of my own time at work.	If I can help, I should help. (90%)	For: I know more than they do. I've been there longer. I've taken more computer classes. Advantages: People will like me if I take care of them. Against: When I put others' needs ahead of my own, I trigger a killer headache. If I put myself out of commission with a headache, I'm no good to myself or others. Disadvantages: I give myself headaches when I always drop what I'm doing to help others.	I'm not worth much. (90–100%)	For: I was always taught to put others' needs ahead of my own. Advantages: At least I have one good thing to offer if I'm unselfish. Against: My family has stayed with me, even with my pain problem, so I must be worth something. Disadvantages: Believing I'm not worth much makes me feel terrible. Believing I'm not worth much makes me act like a doormat.	

FIGURE MOD. 5.4. Jennifer's in-session Changing Beliefs Worksheet.

ten referred to as the "acting as if" exercise. Even if a client does not wholly accept the alternative belief in replacing the original intermediate or core belief, ask her to experiment during the next week with *acting as if* the new belief is true. It is important to help clients be specific about how they plan to act as if their new belief is true. For example, Jennifer held the belief that "I'm not worth much." What, specifically, would she do if she had the alternative belief that "I *am* worth a lot?" How would she behave differently if she really believed in her own self-worth? Get clients to state a specific behavior or activity they can try that will be different for them, and in the spirit of acting as if their new belief is true. Most clients who try this exercise will report at the next session that at least certain elements of their old belief system are challenged when they try the exercise, and invariably, they feel better about themselves in the process.

HOMEWORK ASSIGNMENT

As homework, clients should use the Identifying Beliefs Worksheet to complete the work they began in session with identifying an underlying intermediate belief and core belief in response to a key automatic thought. In addition, they should use the Changing Beliefs Worksheet to practice with identifying and challenging at least one new belief system in response to a different key automatic thought. Often clients will come in with a very similar "new" belief system identified, which is okay. The point is to get them to work with these concepts on their own at home. Any homework should be considered good work!

Clients are also asked to experiment with the "acting as if" exercise. After coming up with an alternative belief to test, they should spend the week behaving *as if* the new belief is true, even if they don't wholly buy into the new belief. They should think of, and experiment with, a variety of ways they can act as if their new belief is true. Clients should note others' reactions to their new behavior, as well as their own.

POSTSESSION PROCESS CHECK

Hand out the Postsession Process Check, and ask clients to fill it out before they leave.

Session 5 Outline for Therapists: Intermediate and Core Beliefs (General)

SESSION OBJECTIVES

- Identify general underlying belief systems.
- Challenge negative, distorted beliefs and construct new beliefs.

NEEDED MATERIALS, HANDOUTS, AND WORKSHEETS

- Session 5 Outline for Therapists (this handout)
- Session 5 Summary for Clients (Client Handout 5.1)
- Presession Process Check (Appendix J)
- Results for each client's Dysfunctional Attitude Scale–24 (DAS-24), completed during assessment (Appendix C)
- Identifying Beliefs Worksheet (Client Handout 5.2)
- Changing Beliefs Worksheet (Client Handout 5.3)
- Postsession Process Check (Appendix J)

PRESESSION PROCESS CHECK

- Hand out Presession Process Check and have clients fill it in.

REVIEW OF PREVIOUS WEEK'S SESSION

- About challenging negative automatic thoughts, remind clients:
  - "Make sure you have listed all the facts supporting and refuting each thought."
  - "Identify the distorted part of the thought."
- About constructing alternative thoughts, remind clients:
  - "Is there an alternative, more realistic thought you could use in place of the original automatic thought?"
  - "It may help to ask yourself what you would tell a friend having your thought or in your situation."

HOMEWORK REVIEW

- Ask several clients: "Pick one automatic thought from your Automatic Thoughts Worksheet (ATW-3), and share what you wrote with the group."
- "What was the alternative response you generated?"
- "What were the results of generating the alternative response? That is, how much did your belief in the automatic thought go down, and what impact did this have on your feelings, physical well-being, and subsequent thoughts?"

(continued)

From *Cognitive Therapy for Chronic Pain* by Beverly E. Thorn. Copyright 2004 by The Guilford Press. Permission to photocopy this handout is granted to purchasers of this book for personal use only (see copyright page for details).

SESSION OBJECTIVE: IDENTIFY GENERAL UNDERLYING BELIEF SYSTEMS

- Underlying belief systems shape our automatic thoughts.
- We have positive as well as negative underlying belief systems.
- Negative belief systems surface in times of stress.
- Intermediate beliefs:
  - Give rise to automatic thoughts.
  - Are the rules and assumptions we hold about the way the world is, or *should* be.
- Core beliefs:
  - Give rise to intermediate beliefs.
  - Are deeply held beliefs about ourselves.
- Have clients review their answers to the DAS-24, to see what kinds of general belief systems they endorsed.

WORKSHEET: IDENTIFYING BELIEFS WORKSHEET

- Give out copies of the Identifying Beliefs Worksheet
- Use the downward-arrow technique to help clients identify a key automatic thought, an intermediate belief, and a core belief. Tell clients:
  - "First, write down a problem situation and a key automatic thought."
  - "Next, ask yourself, 'If that thought were true, what would it mean to me?' " (This helps identify the intermediate belief.)
  - "Next, ask yourself, 'If that thought were true, what would it mean about me?' " (This helps identify the core belief.)
- Get at least one example from each client.

SESSION OBJECTIVE: CHALLENGE NEGATIVE, DISTORTED BELIEFS AND CONSTRUCT ALTERNATIVE BELIEFS

- Tell clients: "Recognize that underlying beliefs are ideas, and that as ideas, they can be tested."
- "Consider the facts supporting and refuting each of your beliefs."
- "Consider the disadvantages and possible advantages to holding onto the belief."
- "Consider creating an alternative belief."
- "Try the 'acting as if' exercise: Act as if your new belief is true."

WORKSHEET: CHANGING BELIEFS WORKSHEET

- Give out copies of the Changing Beliefs Worksheet.
- Say to clients: "Make a list of facts supporting an underlying belief, and a list of facts refuting the underlying belief."
- "Are there any advantages to holding onto the underlying belief?"
- "Are there any disadvantages?"
- "Is there an alternative belief that you can try as a replacement for the underlying belief? Don't create an alternative that is unrealistically positive—just try one that is slightly more positive than the original."

(continued)

155

HOMEWORK ASSIGNMENT

- Tell clients: "Use the Identifying Beliefs Worksheet to identify a key automatic thought, a related intermediate belief, and a core belief. Try to work on this every day."
- "Remind yourself that underlying beliefs are *ideas*, not necessarily facts, and that they can be tested."
- "Use the Changing Beliefs Worksheet to list facts supporting and refuting the underlying beliefs, and to examine possible advantages and disadvantages of holding these beliefs. Then try to construct alternative beliefs."
- "Use the 'acting as if' exercise to experiment with a new belief: For the next week, act as if your new belief is true."
- "Bring your homework to the next session, and be ready to discuss what you have learned with other group members."

POSTSESSION PROCESS CHECK

- Have clients fill out Postsession Process Check before they leave. Glance at responses and troubleshoot if necessary.

Session 5 Summary for Clients: Intermediate and Core Beliefs (General)

THE GOALS OF THIS SESSION

- To identify general underlying belief systems.
- To challenge negative, distorted beliefs and construct alternative beliefs.

REVIEW OF PREVIOUS WEEK'S SESSION

- Challenging negative automatic thoughts:
  - Make sure you have listed all the facts supporting and refuting each thought.
  - Identify the distorted part of the thought.
- Constructing alternative thoughts:
  - Is there an alternative, more realistic thought you could use in place of the original automatic thought?
  - It may help to ask yourself what you would tell a friend having your thought or in your situation.

HOMEWORK REVIEW

- Pick one automatic thought from your Automatic Thoughts Worksheet (ATW-3), and share what you wrote with the group.
- What was the alternative response you generated?
- What were the results of generating the alternative response? That is, how much did your belief in the automatic thought go down, and what impact did this have on your feelings, physical well-being, and subsequent thoughts?

IDENTIFYING GENERAL UNDERLYING BELIEF SYSTEMS

- Underlying belief systems shape our automatic thoughts.
- We have positive as well as negative underlying belief systems.
- Negative belief systems surface in times of stress.
- Intermediate beliefs:
  - Give rise to automatic thoughts.
  - Are the rules and assumptions we hold about the way the world is, or *should* be.
- Core beliefs:
  - Give rise to intermediate beliefs.
  - Are deeply held beliefs about ourselves.
- The Identifying Beliefs Worksheet can help you identify underlying intermediate and core beliefs.
  - First, write down a problem situation and a key automatic thought.
  - Next, ask yourself, "If that thought were true, what would it mean to me?" (This helps identify the intermediate belief.)
  - Next, ask yourself, "If that thought were true, what would it mean about me?" (This helps identify the core belief.)

(continued)

From *Cognitive Therapy for Chronic Pain* by Beverly E. Thorn. Copyright 2004 by The Guilford Press. Permission to photocopy this handout is granted to purchasers of this book for personal use only (see copyright page for details).

CHALLENGING NEGATIVE, DISTORTED BELIEFS
AND CONSTRUCTING NEW BELIEFS

- Recognize that underlying beliefs are ideas, and that as ideas, they can be tested.
- Using the Changing Beliefs Worksheet, make a list of facts supporting an underlying belief, and facts refuting the underlying belief.
- Identify any disadvantages to holding onto the underlying belief
- Are there any advantages?
- Is there an alternative belief that you can try as a replacement for the underlying belief? (Note: Don't create an alternative that is unrealistically positive—just try one that is slightly more positive than the original.)
- Test out your new belief by "acting as if" your new belief is true, and see what happens.

SUMMARY OF KEY POINTS

- Key automatic thoughts (ones that come up again and again) may be linked to underlying beliefs.
- Underlying beliefs about others and yourself can get distorted when things are going poorly.
- Negative, distorted underlying beliefs have a negative impact on thoughts, feelings, and the way we act.
- Identifying negative, distorted underlying beliefs is the first step to changing them.
- You can challenge negative beliefs by looking at the disadvantages (and advantages) of holding onto them.
- Try to create a realistic alternative belief, and try it out by using the "acting as if" exercise.

HOMEWORK ASSIGNMENT

- Use the Identifying Beliefs Worksheet to identify a key automatic thought, a related intermediate belief, and a core belief. Try to work on this every day.
- Remind yourself that underlying beliefs are *ideas*, not necessarily facts, and that they can be tested.
- Use the Changing Beliefs Worksheet to list facts supporting and refuting the underlying beliefs, and to examine possible advantages and disadvantages of holding these beliefs. Then try to construct alternative beliefs.
- Use the "acting as if" exercise to experiment with a new belief: For the next week, act as if your new belief is true.
- Bring your homework to the next session, and be ready to discuss what you have learned with other group members.

CLIENT HANDOUT 5.2

Identifying Beliefs Worksheet

Situation:

Automatic Thought:

Intermediate Belief:

Core Belief:

From *Cognitive Therapy for Chronic Pain* by Beverly E. Thorn. Copyright 2004 by The Guilford Press. Permission to photocopy this handout is granted to purchasers of this book for personal use only (see copyright page for details).

CLIENT HANDOUT 5.3

Changing Beliefs Worksheet

Automatic thought (How much do you believe it? 0–100%)	Intermediate belief (How much do you believe it? 0–100%)	Evidence for/against Advantages/disadvantages	Core belief (How much do you believe it? 0–100%)	Evidence for/against Advantages/disadvantages	Alternative belief* (use questions below to review the evidence and compose alternative)

*What is the evidence that the belief is true? What is the evidence that the belief is not true? What are the advantages and disadvantages of holding this belief? Is the belief still serving you? Is there an alternative belief that can be tested?

From *Cognitive Therapy for Chronic Pain* by Beverly E. Thorn. Copyright 2004 by The Guilford Press. Permission to photocopy this handout is granted to purchasers of this book for personal use only (see copyright page for details).

PAIN-SPECIFIC INTERMEDIATE AND CORE BELIEFS

The sixth treatment session introduces the concept of pain-specific intermediate and core beliefs. Therapist Handout 6.1, found at the back of this module, provides an outline of Session 6 to be used by the therapist. Client Handout 6.1, also at the back of the module, can be copied and used as a session outline to be given to clients at the beginning of the session.

SESSION 6 TREATMENT OBJECTIVES

- Identify pain-related intermediate and core beliefs.
- Challenge negative, distorted pain-related beliefs and construct new beliefs.

PRESESSION PROCESS CHECK AND REVIEW OF PREVIOUS WEEK'S SESSION

As usual, start the session with the Presession Process Check and a review of the previous week's session. Last week's treatment goals were to begin learning to identify and challenge general underlying belief systems. Remind clients that people construct beliefs as a way of making sense of the world around them. Beliefs, just like automatic thoughts, are ideas, and as ideas, they can be tested. People have both positive and negative beliefs; typically, negative core beliefs are not everyday beliefs, but are more likely to be triggered during times of stress. Since chronic pain is considered to be a negative stressor, it certainly has the capacity to trigger negative beliefs. Core beliefs are deeply held ideas about the self, others, and the world, and are thought to give rise to intermediate beliefs. Intermediate beliefs are the "should," "must," and "ought to" ideas that we all tend to hold as rules for ourselves and for others. Intermediate beliefs are said to give rise to automatic thoughts.

HOMEWORK REVIEW

As homework, group members were asked to use the Identifying Beliefs Worksheet to identify an intermediate belief and a core belief from a key automatic thought. Once they identified the beliefs, they were to use the Changing Beliefs Worksheet to examine the facts supporting and refuting the beliefs, as well as to examine the advantages and disadvantages of holding the beliefs. They were then asked to identify alternative beliefs, and to try the "acting as if" exercise during the coming week.

My next vignette involves examining Melissa's homework in session. Melissa is a 32-year-old mother of two children in elementary school. She does not work outside the home, although she was employed as a nurse prior to injuring her neck and back in a motor vehicle accident over 2 years ago. Melissa has gained considerable weight since her accident. In addition to becoming relatively sedentary, Melissa is taking antidepressant medication, which often causes weight gain. A key automatic thought that Melissa identified while doing her Session 5 homework occurred in response to a situation where she was weighed in her physician's office, and found she had gained 5 additional pounds in 3 months. She noticed feeling "deflated" after getting off the scales, and said to herself, "I'm going downhill; why do I bother to try to eat right?" Melissa was able to identify her intermediate belief as "The least I should be able to do is stay slim!" The core belief she identified was "I am weak and unattractive."

The Changing Beliefs Worksheet that Melissa completed as homework is provided in Figure Mod. 6.1.

Without dissecting Melissa's Changing Beliefs Worksheet in detail, it is fair to say that she hit on a key automatic thought that triggered very emotionally charged material. Many patients with chronic pain have issues regarding changed body image, and/or feel betrayed by their bodies because their bodies have "failed" them. Melissa's Changing Belief Worksheet reflected her struggle between trying to do something about maintaining her weight and giving herself permission to quit trying and accept "fate." Key here, though, is that she held a strong core belief that she was weak and unattractive. Incidentally, in addition to filling out the Changing Beliefs Worksheet for homework, Melissa tried the "acting as if" exercise on part of her core belief: She decided to act as if she was not a weak person. Unfortunately, she defined "not weak" as being able to lose 2 pounds in the upcoming week, which may have been an unrealistic goal without a structured plan.

I pointed out to Melissa that she seemed to be basing her beliefs about being unattractive mainly on the fact that she had gained weight. During the previous week, Melissa had tried to act as if she was not "weak" by losing 2 pounds, even though she didn't have a plan set up. This week, I invited Melissa to try the "acting as if" exercise with the other part of her core belief: I invited her to experiment with behaving as if she was attractive, despite her weight. I asked her specifically what she could do differently if she believed she was attractive. She immediately said that she could dress more nicely, take care with her hair, and apply makeup. Happily, she arrived at the next session well groomed and well dressed, feeling like "a million bucks!" What astonished her during the week she behaved as if she was attractive was that people responded to her the way they would respond to an attractive person, even though she had not lost an ounce.

Automatic thought (How much do you believe it? 0–100%)	Intermediate belief (How much do you believe it? 0–100%)	Evidence for/against Advantages/ disadvantages	Core belief (How much do you believe it? 0–100%)	Evidence for/against Advantages/ disadvantages	Alternative belief (use questions below to review the evidence and compose alternative)
I'm going downhill; why do I bother to try to eat right? (95%)	The least I should be able to do is stay slim! (90%)	For: I don't eat very much as it is! My body has betrayed me in every other way. Other chronic pain patients manage to keep the weight off. Against: I don't get to exercise at all any more. They say that antidepressants cause weight gain. Advantages: If I believe I should stay slim, I'll continue to try. If I drop that belief, I'll stop trying altogether. Disadvantages: I feel bad about myself.	I am weak and unattrac- tive. (98%)	For: I've gained 25 pounds in 2 years. None of my nicer clothes fit any more. My husband is unhappy about my weight. Against: None—I think this belief is true! Advantages: NONE!! Disadvantages: I feel worse about myself believing this.	I'm not weak, just human. Everyone gets less attractive as they age.

FIGURE MOD. 6.1. Melissa's Session 5 homework Changing Beliefs Worksheet.

SESSION OBJECTIVE: IDENTIFY PAIN-RELATED INTERMEDIATE AND CORE BELIEFS

In Session 5, clients were helped to make the connection between a key automatic thought and more general underlying intermediate and core beliefs. General underlying beliefs and automatic thoughts in stressful situations can lead to an increase in the stress response, and can trigger a pain episode or exacerbate a pain flare-up. Jennifer's examples of "If I can help, I should help," and "I'm not worth much," used in the previous session, are certainly relevant to individuals with chronic pain, but not necessarily *specific* to someone with a chronic painful condition.

In addition to general belief systems, patients with pain hold entire sets of underlying beliefs, attitudes, and assumptions related to their pain condition and about themselves as persons with chronic pain. When negatively distorted, as they often are, these attitudes and beliefs about the pain (and about the self as someone "in" pain) create a cognitive set that works against the goal of developing pain self-management skills. Negatively distorted pain-related beliefs move patients more quickly down the spiral of pain-related dysfunction and disability. Therefore, it is not only useful, but quite essential, to help patients with chronic pain identify dysfunctional underlying beliefs about their pain, help them challenge these beliefs, and construct more realistic (and more adaptive) alternative underlying belief systems regarding their pain condition.

Negative life events are thought to trigger negative core beliefs. For patients with chronic pain, the pain and the pain-related stressors represent long-term negative life events, so it follows that they would experience more negative core beliefs. In addition, the periodic exacerbation of pain during a pain flare-up is likely to be especially disruptive of a positive sense of self. A very brief session transcript illustrates the point that chronic pain, and particularly a chronic pain flare-up, can trigger negative pain-related core beliefs.

MELISSA: When I have a setback, and my pain is very bad, and I'm into the second or third day of incapacitating pain, it's as if some of the ways I identify myself get all scrambled. Normally, I see myself as a competent and independent person. But when I'm in bad pain, I start to see myself as weak, vulnerable, and needy—definitely needy. And that's something I'm not comfortable being—not being able to meet my own needs.

The concept of pain-related core beliefs is also quite relevant to the manner in which a person with a chronic painful condition identifies himself. As I have discussed in Chapter 1, development of a personal identity as a "chronic pain patient," as distinct from a "well person with pain," can be an unfortunate consequence of dealing with chronic pain. The following "mini-lecture" introduces pain-related intermediate and core beliefs.

Last week we worked with general underlying belief systems that you hold about others, the world, and yourself. I talked about how, when things are going badly in people's lives, negative belief systems tend to come to the surface. Dealing with a chronic painful condition is one of those things that can trigger these negative general belief systems. There are other belief systems that are more specific to the pain situation, and we call these "pain-related beliefs." As we talked about last week, people develop belief systems to make sense of the world. And people with chronic pain develop belief systems in an attempt to make sense of their pain condition. These pain-related beliefs include beliefs about the cause of pain, the meaning of the pain, the amount of control people think they have over the pain, and even beliefs about appropriate and inappropriate means of treating the pain. I label these pain-related beliefs "intermediate pain-related beliefs," because they often are couched in "should," "must," and "ought to" terms.

For example, think about before you came to this group and your original beliefs about the value of psychological approaches to pain management. Many patients with pain who are referred to a psychologist (or some other mental health practitioner) for pain treatment initially see this as an inappropriate referral and a useless approach to their pain management. They equate psychological interventions with a declaration that their pain is not "real." By this point in treatment, I hope you have changed your mind about that! I expect that an original belief something like "My pain cannot be treated with psychological techniques" has already been modified to the belief that "Psychological approaches *can* be used to help me cope with pain."

Discussion of Clients' PBPI and SOPA-R Responses

To help clients identify their pain-related intermediate beliefs, you should provide them with their initial responses to the Pain Beliefs and Perceptions Inventory (PBPI) and the Survey of Pain Attitudes—Revised (SOPA-R). (See Chapter 4 and Appendices E and F.) Remind clients that before the treatment groups began, they filled out several questionnaires that were aimed at examining their belief systems associated with the pain experience. I give clients their individual responses to these measures, including the key matching each item with a category of beliefs. Once again, scores are not important for in-session purposes; the point is to stimulate thinking and generate discussion. The PBPI taps into whether clients understand the nature of their pain, whether they believe that their pain is constant, and whether they believe that their pain is a permanent condition. It also taps into whether clients feel responsible for their pain condition. The SOPA-R assesses a different set of attitudes about pain—those attitudes that involve patients' belief about the appropriate treatment of their pain. Some examples of the attitudes assessed include whether patients believe that emotions play a role in their pain, and whether they believe that a medical cure will be found for their pain, and whether they believe that medication is the best treatment for their pain. Following clients' examination of their PBPI and SOPA-R responses, move back to the "mini-lecture" mode.

> Pain-related beliefs and attitudes, just like general beliefs, are *ideas* that people hold. These ideas may be completely true, partially true, or completely false. When the beliefs are of a negative, global, and all-encompassing nature, they usually involve some amount of distortion that can be examined. Other beliefs are widely accepted in certain cultures, and not necessarily negative in content, but still interfere with the ability to cope effectively with chronic pain. For example, the belief that long-term pain medication is the *best* (and only) treatment for chronic pain is a widely held belief, but one that promotes dysfunction and disability.[1]
>
> Since beliefs and attitudes are ideas, they can be tested as ideas, using the methods we have already learned. But before we work on testing some of these ideas, I want to introduce the idea of "pain-related core beliefs."
>
> As I said earlier, negative life events tend to trigger negative core beliefs. We don't necessarily walk around on a daily basis with beliefs such as "I am unlovable," "I am useless," or "I am not good enough." But when things are going badly, these types of negative beliefs are likely to surface. Think for a moment about how your self-concept has changed since you began experiencing chronic pain. I have heard other people who cope with chronic pain talk about feeling less worthwhile, more unlovable, and less competent. Again, though they don't necessarily feel this way at all times, the negative life circumstance of chronic pain tends to trigger the more negative core beliefs, at least on occasion. Developing a personal identity as a "chronic pain patient" is also certainly related to the idea of a pain-related core belief. Think for a moment about how people refer to pain—often as "*my* pain" rather than "*the* pain." And as people assume a greater and greater role as *patients*, they may grow to believe less and less in themselves as competent to deal with *anything* associated with the pain.

Troubleshooting Tip: The fact that negative core beliefs are often contrary to one's ordinary sense of self (i.e., "ego-dystonic") makes them all the more upsetting when they are recognized and examined. As I have noted in Treatment Module 5, you will find that group members do not like to examine negative core beliefs—pain-related or otherwise. In my experience, clients put up more resistance to this part of the therapy than to any other aspect.

---

[1]*Troubleshooting Tip:* You will find that most of your clients with chronic pain are on multiple long-term pain medications, and they may be quite sensitive to the implication that pain medications are "bad." You will probably need to specify that although physician-prescribed pain medications are not "bad" per se, they are less likely to be useful over long periods of time; they cause a variety of unwanted side effects that can interfere with the quality of life; and exclusive reliance on medication as a means of coping with pain increases reliance on the health care system and decreases one's sense of personal control over aspects of the pain situation.

One client in a recent group claimed not to have understood the assignment, and therefore did not come up with any examples to work on or homework to turn in. After the other group members left, however, she admitted to the group leaders that this part of the treatment was too upsetting for her and she just couldn't "go there" at this point in her life.[2] Remember that core beliefs are usually rigidly held as incontrovertible "truths" about the self. Understandably, none of us *want* to examine what we sometimes interpret to be the harsh reality of our (negative) core being.

Exercise: "Why Me?"

As a first step to helping clients capture a core belief about themselves as patients with pain, I ask group members to ask themselves this question: "Why me?" For one of my clients, Martha Anne, who had been involved in a near-fatal motor vehicle accident with the brand-new car of her dreams, her underlying core belief was "I had no business buying that car—I never *deserved* that car." The fact that she had had such a terrible accident—which totaled her car almost as soon as she got it, and left her to deal with a chronic pain condition—was "proof" that her core belief was actually "fact." It is also interesting to note that when Martha Anne had a pain flare-up, she sometimes caught herself thinking that the flare-up was a kind of payback.

WORKSHEET: IDENTIFYING PAIN BELIEFS WORKSHEET

Client Handout 6.2 is used to help clients identify underlying pain beliefs. First, have clients identify a pain situation, and then help them identify a key automatic thought. Once a key automatic thought is identified, ask, "If that automatic thought were true, what does it mean *to* you?" This helps to identify the pain-related intermediate belief. After identifying an intermediate belief, then ask, "If that automatic thought were true, what does it mean *about* you?" This helps to identify the pain-related core belief. The meaning about the self, based on the automatic thought, is considered the core belief.

To return to David's case (last used as an example in Session 4), it is easy to see how his beliefs related to the meaning of his MRI results ("physical evidence" of spinal pathology) played into his automatic thoughts, subsequent emotions, and behavior. If David believed that the MRI pathology guaranteed that he would perceive pain (i.e., the "tissue damage equals pain" theory), he would be likely to view his MRI results as a sentence to chronic and possibly even worsening pain, over which he would have little control. He would be likely to have considerable fear of engaging in restorative exercises, out of concern that he might do even more damage to his spine. Without having a clear understanding of his doing so, David would be likely to adopt a palliative approach to his pain condition—believing recovery of function to be an impossibility; behaving likewise; and simultaneously increasing the likelihood of additional surgeries, more medications, and ever-decreasing function. In the next section, I use David's example to illustrate how his core beliefs as a person in pain gave rise

---

[2]Incidentally, this particular patient with chronic pain had comorbid panic disorder, generalized anxiety disorder, and agoraphobia. I felt that we had scored a huge success in just getting her to attend the group sessions. She told me that in her past individual therapy for anxiety, during which cognitive restructuring was implemented, she had terminated therapy at the point of examining core beliefs. Obviously, she was not yet ready to "go there."

to pain-related intermediate beliefs, which in turn led to some of the specific automatic thoughts that recurred for him on a day-to-day basis.

Recall from the previous session that David had struggled with creating an alternative belief for his original automatic thought, "The pain is just eating me up!" Although he created a somewhat less noxious alternative response, "The pain is chipping away at me," he still believed the original automatic thought 60%. I therefore worked further with David in session, and asked him to continue his efforts related to this theme as homework. I made a mental note that a common theme in many of David's "facts" refuting his automatic thought had to do with work-related issues. Also, since David was referred to cognitive treatment by his physician after they had discussed his applying for disability, work-related issues were probably paramount for David. I suggested to David that he might think about possible intermediate and core beliefs related to work issues for his in-session assignment.

During our discussion of using the Identifying Pain Beliefs Worksheet, David filled it in as shown in Figure Mod. 6.2.

Obviously, some powerful material is generated by examining pain-related intermediate and core beliefs. Remind clients that although underlying belief systems are harder to challenge than automatic thoughts, they are still ideas, not necessarily facts. Ideas can always be

Situation: Back pain getting worse while at work.

Automatic Thought: I guess I should go ahead and apply for disability; I won't be able to work much longer.

Intermediate Belief: My spine is disintegrating, and I can't do anything about it.

Core Belief: I'm becoming an invalid; I will be worthless.

FIGURE MOD. 6.2. David's in-session Identifying Pain Beliefs Worksheet.

tested. By this point in the treatment program, clients should have experienced success with examining and challenging automatic thoughts, and they should be able to generate alternative responses to negative, distorted automatic thoughts. The next hurdle is to help clients examine and challenge negative, distorted underlying pain-related beliefs and to create alternative belief systems.

SESSION OBJECTIVE: CHALLENGE NEGATIVE, DISTORTED PAIN-RELATED BELIEFS AND CONSTRUCT ALTERNATIVE BELIEFS

Once clients have identified pain-related intermediate and core beliefs, the next step is to challenge the negative, distorted beliefs and construct alternative beliefs.

WORKSHEET: CHANGING PAIN BELIEFS WORKSHEET

Use the Changing Pain Beliefs Worksheet (Client Handout 6.3) to help clients work through an example. First, have clients list the pain-related intermediate and core beliefs, and then have them list the advantages and disadvantages of holding these beliefs. An example of how to use the Changing Pain Beliefs Worksheet in session is given below.

THERAPIST: David, you have listed as an automatic thought "I guess I should go ahead and apply for disability; I won't be able to work much longer," and as an intermediate belief "My spine is disintegrating, and I can't do anything about it." Go ahead and list both on your Changing Pain Beliefs Worksheet, but for now, let's focus on the intermediate belief.

DAVID: Okay. Actually, I don't believe that as much as I did before last week, but I figured it was a good one to keep working on.

THERAPIST: I agree. I think it's critical to keep working on. So at this moment, how much do you hold the belief that "My spine is disintegrating, and I can't do anything about it"?

DAVID: About 40%.

THERAPIST: And you said you don't believe it as much as you did before last week. How much did you believe those thoughts last week?

DAVID: 100%! I didn't even know I *had* that belief until last week! And I had it 100%—I guess ever since my doc brought up the idea of my applying for disability. And he brought out that damn MRI to show me my disc damage . . .

THERAPIST: In reality, two beliefs are listed here: (1) your belief that your spine is disintegrating, and (2) your belief that you can't do anything about it. They are certainly related to each other, but I'm wondering if your second belief—that you can't do anything about it—is just related to your belief that your spine is disintegrating.

DAVID: You lost me, Doc.

ANOTHER GROUP MEMBER: I think she means this: Do you only believe you can't do anything about your spine dissolving, or do you believe you can't do much about your entire situation?

DAVID: Well, they're related. If I didn't think my backbone was going bad on me, I wouldn't feel so helpless. But I kinda see what you mean: I feel helpless about a lot of things related to my situation—not just my spine.

THERAPIST: So if you listed on your chart there "I can't do anything about my pain situation" as your intermediate belief, could you begin to list the facts supporting that belief and the facts not supporting that belief?

DAVID: Well, my doctor thinks I should apply for disability, for God's sake! Plus, I do miss a lot of work, and I can't seem to do anything about that. Plus, I'm holding a position that someone who's more able-bodied could have. That doesn't seem quite fair of me.

ANOTHER GROUP MEMBER: Wait a minute! I'll buy the part about missing a lot of work, but talking about being unfair because you are keeping someone else from being hired isn't a fact—that's an opinion!

THERAPIST: Good call, Tony. David's belief that he is being unfair by holding onto his work position should not be listed in the "Evidence for/against" column. So what about striking that one as a fact supporting your belief, David?

DAVID: Geez, once again, I wasn't even aware I was doing that. These thoughts we have are downright deadly!

THERAPIST: I suspect that as you listed that one on your sheet, you may have caught it. For now, let's get specific about the facts supporting and not supporting your intermediate belief that "I can't do anything about my pain situation."

DAVID: Oh, yeah. Well, actually, since you told me that an MRI's not all that it's cracked up to be, and that lots of people have spine problems without back pain, I don't have that image any more that my spine is disintegrating. I still don't think I have much control over whether or not my spine disintegrates, but at least I don't believe my MRI proves that any more.

THERAPIST: So what are some facts supporting your idea that you can't do much about your pain condition?

DAVID: Well, beside the fact that I miss a lot of work because I feel so bad, I don't really know. Except that nothin' I try seems to help.

THERAPIST: You can go ahead and list that, but you're going to have to be more specific about what you try that doesn't help.

DAVID: You know, operations, medicine.

ANOTHER GROUP MEMBER: I might as well say it before Dr. Thorn does: What about this group? Has it helped?

DAVID: Yeah, this group helps, and swimming helps. I'd have to list them both in the "Evidence for/against" column, under "Against."

THERAPIST: Now you're getting the idea about being specific. Some things you try have worked, while some things you try have not worked. Where does that put you in terms of your belief that "I can't do anything about my pain situation"?

DAVID: A different place, I guess.

THERAPIST: Well, don't give up on your belief quite so readily, but for homework, it sounds like you would do well to add to both columns on that list. Okay?

DAVID: You're the boss.

THERAPIST: Good work. Now let me ask you a tricky question to help you along. What is the advantage of holding onto the belief "I can't do anything about my pain situation"? How does it serve you?

DAVID: I can't see any advantage. It makes me feel terrible about myself—like a real loser!

THERAPIST: That's certainly a disadvantage. Go ahead and list that. But wouldn't there be some benefits of not being able to do anything about your condition?

DAVID: Well, maybe it helps me feel less guilty. If it's not my fault, then maybe I can live easier with the fact that I've brought this burden on my family.

ANOTHER GROUP MEMBER: Hey, it's not like any of us are getting a kick out of making things tougher on our family. It just makes matters worse if you make yourself feel guilty about it.

DAVID: I don't want to feel guilty, but I can't help it.

A DIFFERENT GROUP MEMBER: Believe me, David, I don't want to feel guilty either, and I do sometimes. But isn't the point of this group to teach us that we *can* help it?

THERAPIST: Sounds like some of David's belief systems about the meaning of his pain condition operate for several of you, which isn't surprising. The question I asked is a challenging one: What do we get out of holding the belief systems that we hold? For David, he's told us that by believing he can't do anything about his pain condition, he feels less guilty about burdening his family.

ANOTHER GROUP MEMBER: For me, it's easier to accept this steady decline believing there's nothing I can do about it than if I believed there was something I could be doing about it.

DAVID, AND OTHERS: Oh, yeah. That's true. I can relate to that.

THERAPIST: So, if I understand what many of you are saying, there's a seeming advantage to believing you can't do anything about your pain condition, because you feel less guilty if things get worse or if your family is burdened. It's as if you are telling yourself that if you believed you had control over your condition, then any setback would be your fault—any family burden would be avoidable.

DAVID: You pretty much hit the nail on the head there.

THERAPIST: Okay, how about disadvantages? Are there any disadvantages to believing "I can't do anything about my pain situation"?

DAVID: It's like giving up! Like giving up on life, or at least what I view life as. I've always worked! I've got three kids! I'm supposed to be the provider, not the invalid!

THERAPIST: Now it sounds like we're moving closer to the core belief you had listed: "I'm becoming an invalid; I will be worthless." Let's go backward for a minute: The last part of your automatic thought was "I won't be able to work much longer." When you asked yourself what it would mean to you if that thought were true, you came up with the belief that "I can't do anything about my pain situation." And finally, when you ask yourself what it would mean *about* you if that automatic thought were true, you shared the belief that you are becoming an invalid—that you will be worthless.

DAVID: Actually, I already feel pretty worthless.

THERAPIST: Once again, would you be willing to experiment with this belief? First, to agree that it is a belief, not a fact, and that as a belief, it can be tested?

DAVID: Hey, man, I've been told this all my life. Why should I stop believing it now?[3]

THERAPIST: You will have to decide if that belief is really serving your needs or not. But if, as I suspect, it's getting in the way of your taking control of your life, then it may be one you

Automatic thought (How much do you believe it? 0–100%)	Intermediate belief (How much do you believe it? 0–100%)	Evidence for/ against Advantages/ disadvantages	Core belief (How much do you believe it? 0–100%)	Evidence for/ against Advantages/ disadvantages	Alternative belief (use questions below to review the evidence and compose alternative)
I should apply for disability; I won't be able to work much longer. (85%)	My spine is disintegrating, and I can't do anything about it. (40%) Second: I can't do anything about my pain situation. (90%)	For: My doc thinks I should apply for disability. I miss a lot of work. ~~I'm holding a position that someone else could have.~~ ~~Nothing I try seems to help.~~ Medicines don't help. Surgeries don't help. Against: Swimming helps. The group helps. Advantages: Less guilty. Easier to accept limitations. Disadvantages: Feel bad about myself. Giving up on life.	I'm becoming an invalid; I will be worthless. (100%) I'm already worthless. (90%)		

FIGURE MOD. 6.3. David's revised in-session Changing Pain Beliefs Worksheet.

want to really examine. So now what about listing the facts supporting your belief that "I'm already worthless," and the facts countering this belief?

David's revised, partially completed in-session Changing Pain Beliefs Worksheet is included as Figure Mod. 6.3.

After helping group members list the facts supporting and disproving their pain-related intermediate and core beliefs, and after helping them examine both the disadvantages *and the advantages* of holding onto their beliefs, it is time to ask them to consider whether an alterna-

---

[3]Note that pain-related core beliefs often relate to general core beliefs, which are thought to be generated in childhood. For patients with pain, these general core beliefs may be translated into their self-image as "chronic pain patients," thus exacerbating the disability or distress caused by the condition itself.

tive belief could be adopted and tested. If group members have worked through the Changing Pain Beliefs Worksheet up to this point, it should be fairly easy for them to construct an alternative belief related to the intermediate and core pain-related beliefs. The trick is to help them buy into the newly constructed belief. Remember from Session 5 that clients should not be expected to adopt an unrealistically positive belief, although they often construct alternatives that are too positive and thus not believable. A belief that is moderately more positive, or one that has taken the distorted aspect of the original belief and corrected that part, is usually the easiest to adopt. Even then, clients are often giving "lip service" to the alternative belief until they can actually test it.

HOMEWORK ASSIGNMENT

As homework, ask group members to use the Identifying Pain Beliefs Worksheet to come up with at least one key pain-related thought, and then to identify an intermediate belief and core belief associated with the thought. Once they have done this, clients should use the Changing Pain Beliefs Worksheet to examine the facts supporting and refuting the intermediate and core beliefs, and to identify disadvantages as well as advantages associated with holding onto the negatively distorted beliefs. Next, they should identify an alternative response—one that is not unrealistically positive, but at least somewhat more positive (and more realistic). Even if clients do not wholly accept the alternative belief replacing the original intermediate or core belief, ask them to experiment during the next week with acting *as if* the new belief is true. Most clients who try this exercise will report at the next session that at least certain elements of their old belief system are challenged when they try the exercise, and invariably, they feel better about themselves in the process.

POSTSESSION PROCESS CHECK

Hand out the Postsession Process Check, and ask clients to fill it out before they leave.

Session 6 Outline for Therapists: Pain-Related Intermediate and Core Beliefs

SESSION OBJECTIVES

- Identify pain-related intermediate and core beliefs.
- Challenge negative, distorted pain-related beliefs and construct new beliefs.

NEEDED MATERIALS, HANDOUTS, AND WORKSHEETS

- Session 6 Outline for Therapists (this handout)
- Session 6 Summary for Clients (Client Handout 6.1)
- Presession Process Check (Appendix J)
- Results for each client's Pain Beliefs and Perceptions Inventory (PBPI; Appendix E) and Survey of Pain Attitudes—Revised (SOPA-R; Appendix F), completed during assessment
- Identifying Pain Beliefs Worksheet (Client Handout 6.2)
- Changing Pain Beliefs Worksheet (Client Handout 6.3)
- Postsession Process Check (Appendix J)

PRESESSION PROCESS CHECK

- Hand out Presession Process Check and have clients fill it in.

REVIEW OF PREVIOUS WEEK'S SESSION

- Intermediate beliefs are the rules and assumptions we hold about the way the world is, or *should* be.
- Core beliefs are deeply held beliefs about ourselves and the world.
- Underlying beliefs are ideas that can be tested: What is the evidence that the belief is true or not true?
- What are the disadvantages and advantages of holding these beliefs?
- Are there alternative responses that could be identified and tested?

HOMEWORK REVIEW

- Ask several clients: "Pick one situation in which you identified an automatic thought, an intermediate belief, and a core belief, and share what you wrote with the group."
- "When you used the Changing Beliefs Worksheet to list the facts supporting and refuting your underlying beliefs, and to list disadvantages as well as advantages in holding onto the belief, were you able to construct an alternative belief?"
- "Were you able to try the 'acting as if' exercise?"

(continued)

From *Cognitive Therapy for Chronic Pain* by Beverly E. Thorn. Copyright 2004 by The Guilford Press. Permission to photocopy this handout is granted to purchasers of this book for personal use only (see copyright page for details).

SESSION OBJECTIVE:
IDENTIFY PAIN-RELATED INTERMEDIATE AND CORE BELIEFS

- Pain-related beliefs are often held about the cause of pain, the meaning of pain, and the ability to influence the pain.
  - Use the SOPA-R and the PBPI as discussion guides to get at some of clients' pain-related beliefs.
  - Ask clients: "What are some pain-related beliefs you hold about the cause of pain, its meaning, or your ability to influence pain?"
- Pain-related beliefs are also held about the self as a person in pain. Ask clients:
  - "Do you see yourself as a 'pain patient' or a 'well person with pain'?"
  - "When you ask yourself the question 'Why me?', what do you answer?"

WORKSHEET: IDENTIFYING PAIN BELIEFS WORKSHEET

- Give out copies of the Identifying Pain Beliefs Worksheet.
- Use the downward-arrow method to help clients identify a key pain-related automatic thought, intermediate belief, and core belief. Tell clients:
  - "First, write down a pain-related problem situation and a key automatic thought."
  - "Next, ask yourself, 'If that thought were true, what would it mean to me?' " (This helps identify the intermediate belief.)
  - "Next, ask yourself, 'If that thought were true, what would it mean about me?' " (This helps identify the core belief.)
- Get at least one example from each client.

SESSION OBJECTIVE: CHALLENGE NEGATIVE, DISTORTED PAIN-RELATED
BELIEFS AND CONSTRUCT NEW BELIEFS

- Intermediate and core beliefs are harder to challenge than automatic thoughts.
- Intermediate and core beliefs are beliefs, not facts, and can be tested.

WORKSHEET: CHANGING PAIN BELIEFS WORKSHEET

- Give out copies of the Changing Pain Beliefs Worksheet.
- Say to clients: "What is the evidence that the belief is true?"
- "What is the evidence that the belief is not true?"
- "What are the advantages and disadvantages of holding this belief?"
- "Is the belief still serving you?"
- "Is there an alternative explanation that could be tested?"
- "Don't jump from the extremely negative to the extremely positive. Consider experimenting with a belief that is *relatively* more positive than the original belief."
- "Test the alternative belief."
  - "What is the evidence that supports the alternative belief?"
  - "What is the evidence that does not support the alternative belief?"
- "Use the 'acting as if' exercise to experiment with the new belief."
  - "Even if you don't totally buy into the alternative belief, try acting as if it were true."
  - "Often, changing the behavior (acting as if) helps change the belief."

(continued)

HOMEWORK ASSIGNMENT

- Tell clients: "Use the Identifying Pain Beliefs Worksheet to identify a key pain-related automatic thought, intermediate belief, and core belief. Try to work on this every day."
- "Remind yourself that underlying beliefs are *ideas*, not necessarily facts, and that they can be tested."
- "Use the Changing Beliefs Worksheet to list facts supporting and refuting the pain-related underlying beliefs, to examine possible advantages and disadvantages of holding these beliefs, and to construct alternative beliefs."
- "Use the 'acting as if' exercise to experiment with a new belief: For the next week, act as if your new belief is true."
- "Bring your homework to the next session, and be ready to discuss what you have learned with other group members."

POSTSESSION PROCESS CHECK

- Have clients fill out Postsession Process Check before they leave. Glance at responses and trouble-shoot if necessary.

Session 6 Summary for Clients: Pain-Related Intermediate and Core Beliefs

THE GOALS OF THIS SESSION

- To identify pain-related intermediate and core beliefs.
- To challenge negative, distorted pain-related beliefs and construct new beliefs.

REVIEW OF PREVIOUS WEEK'S SESSION

- Intermediate beliefs are the rules and assumptions we hold about the way the world is, or *should* be.
- Core beliefs are deeply held beliefs about ourselves and the world.
- Underlying beliefs are ideas that can be tested: What is the evidence that the belief is true or not true?
- What are the disadvantages and advantages of holding these beliefs?
- Are there alternative responses that could be identified and tested?

HOMEWORK REVIEW

- Pick one situation in which you identified an automatic thought, an intermediate belief, and a core belief, and share what you wrote with the group.
- When you used the Changing Beliefs Worksheet to list the facts supporting and refuting your underlying beliefs, and to list disadvantages as well as advantages in holding onto the belief, were you able to construct an alternative belief?
- Were you able to try the "acting as if" exercise?

IDENTIFYING PAIN-RELATED INTERMEDIATE AND CORE BELIEFS

- Pain-related beliefs are often held about the cause of pain, the meaning of pain, and the ability to influence the pain.
  - What are some pain-related beliefs you hold about the cause of pain, its meaning, or your ability to influence pain?
- Pain-related beliefs are also held about the self as a person in pain.
  - Do you see yourself as a "pain patient" or a "well person with pain"?
  - When you ask yourself the question "Why me?", what do you answer?

CHALLENGING NEGATIVE, DISTORTED PAIN-RELATED BELIEFS AND CONSTRUCTING NEW BELIEFS

- Intermediate and core beliefs are harder to challenge than automatic thoughts.
- Intermediate and core beliefs are beliefs, not facts, and can be tested.

(continued)

From *Cognitive Therapy for Chronic Pain* by Beverly E. Thorn. Copyright 2004 by The Guilford Press. Permission to photocopy this handout is granted to purchasers of this book for personal use only (see copyright page for details).

- Use the Changing Pain Beliefs Worksheet and list the following:
  - What is the evidence that the belief is true?
  - What is the evidence that the belief is not true?
  - What are the advantages and disadvantages of holding this belief?
  - Is the belief still serving you?
  - Is there an alternative explanation that could be tested?
- Don't jump from the extremely negative to the extremely positive. Consider experimenting with a belief that is *relatively* more positive than the original belief.
- Test the alternative belief.
  - What is the evidence that supports the alternative belief?
  - What is the evidence that does not support the alternative belief?
- Use the "acting as if" exercise to experiment with the new belief.
  - Even if you don't totally buy into the alternative belief, try acting as if it were true.
  - Often, changing the behavior (acting as if) helps change the belief.

SUMMARY OF KEY POINTS

- Just like general beliefs, negative pain-related beliefs can be triggered by things going badly in your life.
- Pain-related intermediate beliefs include acquired beliefs about the cause of pain, the meaning of pain, the appropriate treatment of pain, and your ability to control pain.
- Pain-related core beliefs involve your sense of yourself as a person in pain.
- Pain-related beliefs are ideas that can be tested.
- Once you identify the facts supporting and not supporting your pain-related beliefs, you can challenge the negative distortions and construct new beliefs.

HOMEWORK ASSIGNMENT

- Use the Identifying Pain Beliefs Worksheet to identify a key pain-related automatic thought, intermediate belief, and core belief. Try to work on this every day.
- Remind yourself that underlying beliefs are *ideas*, not necessarily facts, and that they can be tested.
- Use the Changing Pain Beliefs Worksheet to list facts supporting and refuting the pain-related underlying beliefs, to examine possible advantages and disadvantages of holding these beliefs, and to construct alternative beliefs.
- Use the "acting as if" exercise to experiment with the new belief: For the next week, act as if your new belief is true.
- Bring your homework to the next session, and be ready to discuss what you have learned with other group members.

CLIENT HANDOUT 6.2

Identifying Pain Beliefs Worksheet

Situation:

Automatic Thought:

Intermediate Belief:

Core Belief:

From *Cognitive Therapy for Chronic Pain* by Beverly E. Thorn. Copyright 2004 by The Guilford Press. Permission to photocopy this handout is granted to purchasers of this book for personal use only (see copyright page for details).

Changing Pain Beliefs Worksheet

Automatic thought (How much do you believe it? 0–100%)	Intermediate belief (How much do you believe it? 0–100%)	Evidence for/against Advantages/disadvantages	Core belief (How much do you believe it? 0–100%)	Evidence for/against Advantages/disadvantages	Alternative belief* (use questions below to review the evidence and compose alternative)

*What is the evidence that the belief is true? What is the evidence that the belief is not true? What are the advantages and disadvantages of holding this belief? Is the belief still serving you? Is there an alternative belief that can be tested?

From *Cognitive Therapy for Chronic Pain* by Beverly E. Thorn. Copyright 2004 by The Guilford Press. Permission to photocopy this handout is granted to purchasers of this book for personal use only (see copyright page for details).

COPING SELF-STATEMENTS

The seventh treatment session introduces the concept of coping self-statements. Therapist Handout 7.1, found at the back of this module, provides an outline of Session 7 to be used by the therapist. Client Handout 7.1, also at the back of the module, can be copied and used as a session outline to be given to clients at the beginning of the session.

SESSION 7 TREATMENT OBJECTIVE
• Construct and use positive coping self-statements.

PRESESSION PROCESS CHECK AND REVIEW OF PREVIOUS WEEK'S SESSION

As always, begin the session by conducting the Presession Process Check and reviewing the previous week's goals and homework assignment. For Session 6, the treatment goals were to identify underlying pain-related beliefs, assumptions, and attitudes, and to examine these beliefs for ways they might be distorted and maladaptive. The Identifying Pain Beliefs Worksheet and the Changing Pain Beliefs Worksheet were used to accomplish these goals and to construct alternative responses.

HOMEWORK REVIEW

As part of homework review, you should check to see whether group members have made progress with the work they began in the previous session, and also whether they were able to identify any other pain-related beliefs. Ideally, this is the time when clients will begin recognizing and questioning several firmly held assumptions about the nature of their pain, about the way it should be treated, and about themselves as persons in pain.

To illustrate how the homework review might go, recall from our last session that Melissa described her self-concept as getting "scrambled" during particularly difficult pain episodes. Although she generally feels self-sufficient and competent, during periods of pain exacerbation she feels "needy." She commented that "that's something I'm not comfortable being—not being able to meet my own needs."

Melissa brought in a completed Identifying Pain Beliefs Worksheet as part of her homework (see Figure Mod. 7.1).

A brief session transcript follows.

Situation: Bad pain into the third day—can't get out of bed.

Automatic Thought: I can't even do the simplest things for myself any more.

Intermediate Belief: I should not be needy—I'm not allowed to be vulnerable.

Core Belief: I'm becoming an invalid.*

FIGURE MOD. 7.1. Melissa's Session 6 homework Identifying Pain Beliefs Worksheet. *Note that this core belief, "I'm becoming an invalid," could also be viewed as a catastrophic automatic thought. There is probably a more basic core belief imbedded behind this catastrophic prediction. One way to approach this would be to treat the belief "I'm becoming an invalid" as an automatic thought (examining the facts supporting and refuting the thought). Another way to intervene here would be to help the client examine the underlying meaning behind the thought. I chose to do the latter, particularly because of the clue Melissa gave me in the words she used to describe her intermediate belief: "I'm *not allowed* to be vulnerable."

THERAPIST: Melissa, I see you were able to identify a pain-related automatic thought and to trace an intermediate belief and a core belief to it.

MELISSA: Well, now, this wasn't a real-life situation for me during this particular week, but it's happened before, so I thought I'd kind of write it down in retrospect.

THERAPIST: That's excellent! You don't have to wait for a particular situation to occur during the week to be able to work on this stuff.

ANOTHER GROUP MEMBER: Yeah, I'd say we have plenty of history to draw from if we think about it for, oh, say, a second or two! (*Other group members laugh.*)

THERAPIST: So, Melissa, what did you learn about your pain-related beliefs?

MELISSA: Well, I'm surprised at how strongly I feel about this! I actually feel *panicky* when I feel needy and vulnerable. It's as if I'm afraid that something really terrible will happen if I need someone else's help.

ANOTHER GROUP MEMBER: I don't think it's a bad thing at all to be vulnerable. I don't see why you have that listed as a *negative* belief.

THERAPIST: Well, the key is that different people have different sets of "shoulds" and "musts." What might really push someone's emotional buttons may not phase another person at all. Melissa has hit on a very important discovery—that when we identify an important underlying belief, it often makes us feel really anxious or upset. Melissa, do you have a sense of what you are afraid of? What terrible thing would happen if you needed someone else's help?

MELISSA: Mmmmm. (*Melissa gets tearful.*) I have this memory of my mother getting sick and really needing my father to help her with even the basic things. One day when she was crying for help in the bedroom, he literally pushed her away and walked out the door. He came back, of course, but she was changed. She died all closed off inside of her.

THERAPIST: That kind of memory can have a long-term effect on what we believe and how we act. It sounds like what might have been the hardest part is watching your mom be rejected, even temporarily, by your dad.

MELISSA: And the effect that had on her. I don't *ever* want to be that vulnerable.

THERAPIST: And "vulnerable" is the word you used to describe your intermediate belief. You said, "I'm not allowed to be vulnerable."

MELISSA: Well, my mom sure wasn't, even though she was literally dying of breast cancer. I'd rather not ask for help than be rejected that way. In fact, I think being rejected did her in.

THERAPIST: That's a very strong belief if you think that rejection can actually kill you. No wonder you don't want to be vulnerable.

ANOTHER GROUP MEMBER: But Melissa, your mom had terminal cancer. Are you sure it was your dad's behavior that killed her?

THERAPIST: Once again, these beliefs are very strongly held ideas that may or may not be factual. But they sink their teeth into us, and it's hard to shake them.

MELISSA: Well, like others have been saying, I didn't even know I had these beliefs until I began working on this. I just thought I was a fiercely independent person, and that this was a good quality to have.

THERAPIST: I can certainly see why you have such a strong fear of being needy and vulnerable. Does your "fierce independence" get in your way at times?

MELISSA: Oh, well, yeah. My husband says I have a wall around me and I won't let him in. There are times when I am in the bed with the pain and so bad off that I lock him out of the room. I've been telling myself that I do that to spare him the hassle of taking care of me, but I'm beginning to think I do it because I'm terrified that he might be disgusted by me and leave me.

THERAPIST: So one of the *disadvantages* to holding onto the belief that "I should not be needy" is that it hurts your relationship with your husband. And one of the advantages to holding onto the belief is that it spares you from finding out if he will abandon you when you need him most.

MELISSA: (*sobbing*) Yes.

THERAPIST: These beliefs are really tough. They bring up a lot of emotions—deep feelings we may have been carrying around with us for a long, long time, without even being fully aware of it. The important thing to remind yourself is that once you identify the beliefs, you can begin to examine them to see whether they are completely true, partially true, or quite distorted.

ANOTHER GROUP MEMBER (KIM): I just don't think I can do this part of the therapy. It's too creepy, and I just can't handle that much emotion right now.

THERAPIST: Well, Kim, strong negative emotions are difficult to experience. But worse yet is when we let our thoughts and emotions boss us around and prevent us from experiencing life fully, because we are afraid of the hold they have over us. As an experiment, Kim, I'd like you to write down on one of your Automatic Thought Worksheets, "I just can't handle that much emotion right now," and during the next week, consider examining the facts behind that automatic thought. Okay?

KIM: I guess I can do that part.

THERAPIST: How likely do you think you are to do that part?[1]

KIM: I can do that. I will do that part. I just don't want to go farther with it, in terms of those deep-down core beliefs.

THERAPIST: That's fair enough. I'd just like you to examine the automatic thought "I can't handle that much emotion right now." Okay?

KIM: Okay.

THERAPIST: And Melissa, I'd like you to continue adding to your list of the disadvantages and advantages of holding the belief that "I should not be needy—I'm not allowed to be vulnerable." Okay?

MELISSA: Yeah, I can do that part.

THERAPIST: And while you're at it, Melissa, take a look at the thought "I'm becoming an invalid," and write down the facts supporting and refuting that thought. Okay?

MELISSA: Okay.

Following the homework review, it is time to move on to the new material presented in Session 7: constructing and using positive coping self-statements.

---

[1]*Troubleshooting Tip:* It's best not to leave a homework assignment hanging with an uncertain or resistant client. If you ask her to do something specific, and she seems unwilling, it is better to honor her resistance and remove the homework assignment than to set her up for a failure experience. As a rule of thumb, if the client is not at least 80% sure that she will do the assigned work, consider explicitly removing the assignment, giving her an alternative assignment, and discussing her hesitance in more depth (either during the session or during a between-session consultation).

SESSION OBJECTIVE: CONSTRUCT AND USE POSITIVE COPING SELF-STATEMENTS

Coping self-statements are broader than the alternative responses clients have already learned to construct in response to distorted automatic thoughts and beliefs. Coping self-statements are cognitive cues, or shortcuts, to a positive cognitive process that can be used in a variety of situations to facilitate adaptive coping responses. In short, coping self-statements are the emotional "cheerleaders" of the coping repertoire.

Today we are going to learn about constructing more global coping self-statements. These go beyond simple alternative responses to negative automatic thoughts, as you will see.

As people go through life and deal with the various challenges presented to them, they develop beliefs about their ability to control what happens around them. Most people with chronic pain feel at least some amount of helplessness when it comes to controlling their situation, particularly as it relates to pain. From this pain management group, you've learned that there are some aspects of the situation that you do have the ability to influence or control. So the ability to control your surroundings is not a black-or-white, yes-or-no occurrence, but more specific to certain aspects of the situation.

There are various parts making up your pain situation, and you might judge yourself to have control over some of them, but not to be in control of others. We call these kinds of judgments "locus of control" beliefs. People can be internally directed (look to the self), externally directed (looking to others), or both when it comes to their locus of control judgments of their pain situation. For example, at first glance, most patients with pain state that they do not have personal control over their pain level. Instead, they might feel that pain medications are the only thing that can help them control their pain. You've already learned that increased stress or emotional upset can very definitely raise your pain level, and ideally, you are beginning to learn that reducing stress and emotional upset can lower your pain level. In this way, your judgment of your locus of control is changing from outside yourself (external) to inside yourself (internal). Another example of a locus of control belief would be your judgment about your ability to control the number of pain flare-ups or pain episodes you have. And another example might be your personal sense of being able to calm your emotions when you get upset.

A different kind of sense of control we have is the part of us that believes we can accomplish some particular goal. We call these kinds of judgments "self-efficacy" beliefs. These could include your belief in your ability to do the homework assigned to you in this group, or your belief that you can recognize a distorted thought and replace it with a more realistic, positive alternative. Another self-efficacy belief could involve your judgment about whether you can do the exercises prescribed to you by your physical therapist.

The more we believe in ourselves, the better able we will be to cope with the stressors associated with the pain. One way to believe in ourselves more is to construct positive coping statements that we can use throughout the day as reminders, or cognitive cues. These coping self-statements serve as the emotional "cheerleaders" in the coping repertoire. Coping self-statements can be pain-specific (meaning that they can be statements specifically about the pain level or our ability to deal with the pain), or they can be much more general (meaning that they can be statements about our ability to deal with emotions or stress, or about our self-concept in general). This is a good time to take a look at a few pain-specific coping self-statements, and to come up with others that are most relevant to your situation.

Discussion of Coping Self-Statements

In order to stimulate discussion, I provide group members with a list of coping self-statements (see Client Handout 7.2 at the back of the module). These statements have been selected from the Cognitive Coping Strategies Inventory—Revised (CCSI-R; Thorn, Ward, & Clements, 2003; see Appendix H) and the Coping Strategies Questionnaire—Revised (CSQ-R; Riley & Robinson, 1997; see Appendix I).

Using this brief list, I give clients an idea of what I am talking about, but I also provide an opportunity for them to construct their own, more personally relevant examples. It is helpful to bear in mind the various themes particular clients have been presenting in the context of their in-session work and homework. Helping each client construct coping self-statements around the topic of a particularly relevant theme may provide the most therapeutic gain for the client. How deeply you go into the belief system of a client with a coping self-statement depends partly on the client and partly on your therapeutic judgment. In earlier sessions, for example, David brought in numerous automatic thoughts with associated work-related themes. These automatic thoughts probably stemmed from intermediate beliefs that he is a worthwhile husband and father only if he is the financial provider ("I 'must' be the provider"), and these intermediate beliefs probably stemmed from a core belief regarding his worth as a person ("I'm worthless"). In the example below, I took my cue from David and helped him construct coping self-statements that would encourage him to stay physically active (both at work and at home) despite the pain, rather than steering him toward coping self-statements regarding his worth as a husband, as a father, or as a person in general. However, with Jennifer, I moved toward coping self-statements about her intermediate belief that "If I can help, I should help."

After giving group members the list of examples of coping self-statements, I provide opportunities for their reactions to the examples, as well as guiding clients toward generating their own coping self-statements. A session transcript illustrates this procedure. Clients will sometimes relate to a particular coping self-statement provided in the handout as a good one for them, and will sometimes react negatively to one or more other examples provided. The point is to get them to generate coping self-statements that are of most relevance to them. At first, I just have them jot their ideas down on a sheet of paper. Shortly thereafter, I have them transfer their coping statements to cards they can carry with them or post at strategic locations around their environment.

THERAPIST: Did anyone relate to any of the coping self-statements on the list?

MARTHA ANNE: Well, I thought about the one that says, " . . . for some reason it is important for me to endure the pain," but since we've already decided that I should not feel like the accident was a message from God that I've been bad, I'm not going to use that one.

THERAPIST: Good idea, Martha Anne. I agree that for you, using that one would be buying into your distorted negative thoughts about blame and punishment. We'll come up with a better one for you. Anyone else?

DAVID: I liked the one about carrying on despite the pain. The "be brave" part is a little dramatic for me, but I could use "Carry on despite the pain."

THERAPIST: Okay, great. Write that one down, and we'll fine-tune it in a few minutes. What did other folks come up with?

JENNIFER: : Well, I can relate to " . . . there are others who are much worse off than me."

THERAPIST: In terms of pain, or in general?

JENNIFER: : Oh, well, I was thinking in general. Is that supposed to be about the pain?

THERAPIST: That example was written about others in pain being worse off. You could use it as a general statement too, but I think for you, Jennifer, using it might buy into your "should" statements that you "should" always help others who are worse off.

JENNIFER: : How about if I said that "Just because others are worse off, I don't always have to help them"?

THERAPIST: Go ahead and write that one down, and we'll work with that statement too.

KIM: None of those fit for me. I'm gonna make up my own.

THERAPIST: That's fine, Kim, and these are meant to be examples to get you thinking. The point is to make up your own—ones that are most relevant for you and your particular situation.

COPING CARDS

This week's session utilizes blank, colored 3" × 5" index cards instead of the typical worksheet. Hand each client five index cards (they can pick their favorite colors). They will be picking one of the coping statements they generated during their discussion and (soon) transferring it to an index card. Before they do, you will want to go over the group members' coping self-statements, as they may need some adjustments. By way of illustration, the session transcript that was begun above continues.

THERAPIST: Okay, now let's begin taking some of the ideas you've come up with, and refining them so that you can come up with some good coping self-statements. Remember that the idea is to have some good coping self-statements ready and waiting, so that when you're feeling bad, you can use them to outwit those negative thoughts that tend to creep in. David, can we start with yours? You had "Carry on despite the pain."

DAVID: Yeah, I like that one. It seems like when the pain gets bad, my negative thoughts try to get me to give up and give in to it. I tell myself that I can't keep going if I'm in pain.

THERAPIST: I remember you saying before that you feel better being at work than sitting at home doing nothing.

DAVID: Yup, and either way, I'm going to have the pain. There's stuff I can do at work that doesn't make it worse—like I shouldn't keep standing in one place for more than 15–20 minutes. But I can move around a lot, and at least I'm occupied and feeling worth a damn.

THERAPIST: Okay, then. Do you want to add anything to your coping statement, "Carry on despite the pain"?

DAVID: No, I like it just like that. It's short and sweet. I can use it as a motto, and I can remember it, even if I don't have the card with me.

THERAPIST: Okay, great. Let's move on to Jennifer.

JENNIFER: : Mine was "Just because others are worse off, I don't always have to help them."

THERAPIST: At what times would you use this coping statement?

JENNIFER: : When I feel that angry feeling—that I have to drop what I'm doing and clean up someone else's mess for them.

ANOTHER GROUP MEMBER: I don't like that one as well as an alternative thought you came up with earlier. It was something like "I can and will take care of myself," or something like that. It sounded more positive.

JENNIFER: : Jeesh, it's so hard for me to say that. What I really need on a coping card is "I am worth taking care of myself."

THERAPIST: I think you've hit the nail on the head. How would it feel to read that in your own handwriting?

JENNIFER: : I think darn good, actually!

THERAPIST: Great! Get that one down. Kim, have you come up with an idea yet?

KIM: Well, my problem is that when I have pain, I slink off to bed. I have "When I'm in pain, there's lots I can do besides go to bed." Then I've listed some things: I can take a bubble bath or hot shower. I can go for a walk. I can call my sister. I can go to the crafts store. I can try a new recipe.

THERAPIST: That's great, Kim. This gives you a list of behaviors that you can try as alternatives to going to bed when you are in pain. You've already realized that for you, going to bed when you're in pain just makes matters worse, because you get lonely and depressed. The coping card gives you the cognitive cue to consider alternative behaviors.

HOMEWORK ASSIGNMENT

For homework, group members are asked to come up with at least three coping self-statements that they can use to short-circuit thematic negative distortions. Remind clients that coping self-statements are a bit different from the alternative responses they generated for distorted automatic thoughts, because coping self-statements are geared toward motivating the clients to feel that they can and will make some positive coping response. Thus coping self-statements are the bridge between thoughts and actions. Also discuss with clients the need to post the coping cards in strategic locations where they will see them frequently. One of my favorite locations is the sun visor of my car, because I flip it up and down several times each day. Other popular locations are over the kitchen sink, on the refrigerator, on the telephone receiver, and on the computer monitor. Coping cards should be prominently displayed and used several times each day. Tell clients that coping cards may be habit-forming, but happily, they are without negative side effects!

POSTSESSION PROCESS CHECK

As usual, hand out the Postsession Process Check, and ask clients to fill it out before they leave.

Session 7 Outline for Therapists: Coping Self-Statements

SESSION OBJECTIVE

- Construct and use positive coping self-statements.

NEEDED MATERIALS, HANDOUTS, AND WORKSHEETS

- Paper and pencils for group members
- 3" × 5" index cards of various colors
- Session 7 Outline for Therapists (this handout)
- Session 7 Summary for Clients (Client Handout 7.1)
- Presession Process Check (Appendix J)
- Examples of Pain-Related Coping Self-Statements (Client Handout 7.2)
- Postsession Process Check (Appendix J)

PRESESSION PROCESS CHECK

- Hand out Presession Process Check and have clients fill it in.

REVIEW OF PREVIOUS WEEK'S SESSION

- Pain-specific beliefs are often held about the cause of pain, the meaning of pain, and the ability to influence the pain.
- Pain-related beliefs are also held about the self as a person in pain.
- Pain-related beliefs are ideas, and just like all ideas, they can be examined.
- Remind clients: "One way to examine pain-related beliefs is to consider whether (and how) they are serving you."
- "If pain-related beliefs are not serving you now, consider experimenting with an alternative belief by using the 'acting as if' exercise."

HOMEWORK REVIEW

- Ask several clients about using the Identifying Pain Beliefs Worksheet:
  - "What did you learn about how your pain-related automatic thoughts are connected to your pain beliefs and your beliefs about yourself as a person in pain?"
- Ask several clients about using the Changing Pain Beliefs Worksheet:
  - "It's usually easy to identify the disadvantages to holding onto a negative pain-related belief."
  - "It's hard to identify the *advantages* of holding onto a negative pain-related belief. What did you learn?"
- Ask several clients about using the "acting as if" exercise to experiment with a new belief:
  - "What happened when you acted as if your new belief was a reality?"
    - "Did others respond differently to you?"
    - "Did you feel differently about yourself?"

(continued)

From *Cognitive Therapy for Chronic Pain* by Beverly E. Thorn. Copyright 2004 by The Guilford Press. Permission to photocopy this handout is granted to purchasers of this book for personal use only (see copyright page for details).

SESSION OBJECTIVE:
CONSTRUCT AND USE POSITIVE COPING SELF-STATEMENTS

- Say to clients: "Coping self-statements are the emotional 'cheerleaders' in the coping repertoire, and can help to increase your sense of personal control and efficacy."
- " 'Locus of control' (or 'LOC') beliefs are judgments about whether you have an internal (within yourself) or external (outside yourself) sense of control over your pain situation."
- " 'Self-efficacy' beliefs are judgments about your ability to accomplish a goal related to pain management."
- "Coping self-statements can be very general positive self-statements, or they can be specific to particular problem areas or 'frequent flyer' automatic thoughts and beliefs."

COPING CARDS

- Tell clients: "Coping cards are used to record and display coping self-statements."
- "Construct a coping self-statement relevant to your pain situation."
- "Write it on a 3" × 5" index card."
- "Pick a place to display the card, and refer to it often."

HOMEWORK ASSIGNMENT

- Tell clients: "Construct at least three additional coping self-statements, and put them on separate coping cards."
- "Pick meaningful places to post them, and display them prominently."
- "Bring your homework to the next session, and be ready to discuss what you have learned with other group members."

POSTSESSION PROCESS CHECK

- Have clients fill out Postsession Process Check before they leave. Glance at responses and troubleshoot if necessary.

Session 7 Summary for Clients: Coping Self-Statements

THE GOAL OF THIS SESSION

- To construct and use positive coping self-statements.

REVIEW OF PREVIOUS WEEK'S SESSION

- Pain-specific beliefs are often held about the cause of pain, the meaning of pain, and the ability to influence the pain.
- Pain-related beliefs are also held about the self as a person in pain.
- Pain-related beliefs are ideas, and just like all ideas, they can be examined.
- One way to examine pain-related beliefs is to look at whether (and how) they are serving you.
- If pain-related beliefs are not serving you now, consider experimenting with an alternative belief by using the "acting as if" exercise.

HOMEWORK REVIEW

- Using the Identifying Pain Beliefs Worksheet:
  - What did you learn about how your pain-related automatic thoughts are connected to your pain beliefs and your beliefs about yourself as a person in pain?
- Using the Changing Pain Beliefs Worksheet:
  - It's usually easy to identify the disadvantages to holding onto a negative pain-related belief.
  - It's hard to identify the *advantages* of holding onto a negative pain-related belief. What did you learn?
- Using the "acting as if" exercise to experiment with a new belief:
  - What happened when you acted as if your new belief was a reality?
    - Did others respond differently to you?
    - Did you feel differently about yourself?

CONSTRUCTING AND USING POSITIVE COPING SELF-STATEMENTS

- Coping self-statements are the emotional "cheerleaders" in the coping repertoire, and can help to increase your sense of personal control and efficacy.
- "Locus of control" or ("LOC") beliefs are judgments about whether you have an internal (within yourself) or external (outside yourself) sense of control over your pain situation.
- "Self-efficacy" beliefs are judgments about your ability to accomplish a goal related to pain management.
- Coping self-statements can be very general positive self-statements, or they can be specific to particular problem areas or "frequent flyer" automatic thoughts and beliefs.
- Coping cards are used to record and display coping self-statements.
  - Construct a coping self-statement relevant to your pain situation.
  - Write it on a 3" × 5" index card.
  - Pick a place to display the card, and refer to it often

(continued)

From *Cognitive Therapy for Chronic Pain* by Beverly E. Thorn. Copyright 2004 by The Guilford Press. Permission to photocopy this handout is granted to purchasers of this book for personal use only (see copyright page for details).

SUMMARY OF KEY POINTS

- Coping self-statements are general positive self-statements.
- Coping self-statements can be used to increase your sense of personal control over aspects of your pain situation.
- Coping cards can be used to record and display coping self-statements.

HOMEWORK ASSIGNMENT

- Construct at least three additional coping self-statements and put them on separate coping cards.
- Pick meaningful places to post them, and display them prominently.
- Bring your homework to the next session, and be ready to discuss what you have learned with other group members.

Examples of Pain-Related Coping Self-Statements

- I tell myself that there are others who are much worse off than me.

- I tell myself to be brave and carry on despite the pain.

- I tell myself that I can overcome the pain.

- I "psych" myself up to deal with the pain, perhaps by telling myself that it won't last much longer.

- I try and imagine that for some reason it is important for me to endure the pain.

- I tell myself I can't let the pain stand in the way of what I have to do.

- I tell myself that I can cope with the pain without imagining or pretending anything.

- I concentrate on convincing myself that I will deal with the pain and that it will get better in the near future.

Copyright 1985 of original CCSI by Robert W. Butler. Copyright 2003 of CCSI-R by Beverly E. Thorn, L. Charles Ward, and Kristi L. Clements. Copyright 1983 of original CSQ by Anne K. Rosenstiel Gross. Copyright 1997 of CSQ-R by Joseph L. Riley and Michael E. Robinson. From *Cognitive Therapy for Chronic Pain* by Beverly E. Thorn. Copyright 2004 by The Guilford Press. Permission to photocopy this handout is granted to purchasers of this book for personal use only (see copyright page for details).

EXPRESSIVE WRITING

The eighth treatment session teaches clients an expressive writing exercise. Therapist Handout 8.1, found at the back of this module, provides an outline of Session 8 to be used by the therapist. Client Handout 8.1, also at the back of the module, can be copied and used as a session outline to be given to clients at the beginning of the session.

SESSION 8 TREATMENT OBJECTIVE
- **Learn and practice expressive writing.**

PRESESSION PROCESS CHECK AND REVIEW OF PREVIOUS WEEK'S SESSION

The session begins with the Presession Process Check and a review of the rationale behind constructing and using coping self-statements. Remind group members that coping self-statements are used as emotional motivators: They are general positive statements used to help clients feel that they have personal control over some aspects of their pain problem (locus of control) and that they can perform the kind of coping tasks that will make a difference in their pain problem (self-efficacy). Since the aim is for clients to use this as an ongoing cognitive coping technique, suggest to group members that they should switch their coping cards every couple of weeks. Encourage them to try a new color or a new saying, so that they will continue to take notice of the cards, and continue to use them.

HOMEWORK REVIEW

Group members were asked to come up with at least three coping self-statements for homework. In reviewing the homework, you want clients to report on the content of the statements they constructed, but you also want to hear about how and where they chose to display their coping cards. A brief session transcript follows.

THERAPIST: How did folks do with their coping cards? I'd like to hear about at least one new coping card you made for yourself. And where did you put your cards?

MARTHA ANNE: Well, I've been thinking about that one on the list you gave us—the one that said, "I try to imagine that for some reason it is important for me to endure the pain." There's really two ways to look at that one: first, that it could be a punishment and you're "sentenced" to suffer. Or another interpretation is that it's important to "endure" in order to not get sucked into the pain.

THERAPIST: Keep talking, Martha Anne. I think you're onto something.

MARTHA ANNE: Well, I changed the meaning of the word "endure," actually. I came up with "It's really important to go on with what's important in life, in spite of the pain." That's kind of a long one, I know.

DAVID: Sounds similar to the one I came up with: "Carry on despite the pain."

MARTHA ANNE: Yeah, but I want mine to be more toward the "what's important in life" part.

KIM: How about "Keep your focus on what's important in life"?

MARTHA ANNE: I like that, and then I could even list those things that *are* important to me in my life.

THERAPIST: Excellent idea, Martha Anne. And good work.

MELISSA: Lord, listen to us. We sound like the walking wounded!

MARTHA ANNE: Hmmm. We may be wounded, but we're walking! Hey, there's a slogan! (*Group laughs.*)

THERAPIST: Actually, Martha Anne, that's not a bad coping card for everyone, is it? It's catchy, and it puts a totally different spin on the "walking wounded" saying.

JENNIFER: Making lemonade out of lemons, my mom used to say.

THERAPIST: Not a bad thing to do with lemons, actually. Now how about places for the coping cards? Did anyone get creative?

JENNIFER: I pinned each one to a different throw pillow in the living room. I spend a lot of time in there, and I'm always picking up throw pillows. I told my kids they better not remove them or make fun of them!

THERAPIST: That's great, Jennifer! Now one thing about coping cards I didn't tell you earlier is that you should replace them with new ones every couple of weeks, or whenever a new situation comes up for you. Experiment with changing the colors of the cards, and changing where you post them, in order to keep noticing them. Coping cards can serve as a great positive reminder to you, as long as you keep working with them, and keep it so that you notice them. Now let's move on to the next topic.

After the homework review, it is time to move on to presenting the new treatment objective for Session 8: learning and practicing the expressive writing technique.

SESSION OBJECTIVE: LEARN AND PRACTICE EXPRESSIVE WRITING

Expressive writing exercises involve having clients write about their deepest thoughts and feelings regarding trauma, loss, or illness. Since the instructions for the exercise presented in this module ask clients to write about their deepest thoughts and feelings, this exercise specifically includes *emotions* as well as thoughts, and encourages their expression. Therefore, the expressive writing exercise processes emotions as well as cognitions. Directly targeting and processing emotions are another means by which patients can cope with the stress of long-term, potentially debilitating pain. In addition, as I have noted in Chapter 3, expressive writing may provide an appropriate outlet for venting without risking negative responses from others.

> The purpose of this week's session is to introduce something called "expressive writing." Scientific research has shown that writing about emotional circumstances in our lives can actually help us to function better, both physically and emotionally. And expressive writing exercises have been shown to be particularly useful for patients with a variety of serious medical problems. Expressive writing may help us to make sense out of our deepest thoughts and emotions regarding seriously stressful life events. Also, expressive writing is a way to "get it off our chests" without burdening our loved ones with our negative thoughts and feelings.
>
> You've already seen that people have negative thoughts they might not even be aware of, and once they become aware of them, they can learn to challenge the distorted part and construct alternative thoughts. The expressive writing exercise you will be learning today focuses more on your emotions, but asks you to write about both your deepest emotions and your deepest thoughts. When you write down your deepest thoughts and emotions, you may be aware that they are not necessarily "facts," especially since you've learned about distorted thoughts in earlier sessions. However, writing down your thoughts and feelings helps you to begin dealing with them instead of denying their existence. Although many people report that expressive writing initially makes them feel sad or even depressed, these feelings usually go away fairly soon. Especially with your new tools for recognizing and challenging distortions, you may find it quite easy by now to vent negative thoughts and emotions, and be done with them for a period of time.
>
> Let's start with an in-session exercise. First, rest assured that your writing is for you and you alone. You don't need to share the content of your writing with the group, and we will not ask to look at your writing—you can throw it away as soon as you're finished, if you like. Sometimes people censor what they write if they know that someone else is going to read it, and we don't want you to censor anything in this exercise. We are going to take 10 minutes now, and I'd like you to write about your deepest thoughts and feelings regarding your chronic pain condition. Really let go, and allow yourself to explore all of your emotions and thoughts about it. You might tie your thoughts and feelings regarding your pain condition to other aspects of your life—to changes that you may not have discussed in great detail with others; to your childhood; to your loved ones; or to your concept of yourself and who you want to be. The most important part of this exercise is to really explore your deepest thoughts and feelings. It is natural to feel a broad range of

emotions, including sadness or grief, when you do this exercise. If you find yourself getting extremely upset about what you are writing, just change topics. The only rule is to write continuously for 10 minutes. If you run out of things to write, go ahead and repeat what you have already written. Don't bother erasing or crossing stuff out. Just write. Don't worry about grammar, or spelling, or sentences. Just write.[1]

Troubleshooting Tip: Clients have different reactions to the expressive writing exercise, and some group members may get tearful. Usually by this time in the group, members are comfortable with each other's occasional tears. Sometimes group members will want to discuss the content of their writing; this is acceptable, but it is not the point of the exercise, and clients should in no way feel obligated to do so. Although some people find it therapeutic to share what they have written, and we are not trying to forbid them to do so, the point of the expressive writing exercise is to encourage the clients to write without concerns regarding who might read it and what they might think—to express their thoughts and feelings with abandon.

After the exercise, ask clients to discuss how they responded to the exercise itself, and explain to them how this is different from sharing the *content* of their writing. Remind clients that expressive writing goes beyond the cognitive restructuring exercises that they practiced in earlier sessions, because expressive writing focuses more on emotions than on thoughts, and provides an avenue to vent these emotions. An example from a session transcript appears below.

THERAPIST: Now that you've completed your first expressive writing exercise, I'd like to spend a few minutes checking to see how it was for you. I'm not asking you to share the contents of your writing, but instead to talk about how the exercise made you feel.

JENNIFER: I'm shocked at how furious I must be under the surface. No wonder I get angry at others so much of the time. I seem to be mad at the world!

THERAPIST: So for you, Jennifer, the exercise opened your eyes to a real anger you're carrying around with you.

JENNIFER: Yes, and it's not doing me a bit of good, I can see that. I don't think my anger caused my pain problem, but it's not helping my pain, either.

THERAPIST: We're not about figuring out what caused your pain. We *are* about figuring out how your thoughts and emotions can have a powerful impact on your pain problem, and figuring out how to channel your thoughts and emotions in a way that can do you powerful good.

DAVID: Boy, this writing made me sad. Talk about being the walking wounded! I must be the poster child!

THERAPIST: When folks do these writing exercises, they often say that they feel sad or even depressed afterward, but that the sadness soon leaves. A very common reaction, though, is also surprise—that we carry around such deep emotions without being fully aware that they are weighting us down. It's almost as if we tell ourselves that if we deny the emo-

---

[1]Instructions for the expressive writing exercise are based on James W. Pennebaker's typical instructions (*http://www.homepage.psy.utexas.edu/homepage/faculty/home2000/JWPhome.htm*), as well as Annette L. Stanton's instructions used in her clinical research on patients with cancer (Stanton, personal communication, August 20, 2003).

tions, they'll go away. But there they are, stuck under the surface, where we can't do
much about them.

KIM: I said it before, and I'll say it again. I don't want to go this deep with the emotional stuff!
I spent my 10 minutes writing about how I was mad at you for making me try!

THERAPIST: That's absolutely fine, Kim. It's okay to be mad at me, and it's okay to use your
expressive writing time to write about being mad at me. The point of the exercise is *not*
to get anyone to write about emotions that are too upsetting for them. And, remember,
one suggestion is that if you find yourself becoming extremely upset about your writing
topic, simply switch topics. You are in charge. And we are not assuming that everyone
has terrible, pent-up emotions boiling beneath their surface that *must* be expressed. The
exercise is there for you to use as you see fit.

Troubleshooting Tip: As you can see from the transcript above, Kim was quite resistant
to the process of going deep into her emotions. This sort of resistance should be honored with
a permissive stance. Remember that if it appears that a client is unlikely to comply with a particular homework assignment, it is better to remove the assignment altogether, or substan-
tially adapt it, than to set the client up for a failure experience. At the end of the session, I
checked in with Kim to see how she was feeling about the assignment. She was still angry,
and said that the chances were only "50–50" that she would do the assignment (and there was
a similar unstated implication regarding her attendance at the next session). Given this, I suggested to Kim that she continue with the coping card assignment rather than participate in
the expressive writing assignment. Alternatively, she could choose to write, but choose a topic
that was not based on her emotions. She decided to choose the latter assignment. (What she
did with this is described in a session transcript in Treatment Module 9.) You will sometimes
find that once you remove the need for client resistance (via a permissive stance), the client
stops resisting.

HOMEWORK ASSIGNMENT

For homework, group members are asked to practice the expressive writing exercise for 10
minutes each day, for a minimum of 3 consecutive days during the coming week. The subject
of their writing should be the same as the in-session topic; that is, they should write about
their deepest thoughts and feelings about their chronic pain condition. See Therapist Handout 8.2 and Client Handout 8.1 for specific instructions.

It is also up to the individual clients whether they choose to share their writing with another person or persons. While sharing the writing should not by any means be forbidden,
the point is for the clients to write without censoring—and often when people expect others
to see their writing, they temper or justify what they write, in a way that sabotages this particular exercise.

Some group members will quickly recognize that much of what they write down will include negative, distorted automatic thoughts and beliefs, and since they have had the opportunity to incorporate cognitive restructuring into their coping repertoire, they will catch
themselves as they are writing down the distorted thoughts. The point of this exercise,
though, is not necessarily to get clients to challenge the thoughts and emotions, but to give

them an opportunity to voice those emotions without being criticized or punished for them, and without turning others off or away.

    Troubleshooting Tip: Sometimes a client with a lot of anger built up at a particular person (often a spouse) may want to use this opportunity to "dump" anger on the spouse or partner by writing it all down, and then "requiring" that the spouse read and respond to it, justifying the ultimatum as part of the therapy. Expressive writing is *not* meant to be a communication exercise (the communication exercise is the topic of the next session). So, although you do not want to forbid clients to share their writing, you also want to caution them that this exercise is *not* intended as a means of communication. Assure them that you will be providing them a means for them to communicate effectively during the next session.

POSTSESSON PROCESS CHECK

As always, hand out the Postsession Process Check, and ask clients to fill it out before they leave.

Session 8 Outline for Therapists: Expressive Writing

SESSION OBJECTIVE

- Learn and practice expressive writing.

NEEDED MATERIALS, HANDOUTS, AND WORKSHEETS

- Paper and pencils for group members
- Session 8 Outline for Therapists (this handout)
- Session 8 Summary for Clients (Client Handout 8.1)
- Presession Process Check (Appendix J)
- General Instructions for Expressive Writing (Client Handout 8.2)
- Postsession Process Check (Appendix J)

PRESESSION PROCESS CHECK

- Handout Presession Process Check and have clients fill it in.

REVIEW OF PREVIOUS WEEK'S SESSION

- Remind clients: "Coping self-statements are the emotional 'cheerleaders' in the coping repertoire."
- "Coping self-statements increase your sense of personal control over some aspects of your chronic pain situation."
- "Coping self-statements increase your sense that you *can* do the things you need to do to better manage the pain and the stress associated with the pain situation."
- "Coping self-statements can be very general positive self-statements, or they can be specific to a particular situation that you need help dealing with."
- "Coping self-statements are particularly useful for 'frequent flyer' automatic thoughts and beliefs."
- "Coping cards are used to record and display coping self-statements."

HOMEWORK REVIEW

- Ask several clients: "What coping self-statements did you put on your coping cards?"
- "Where did you display your coping cards?
- "What did you learn from using the coping cards?"

(continued)

From *Cognitive Therapy for Chronic Pain* by Beverly E. Thorn. Copyright 2004 by The Guilford Press. Permission to photocopy this handout is granted to purchasers of this book for personal use only (see copyright page for details).

SESSION OBJECTIVE: LEARN AND PRACTICE EXPRESSIVE WRITING

- Say to clients: "Writing about emotional experiences in our lives can help us function better and feel better."
- "Expressive writing focuses on emotions more than thoughts, but it is a tool for self-expression of your deepest feelings *and* thoughts."
- "You may not even be aware of some deep feelings associated with your pain situation. If so, writing about your feelings can help you identify them."
- "You may be aware of some feelings, but think you should not express them for fear of getting 'carried away' with your emotions. If so, writing about them can help show you that you have more control over negative emotions than you thought you did."
- "You may be concerned that expressing negative emotions might hurt others, or might drive them away. If so, writing about them can allow you to express them without burdening others or hurting them, but to honor your feelings at the same time."
- "You may discover that your deep thoughts and feelings have distortions (just like your automatic thoughts and beliefs sometimes do). If so, writing about them anyway can help you vent them and be done with them for a time."

EXPRESSIVE WRITING EXERCISE

- Tell clients: "Take 10 minutes and write about your deepest thoughts and feelings regarding your pain situation."
- "When you write, write just for yourself—not as if you were going to share it with someone. This allows you to write anything you want without censoring it."
- "You might tie your thoughts and feelings regarding your pain condition to other aspects of your life—to changes that you may not have discussed in great detail with others; to your childhood; to your loved ones; or to your concept of yourself and who you want to be."
- "Write continuously for 10 minutes—don't worry about spelling, grammar, or repeating yourself. If you run out of things to say, simply repeat what you have said."
- "It's natural to experience a wide range of emotions, including sadness and anger, and it's okay to express them."
- "If you find yourself getting extremely upset about what you are writing about, simply switch topics and continue writing."

(continued)

HOMEWORK ASSIGNMENT

- Say to clients: "Practice the expressive writing exercise for 10 minutes each day, for a minimum of 3 consecutive days during the coming week. Again, write about your deepest thoughts and feelings about your chronic pain condition. You might tie your thoughts and feelings regarding your pain condition to other aspects of your life—to changes that you may not have discussed in great detail with others; to your childhood; to your loved ones; or to your concept of yourself and who you want to be. You can write either in longhand or on a computer. If you can't write, you can talk into a tape recorder. You can choose to write about the same thing every day, or you can write about a different aspect of your pain condition on each day. The goal is to explore your deepest thoughts and feelings about your pain condition, and to write continuously for 10 minutes for at least 3 consecutive days. If you run out of things to say before the 10 minutes are up, you can just repeat what you have said. If you find yourself getting extremely upset about what you are writing, simply switch topics. Don't worry about grammar, or erasing, or crossing out. The goal is to just write.

  "Your writing is meant for you and you alone. It is up to you whether you keep what you have written or throw it away. Some people choose to keep what they have written, so that they can look back over their writing and see how their thoughts and feelings change over time. Other people make a ceremony out of destroying their writing samples—by burning them; tearing them into pieces and 'offering' them to a lake or ocean; erasing them; or running them through a paper shredder. The choice is yours."

POSTSESSION PROCESS CHECK

- Have clients fill out Postsession Process Check before they leave. Glance at responses and troubleshoot if necessary.

Session 8 Summary for Clients: Expressive Writing

THE GOAL OF THIS SESSION

- To learn and practice expressive writing.

REVIEW OF PREVIOUS WEEK'S SESSION

- Coping self-statements are the emotional "cheerleaders" in our coping repertoire.
- Coping self-statements increase your sense of personal control over some aspects of your chronic pain situation.
- Coping self-statements increase your sense that you *can* do the things you need to do to better manage the pain and the stress associated with the pain situation.
- Coping self-statements can be very general positive self-statements, or they can be specific to a particular situation that you need help dealing with.
- Coping self-statements are particularly useful for "frequent flyer" automatic thoughts and beliefs.
- Coping cards are used to record and display coping self-statements.

HOMEWORK REVIEW

- Ask clients: "What coping self-statements did you put on your coping cards?"
- "Where did you display your coping cards?"
- "What did you learn from using the coping cards?"

EXPRESSIVE WRITING EXERCISE

- Take 10 minutes and write about your deepest thoughts and feelings regarding your pain situation.
- When you write, write just for yourself—not as if you were going to share it with someone. This allows you to write anything you want without censoring it.
- You might tie your thoughts and feelings regarding your pain condition to other aspects of your life—to changes that you may not have discussed in great detail with others; to your childhood; to your loved ones; or to your concept of yourself and who you want to be.
- Write continuously for 10 minutes—don't worry about spelling, grammar, or repeating yourself. If you run out of things to say, simply repeat what you have said.
- It's natural to experience a wide range of emotions, including sadness and anger, and it's okay to express them.
- If you find yourself getting extremely upset about what you are writing about, simply switch topics and continue writing.

(continued)

Adapted by permission of Annette L. Stanton in *Copyright Therapy for Chronic Pain* by Beverly E. Thorn. Copyright 2004 by The Guilford Press. Permission to photocopy this handout is granted to purchasers of this book for personal use only (see copyright page for details).

SUMMARY OF KEY POINTS

- Expressive writing helps you recognize and process emotions as well as thoughts.
- Expressive writing gives you an outlet for venting strong emotions without overwhelming others or risking their criticism.
- Expressive writing is meant for *you*, rather than as a tool for communicating with others.
- You can keep what you write, or you can throw it away.
- If you find yourself getting too upset by a writing topic, simply switch topics—you are in charge!

HOMEWORK ASSIGNMENT

- Practice the expressive writing exercise for 10 minutes each day, for a minimum of 3 consecutive days during the coming week. Write about your deepest thoughts and feelings about your chronic pain condition. You might tie your thoughts and feelings regarding your pain condition to other aspects of your life—to changes that you may not have discussed in great detail with others; to your childhood; to your loved ones; or to your concept of yourself and who you want to be. You can write either in longhand or on a computer. If you can't write, you can talk into a tape recorder. You can choose to write about the same thing every day, or you can write about a different aspect of your pain condition on each day. The goal is to explore your deepest thoughts and feelings about your pain condition, and to write continuously for 10 minutes for at least 3 consecutive days. If you run out of things to say before the 10 minutes are up, you can just repeat what you have said. If you find yourself getting extremely upset about what you are writing, simply switch topics. Don't worry about grammar, or erasing, or crossing out. The goal is to just write.

  Your writing is meant for you and you alone. It is up to you whether you keep what you have written or throw it away. Some people choose to keep what they have written so that they can look back over their writing and see how their thoughts and feelings change over time. Other people make a ceremony out of destroying their writing samples—by burning them; tearing them into pieces and "offering" them to a lake or ocean; erasing them; or running them through a paper shredder. The choice is yours.

ASSERTIVE COMMUNICATION

The ninth treatment session introduces assertive communication. Therapist Handout 9.1, found at the back of this module, provides an outline of Session 9 to be used by the therapist. Client Handout 9.1, also at the back of the module, can be copied and used as a session outline to be given to clients at the beginning of the session.

SESSION 9 TREATMENT OBJECTIVES

- **Learn about assertive communication.**
- **Plan an assertive communication.**

PRESESSION PROCESS CHECK AND REVIEW OF PREVIOUS WEEK'S SESSION

After the Precession Process Check is completed, review what was covered in Session 8. Last week's treatment session introduced a new avenue for helping clients cope with their chronic pain—the expressive writing exercise. In reviewing the rationale for the exercise, focus on two things: first, that this tool has been shown to be of therapeutic benefit to individuals with a variety of medical problems; and second, that people often ignore or deny their deep feelings without honoring them and allowing them to be expressed. The idea behind expressive writing is that it is a tool for processing (and venting) a person's deepest thoughts and emotions. The way we use it in this treatment program, it is a means for clients to really let go and express feelings about their chronic pain condition, without fear of being judged or turning anyone off.

HOMEWORK REVIEW

In checking in about the homework, bear in mind that the point is not to get people to share what they have written, but to share what they have *learned* in doing the writing exercise, particularly after having done the exercise for 3 or more consecutive days. Clients will often say that after they wrote for several days in a row, their feelings began to change. The intense emotions they may have been surprised by at first are now in their immediate awareness, and are not unknown "monsters." At times, an issue will surface that may necessitate individual sessions in order to process more completely than is appropriate for the group format. Needing to do so in no way negates the value of the exercise, nor does it require removing such clients from the group while helping them process their strong emotions. Finally, clients will often state that after writing for 3 days, they don't feel a need to continue the exercise, at least not for the topic they were writing about. This is fine; in fact, it is a natural consequence of writing and processing their emotions. Now that they have another tool to use, they can file it away for future use when it seems appropriate. An example of the homework review from a session transcript is provided below.

THERAPIST: I would like to hear how the expressive writing exercise went. I'm interested in knowing how you responded to the exercise, rather than necessarily hearing about the content of your writing.

JENNIFER: You know, now that I realize how mad I am, I'm not so mad any more! Go figure that!

THERAPIST: Can you give us an example of how or when you noticed you weren't so mad this week?

JENNIFER: Yeah, at work. My supervisor came up to me and very rudely interrupted what I was doing. In the past, I would have gotten my hackles up for sure (not to mention gotten a killer headache). I actually found it amusing! It was like I was observing her from afar, and observing that I didn't have to get all in a sweat just because she was excited. I found myself saying, "There's really no problem here; you didn't do anything wrong." And I'll be darned—when I didn't get upset, she calmed down, too.

THERAPIST: Great example, Jennifer. Thank you for sharing that. I really liked the part about you actually being amused by the situation. That's new for you, eh?

JENNIFER: Oh, yeah! (*grinning*)

THERAPIST: Anyone else?

KIM: All right, I know everyone will be shocked, but I did the exercise, and it wasn't so bad. It made me sad, but I didn't die or anything. I had a good cry about my pain, and I found out that I'm mostly afraid—afraid of getting to the point where there are no more medicines that work, or afraid of getting addicted to them, or both.[1]

THERAPIST: Kim, it sounds like you got in touch with some fears that you might have been avoiding, because they're so, well, scary. Sometimes expressing them is the first step to

---

[1]Notice that although I had removed the assignment for Kim to do an expressive writing exercise regarding her emotions, she chose to do so anyway. When that happens, you don't need to make a special point about clients' doing so. They're already aware of it.

them not being so scary. Did you find your thoughts and feelings, particularly the scared part, change at all over the time you did the exercise?

KIM: Well, it renewed my resolve to cut down on the amount of medicines I take, and lessen my reliance on them. Sometimes I'm just too quick to pop a pill, because I'm afraid my pain might get bad. I'm going to talk to my doctor more about this.

THERAPIST: Great. And, with your permission, I'll drop him a note letting him know that you talked about wanting to reduce your meds if possible. Okay?

KIM: That'd be good.

THERAPIST: Anyone else?

MARTHA ANNE: I'm just feeling much more philosophical about this "God is punishing me" business. It's just a whole lot less "doomsday" than it was.

THERAPIST: That's so good to hear. Now you guys know that you have another tool in your toolbox, especially when you feel strong emotional upset and aren't sure what to do. You can keep on doing the expressive writing exercise as long as it serves you. And come back to it when you feel the time is right.

Following the homework review, introduce the new treatment goal for today's session, which is assertive communication training.

SESSION OBJECTIVE: LEARN ABOUT ASSERTIVE COMMUNICATION

This treatment module offers some practical suggestions for expressing one's needs in an assertive and more effective fashion. Patients with chronic pain—especially those individuals who engage in a lot of catastrophic thinking—may have a high need for emotional support, but insufficient communication skills to express themselves in an assertive manner. Individuals dealing with chronic pain, like everyone else, need to be able to ask for what they want and need in a straightforward, unapologetic, and honest manner. Assertiveness skills provide just such a means.

> As we all know, there is a big difference between *short-term* pain and *long-term* pain. In the short run, doctors seem motivated to find out what's wrong, and loved ones are eager to give us emotional support. However, as pain drags on and becomes a chronic, ongoing problem, physicians can become less attentive, and loved ones may grow weary of the daily pain reports and distress. To make matters worse, when our distress is really high, we tend to express ourselves in a *really* negative emotional manner, and we can actually do the opposite of what we intend to do—that is, overwhelm others and drive them away.
>
> Since the pain doesn't go away just because others get tired of hearing about it, people experiencing chronic pain are in a real bind. They still need emotional support and understanding. They may also sometimes need others to help them with daily responsibilities. In addition, people with pain, just like everyone else, have general (non-pain-related) wants and needs, and they have a right to be able to ask for what they want. The point of this session is to help you express your wants and needs in an assertive way that increases the likelihood of getting you what you need, but does not drive others away in the process.
>
> Often people are able to respond assertively in some situations, but not others. For example, they may have a difficult time asking for what they want and need from people

who are close to them, like family members. But when people feel unable to assert themselves, or lack the skills to be assertive, communication breaks down and relationships suffer. Sometimes unassertive individuals switch back and forth between passive and aggressive behavior in dealing with others. Passive or submissive behavior tends to discount your own needs while putting other's needs first. This style avoids confrontation and rejection, but can make you feel like a doormat. Aggressive behavior involves demanding what you want in a hostile, angry, or accusatory manner. People who use this style of communication avoid getting pushed around, but others avoid them.

Assertiveness involves asking for what you want or saying no to something in a simple, direct, and honest manner. Sometimes it's hard to know what it is that you want. We often have an easy time figuring out what is bothering us about another person, but we may have a harder time figuring out what we want instead. You have the right to express your feelings, to ask for what you want, and to say no. Assertiveness involves the skill of doing that without disrespecting others, but at the same time standing up for yourself without guilt or apology. Bear in mind that other people are not mind readers. Most people are caught up in their own thoughts and problems; they don't focus on what's going on with you unless you tell them directly. Most people respond very favorably to assertive behavior, because it's clear where you stand and what you want.

Assertiveness also involves nonverbal behaviors. Nonverbal assertive behaviors include looking directly at a person when you are speaking to her, remaining calm, and standing your ground (that is, not backing off or moving away from the person as you are speaking to her). It's also important to hold an open, rather than closed, posture (that is, have your body turned toward the other person and your arms resting easily at your side or on your lap, rather than turning your body away, hunching over, or crossing your arms in front of you).

SESSION OBJECTIVE: PLAN AN ASSERTIVE COMMUNICATION

After introducing the concept of assertiveness, help group members work through the steps of assertiveness by providing an in-session exercise.

WORKSHEET: ASSERTIVENESS WORKSHEET

Hand each group member the Assertiveness Worksheet (Client Handout 9.2), and begin working through the steps with group members. The point of the in-session work is to help clients plan for an actual attempt at an assertive response to a problematic situation during the upcoming week. It often helps to provide an example for clients to refer to while learning how to plan an assertive response using the worksheet. An example is included as Client Handout 9.3 at the back of this module. You can make up your own if you need a more representative vignette for a particular population with pain.

Troubleshooting Tip: Working through the assertiveness exercise takes some time, but is quite informative for the group members. They are often surprised to recognize that their typical response patterns have been passive, aggressive, or both. They are also taken aback at how difficult constructing an assertive response seems to be. And they will sometimes put up resistance to the entire exercise as being contrived or unnatural, and thus not applicable to real life. A representative in-session transcript illustrates some common reactions.

MARTHA ANNE: You know, it's funny, but doing this exercise makes me realize that I always thought I was being "nice" when I didn't ask for what I wanted directly. Here I've been thinking it's a virtue, and instead it's a liability!

KRISTI: But it is important to be nice. And I sure don't want to be seen as a "pushy broad"!

THERAPIST: The difference between begin pushy and being assertive is that assertiveness is not being bossy or demanding. Assertiveness is making a straightforward request. But it does require that you ask for what you want directly.

KRISTI: Sometimes I don't even know what I want. I want someone else to figure it out for me.

THERAPIST: There are two problems with that. First, it means that you'll be receiving what the other person may think you want or need, not necessarily what *you* want or need. Second, it puts the other person in the position of being a mind reader.

TONY: Yeah. I can't stand it when my wife gets mad at me for something I didn't even know she wanted me to do, and then she says, "If you really cared about my feelings, you would know that going out to dinner on Friday was important to me," or some such thing like that!

THERAPIST: We all do a bit of that to our loved ones at times, but being on the receiving end never feels good. What if your wife stated up front that going out to dinner on Friday was important to her, and that it would make her feel happy and cared for if the two of you went?

TONY: Honestly, it would make me nervous, 'cause we don't have the money. But if I knew it was that important to her, we could find a way. I couldn't hardly just avoid the issue if she was that honest.

MARTHA ANNE: But, see, there's no guarantee that the other person is going to do what you want them to do, even if you go out on a limb and risk asking directly.

THERAPIST: You're right, Martha Anne. There are no guarantees that your request *will* be granted. But at least this way, you've got a better chance. And the person hearing your request knows exactly what you want. Everyone knows where they stand.

PAT: I have a problem with the whole exercise bit to this. It's not as if we're going to have the time to run into a problem situation, go to our rooms for 30 minutes, sketch out a response, and then come back and deliver it. That's just not real-life—it's dorky!

THERAPIST: Learning any new skill can feel awkward and unnatural. Remember learning to ride a bike or skate? "Dorky" is the exact word I'd use to describe myself at that time. But there's something to going through the steps in a systematic way that helps us learn to put the skill into real-life practice.

PAT: I'm just afraid I can't pull this off. My family won't know what to do with me if I start asking for what I want. They already see me as the big drain on the family fun. They'll probably get mad at me!

MELISSA: Oh, oh. I think Pat needs to get out her Automatic Thoughts Worksheet! (*Group laughs.*)

THERAPIST: It does sound like there were some automatic thoughts that slipped in there. Dealing with them may reduce your apprehension about this exercise, Pat. But it's okay to be apprehensive. This is a new skill for you, and our loved ones do respond differently when we change. Sometimes they don't like it when we change, because it frightens them at first. It's important to know that most people report a *very positive* shift in their relationships as they learn to become assertive. And people tend to respect you more when you're assertive.

HOMEWORK ASSIGNMENT

As homework, ask group members to use their Assertiveness Worksheet to work on at least one problem situation in which they would like to respond assertively. Although it is fine for them to continue working on the problem situation they identified in session, ask them to identify and write out at least one additional problem situation and assertiveness response, using their worksheet. In addition to *planning* an assertive response, ask clients to *practice* an assertive response during the week. Remind clients that assertive responses do not always produce the desired outcome, but even so, people tend to feel much better about themselves if they have been assertive instead of passive or aggressive. Let clients know that once they have tried out an assertive response, you will be able to help them problem-solve during the homework review the following week.

Since the next session is the last session, also ask clients to begin thinking about the last session, what they'd like to get out of it, and questions or concerns they may still have.

POSTSESSION PROCESS CHECK

Once again, hand out the Postsession Process Check, and ask clients to fill it out before they leave.

Session 9 Outline for Therapists: Assertive Communication

SESSION OBJECTIVES

- Learn about assertive communication.
- Plan an assertive communication.

NEEDED MATERIALS, HANDOUTS, AND WORKSHEETS

- Session 9 Outline for Therapists (this handout)
- Session 9 Summary for Clients (Client Handout 9.1)
- Presession Process Check (Appendix J)
- Assertiveness Worksheet (Client Handout 9.2)
- Example: Brian's Completed Assertiveness Worksheet (Client Handout 9.3)
- Postsession Process Check (Appendix J)

PRESESSION PROCESS CHECK

- Hand out Presession Process Check and have clients fill it in.

REVIEW OF PREVIOUS WEEK'S SESSION

- Expressive writing has been shown to help people with a variety of medical disorders.
- Often we are unaware of, or even deny, our deepest thoughts and feelings. If so, expressive writing helps us to identify them, honor them, and understand them.
- Expressive writing allows us to vent our negative feelings without burdening others or turning them off.
- Expressive writing teaches us that even strong negative emotions do not have a hold over us. Identifying them and expressing them help us to be in charge of them.
- Expressive writing may help us identify negatively distorted emotions. Writing them down may clarify the distortions, and may help us be rid of them for a time.

HOMEWORK REVIEW

- Ask several clients: "What did you learn about the process of expressive writing, particularly after doing it for at least 3 days in a row?"
  - "Did the topics you wrote about change over time?"
  - "Did your feelings change as you continued to write?"
- "Is this a tool that has value on a continuing basis, or on a periodic basis, for you?"
- "Remember that you can share or not share your writing, and can keep or not keep your writing—the choice is yours in each case."

(continued)

From *Cognitive Therapy for Chronic Pain* by Beverly E. Thorn. Copyright 2004 by The Guilford Press. Permission to photocopy this handout is granted to purchasers of this book for personal use only (see copyright page for details).

SESSION OBJECTIVE: LEARN ABOUT ASSERTIVE COMMUNICATION

- Provide clients with the rationale for assertiveness:
  - "Most of us are unskilled when it comes to assertiveness."
  - "You may act assertively in some situations, but have difficulty making requests or saying no to family members or close friends."
  - "Many clients with chronic pain problems have special needs for support from others, but often do not ask for it."
  - "You have the right to express your feelings, to ask for what you want, and to say no."
- Give clients this definition of assertiveness: "A way of communicating and behaving in any situation where you would like to express your feelings, ask for what you want, or say no to something you don't want."
- Tell clients that learning to be assertive involves the following:
  - "Becoming aware of your own unique feelings, needs, and wants."
  - "Communicating your feelings, wants, and needs to others (remember that other people are not mind readers)."
  - "Developing nonverbal assertive behaviors (looking directly at another person, holding an open posture, standing your ground, and staying calm)."
  - "Developing assertive verbal behaviors (using simple and direct 'I' statements to object to behaviors, state your feelings, and make requests)."

SESSION OBJECTIVE: PLAN AN ASSERTIVE COMMUNICATION

Worksheet: Assertiveness Worksheet

- Give out copies of the Assertiveness Worksheet.
- Tell clients: "Using the steps outlined in the worksheet, plan an assertive communication in response to a problem situation. Writing out a plan ahead of time increases the chances of success."
  - "Identify a problem situation."
  - "Plan your assertive communication of the problem to the person involved."
  - "Plan your assertive request (or response)."

HOMEWORK ASSIGNMENT

- Tell clients: "During the coming week, make at least one additional assertiveness plan in response to an identified problem situation. Then *try out* at least one planned assertive communication with the person who is involved in the problem."
- "Remember to choose a problem situation that has meaning for you, but not the most challenging problem situation that you can identify. Starting the process of assertive communication gradually, with a less challenging situation, increases your chances of success and boosts your self-confidence. Come to the next group ready to discuss how it went."
- "Also, since next week is our last treatment session, think about questions you might have regarding the group, or how to proceed from here. Think about what you particularly liked about the group, and what didn't fit as well for you. We will discuss these things next week."

POSTSESSION PROCESS CHECK

- Have clients fill out Postsession Process Check before they leave. Glance at responses and troubleshoot if necessary.

Session 9 Summary for Clients: Assertive Communication

THE GOALS OF THIS SESSION

- To learn about assertive communication.
- To plan an assertive communication.

REVIEW OF PREVIOUS WORK'S SESSION

- Expressive writing has been shown to help people with a variety of medical disorders.
- Often we are unaware of, or even deny, our deepest thoughts and feelings. If so, expressive writing helps us to identify them, honor them, and understand them.
- Expressive writing allows us to vent our negative feelings without burdening others or turning them off.
- Expressive writing teaches us that even strong negative emotions do not have a hold over us. Identifying them and expressing them help us to be in charge of them.
- Expressive writing may help us identify negatively distorted emotions. Writing them down may clarify the distortions, and may help us be rid of them for a time.

HOMEWORK REVIEW

- What did you learn about the process of expressive writing, particularly after doing it for at least 3 days in a row?
  - Did the topics you wrote about change over time?
  - Did your feelings change as you continued to write?
- Is this a tool that has value on a continuing basis, or on a periodic basis, for you?
- Remember that you can share or not share your writing, and can keep or not keep your writing—the choice is yours in each case.

LEARNING ABOUT ASSERTIVE COMMUNICATION

- This is the rationale for assertiveness:
  - Most of us are unskilled when it comes to assertiveness.
  - You may act assertively in some situations, but have difficulty making requests or saying no to family members or close friends.
  - Many clients with chronic pain problems have special needs for support from others, but often do not ask for it.
  - You have the right to express your feelings, to ask for what you want, and to say no.
- Here is a definition of assertiveness: A way of communicating and behaving in any situation where you would like to express your feelings, ask for what you want, or say no to something you don't want.

(continued)

From *Cognitive Therapy for Chronic Pain* by Beverly E. Thorn. Copyright 2004 by The Guilford Press. Permission to photocopy this handout is granted to purchasers of this book for personal use only (see copyright page for details).

- Learning to be assertive involves the following:
  - Becoming aware of your own unique feelings, needs, and wants.
  - Communicating your feelings, wants, and needs to others (remember that other people are not mind readers).
  - Developing nonverbal assertive behaviors (looking directly at another person, holding an open posture, standing your ground, and staying calm).
  - Developing assertive verbal behaviors (using simple and direct "I" statements to object to behaviors, state your feelings, and make requests).

PLANNING AN ASSERTIVE COMMUNICATION

- Using the steps outlined in the Assertiveness Worksheet, plan an assertive communication in response to a problem situation. Writing out a plan ahead of time increases the chances of success.
  - Identify a problem situation.
  - Plan your assertive communication of the problem to the person involved.
  - Plan your assertive request (or response).

SUMMARY OF KEY POINTS

- You have a right to express your wants and needs in a straightforward and unapologetic manner.
- Assertive communication helps you to do so.
- Assertive communication is not mean or selfish—it helps people to know exactly where you stand.
- Your loved ones may not be used to assertive communication, but most people respond very well to it.

HOMEWORK ASSIGNMENT

- During the coming week, make at least one additional assertiveness plan in response to an identified problem situation. Then *try out* at least one planned assertive communication with the person who is involved in the problem.
- Remember to choose a problem situation that has meaning for you, but not the most challenging problem situation that you can identify. Starting the process of assertive communication gradually, with a less challenging situation, increases your chances of success and boosts your self-confidence. Come to the next group ready to discuss how it went.
- Also, since next week is our last treatment session, think about questions you might have regarding the group, or how to proceed from here. Think about what you particularly liked about the group, and what didn't fit as well for you. We will discuss these things next week.

Assertiveness Worksheet

STEP 1: IDENTIFY A PROBLEM SITUATION

Think of one situation that is a problem for you right now—one that you'd like to handle assertively. Choose a situation that's not too overwhelming, but one that has meaning for you. Write down your answers to the following questions:

• What is the problem?

• Who is involved?

• How does it make you feel?

• What do you want?

• How would you normally handle the problem?

• What do you think would happen if you gave an assertive response?

STEP 2: PLAN THE ASSERTIVE RESPONSE

Reminding yourself what you want, and that you have the right to ask for it, list the steps involved in making an assertive response. Writing out your response ahead of time, especially when you are first learning assertiveness, increases your chances of success:

• Think of a time and place convenient for both of you. (Note: You may have to ask the other person when you could have 15 minutes to talk.) Write this down.

(continued)

From *Cognitive Therapy for Chronic Pain* by Beverly E. Thorn. Copyright 2004 by The Guilford Press. Permission to photocopy this handout is granted to purchasers of this book for personal use only (see copyright page for details).

- Now write down the problem, the way you want to describe it to the other person.
  - State the problem objectively, and avoid accusing or blaming with "you" statements. ("You" statements often put others on the defensive, and then they don't listen.)
  - Object to the person's behavior, not the person.
  - State your feelings about the situation, using "I" rather than "you." ("I" statements acknowledge that you are responsible for your feelings.)
  - *Example*: "I feel left out when you and the kids go to the movies without asking me," *rather than* "You don't care about me or my feelings—you take the kids to the movies without even asking me."
- **My Problem:**

STEP 3: WRITE DOWN YOUR REQUEST

- Keep the request short and simple.
- Be specific.
- Use "I" statements.
- Ask for one thing at a time.
- Don't explain why you deserve it, or state why the other person should feel obligated to grant your request.
- Don't apologize for making the request.
- Don't demand, command, or make ultimatums. (Demands are aggressive, cause defensiveness and resistance, and are based on the distorted belief that you are always right or always entitled to get what you want or need.)
- State the consequence of getting your request granted. (State positive emotions or other results of having your request granted, or negative emotions or other natural negative consequences of not having your request granted—not threats.)
  - *Example:* "If you are thinking about going to the movies, I'd like you to ask me if I would like to go. Even if I say no, if you asked it would make me feel more like part of the family," *as a substitute for* "I'm a member of this family too, even if I have chronic pain. I know you think I'm an invalid, and I say no most of the time, so it's probably stupid to bring it up, but it's about time you showed me some respect and considered my feelings! If you don't, I may not be here when you get back!"
- If you want to decline a request, do so as simply and straightforwardly as you would make a request.
  - *Example:* "No, thank you," "No, I'm not interested," or "No, I'm not able to do that," *instead of* "Why do you always ask me to do things like that? You know I'm not able to do that kind of thing with my back the way it is. You must be getting some kind of pleasure out of adding to my suffering!"
- **My Request (or Response):**

Example: Brian's Completed Assertiveness Worksheet

Brian is 57 years old, married, with two grown kids and three grandchildren. Brian has had low back pain on and off for over 10 years. He has been retired since the age of 55, although his wife, who is 49, still works. Brian has taken over the cooking duties on the weekdays. His daughter, with two young children, often stops by about dinnertime, and his wife usually invites them all to stay. Here is Brian's completed Assertiveness Worksheet (most of the instructions have been omitted).

STEP 1: IDENTIFY A PROBLEM SITUATION

- *What is the problem?*

My wife invites my daughter and grandkids to stay for dinner without asking me.

- *Who is involved?*

My wife, my daughter, my two grandkids.

- *How does it make you feel?*

Disrespected, taken for granted, and mad.

- *What do you want?*

I don't mind if they come to dinner sometimes, but I want to know beforehand.

- *How would you normally handle the problem?*

I usually don't say anything, but then my wife asks me later on why I was so grumpy. I tell her my back was acting up, which it usually is anyway.

- *What do you think would happen if you gave an assertive response?*

I might not be as mad inside. I could plan instead of being surprised. I'd enjoy my grandkids' visit more. My wife might get mad at me.

STEP 2: PLAN THE ASSERTIVE RESPONSE

- Think of a time and place convenient for both of you. (Note: you may have to ask the other person when you could have 15 minutes to talk.) Write this down.

Over morning coffee, before my wife leaves for work.

(continued)

From *Cognitive Therapy for Chronic Pain* by Beverly E. Thorn. Copyright 2004 by The Guilford Press. Permission to photocopy this handout is granted to purchasers of this book for personal use only (see copyright page for details)

Example: Brian's Completed Assertiveness Worksheet *(page 2 of 2)*

- *Now write down the problem,* the way you want to describe it to the other person.
- **My Problem:**

It makes me mad when you invite Cindy and the kids to stay for dinner on the spur of the moment without asking me.

STEP 3: WRITE DOWN YOUR REQUEST

- **My Request (or Response):**

I want you to talk to me before you ask Cindy and the kids to stay for dinner—preferably before I start cooking. If we could plan it ahead of time, I'd be more relaxed and less grumpy.

FINAL SESSION

The 10th treatment session is the final session in this treatment manual. Therapist Handout 10.1, found at the back of this module, provides an outline of Session 10 to be used by the therapist. Client Handout 10.1, also at the back of the module, can be copied and used as a session outline to be given to clients at the beginning of the session.

SESSION 10 TREATMENT OBJECTIVES

- **Review concepts taught and skills learned in this program.**
- **Provide feedback about helpful and challenging aspects of treatment.**
- **Continue to practice and include these techniques in everyday life.**

PRESESSION PROCESS CHECK AND REVIEW OF PREVIOUS WEEK'S SESSION

The final session begins with the typical Presession Process Check and session review. The treatment goal for last week's session was to teach group members the principles of assertiveness and to help them begin planning an assertive communication. Remind clients that most of us are unskilled when it comes to assertiveness, but that a lack of assertiveness leads to communication breakdowns and sometimes to relationship problems. It is particularly important for people with chronic pain to communicate assertively, because (1) sometimes passive communication of pain via pain expressions and catastrophic language has the opposite effect of getting the support desired (i.e., it turns loved ones off and away); and (2) people in chronic pain have legitimate needs for emotional support and practical help, and assertive communication increases the chances of getting those needs met.

During the session, the Assertiveness Worksheet was used to lead group members through the steps of planning an assertive communication with another person regarding a problem situation. Those steps included describing the problem to oneself in detail, writing down a planned communication of the problem to another individual, and writing down an assertive request or an assertive response to the situation.

HOMEWORK REVIEW

For homework, clients were asked to choose a problem situation and write out an assertiveness plan, as well as to practice at least one assertive communication after having planned it out beforehand. Group members were also asked to think about concerns or questions they might have for the group leaders, what they'd like to get out of the final session, and feedback for the group leaders regarding the aspects of treatment that were most and least helpful.

Troubleshooting Tip: In reviewing the homework, you can expect that some clients will not have actually carried out an assertiveness plan, that some will have attempted assertiveness without planning it ahead of time, that some will have tackled an exceptionally challenging issue, and that a few will have followed your instructions to the letter. Remember the principle that all homework is good work, because it is at least an approximation of what you want clients to do, and it provides an opportunity for corrective feedback.

The session transcript below illustrates some of the more common issues encountered during homework review.

THERAPIST: So the homework was for each of you to come up with at least one assertive communication plan in addition to the one you had begun to work through in session, and to actually carry out an assertive communication after planning it. Let's discuss how that went for folks.

TONY: Well, I learned that I'm a miserable failure at this. Here I was complaining bout my wife last week, and I found out that I'm probably worse than she is! When I'm in pain, I want everyone to read my mind that they should leave me alone, but I don't ever tell them directly.

THERAPIST: Before we agree that you are a "miserable failure," you'll have to give us some specifics. What was the situation and the plan, and how did you carry it out?

TONY: Well, I didn't get to the carrying-out stage. My wife wanted to go to dinner. I was in pain and wanted to stay home. I gritted my teeth and went anyway—had a miserable time. Later we had a fight, because I was apparently a jerk all through dinner. End of story.

THERAPIST: First of all, Tony, I'm hearing some thoughts and beliefs in that scenario that might contain some distortions. For example, it sounds as if you hold the belief that you don't have the right to say no to a request to go out to dinner.

TONY: Well, I owe it to her, for God's sake!

KRISTI: Wait, that's another distorted belief, isn't it? How come you couldn't tell her that you guys could go another day?

TONY: That's just it—you see that I didn't do it right.

THERAPIST: The point of these exercises is not to "get it right," especially at first. The point is to learn something in the process of making the attempt. Remember that just last week, you folks were surprised to learn about passive and aggressive modes of communication, and that you recognized yourself in those descriptions. This is new stuff. And by the way, most people have difficulty with assertive communication. So, instead of condemning yourself, let's see how you can plan a more assertive response for the next time. [Works with Tony to construct a planned response, then moves on to other group members.] Okay, how about someone else? What was your situation, what was your plan, and how did it go?

PAT: Well, I was amazed! I actually told my family that I wanted more help with the household chores. I didn't apologize, or whine that I was in too much pain to do them all by myself. I just stated my request! It was really interesting. My oldest kid started trying to guilt-trip me, saying stuff like "Well, you don't work, Mom, after all," but I didn't take the bait. I just repeated my request.

THERAPIST: That's excellent, Pat! Sometimes when we make our assertive request, we have to repeat ourselves more than once, and sometimes it feels like we're being a broken record. But not wavering from the simple, nondefensive request is very important.

KIM: Yeah, but so what happened anyway? Sooner or later, the other person has to either say yes, or flat-out say no, and then where does that leave you?

THERAPIST: It leaves you knowing exactly where you stand. Sometimes that's more difficult to know than not knowing. But it's clear. Then you can work from there. Again, there are no guarantees that you will get exactly what you want. But the point of assertive communication is learning that you can be clear about what you want and need and that you have a right to ask for it, or to say no.

PAT: Well, I don't have the problem solved once and for all, by any means. But I did tell the kids that if they wanted their clothes washed, the clothes would have to arrive in the laundry room—no more me picking them up off the floors of their rooms. I was tempted to justify that by saying that with my back the way it is, I can't bend over, but I didn't. I just said that if the clothes weren't there, they wouldn't get washed.

THERAPIST: Which is exactly what I meant about stating a natural consequence of not getting your request met. You weren't threatening the kids; you were just telling them what would happen if they did not comply—a natural consequence. Now assume that at least one of them will test this, and you'll want to be able to follow through and let them have dirty clothes. It may be hard to watch them walk out the door with a dirty shirt on, but it's important to follow through. Okay?

PAT: Yeah, I've thought about that. And I know just who will test me first. It'll be Frank, my *husband!* (*Pat and others laugh.*)

THERAPIST: Okay, good work, Tony and Pat. You both learned things from this exercise, and you learned that it's not all taken care of with one try at a new skill. Keep practicing! Let's move now to the goals for this session—our final session.

SESSION OBJECTIVE:
REVIEW CONCEPTS TAUGHT AND SKILLS LEARNED IN THIS PROGRAM

During this final phase of treatment, the important concepts presented during the treatment sessions are reviewed. Client Handout 10.2 provides a list of these concepts. I also enlarge the list and put it up on a flipchart, going over the concepts one at a time.

SESSION OBJECTIVE:
PROVIDE FEEDBACK ABOUT HELPFUL AND CHALLENGING ASPECTS OF TREATMENT

Once you have gone over the concepts as noted above, it is time to ask group members to give you feedback about which aspects of the treatment they found particularly helpful and which they found less helpful, especially challenging, or difficult. This will sometimes occur as you are going through the concepts in Client Handout 10.2, which you can then integrate more fully into this phase of the session.

Troubleshooting Tip: You will find that different clients will respond positively (and negatively) to certain aspects of treatment; what was a difficult concept for one client is something that another quickly mastered. Beyond the positive and negative feedback, I listen for the subtleties about what clients seemed to be responding to when they found something particularly useful or difficult. This can give you a special insight into the cognitive processes of the client. Although your time is now limited in terms of being able to conduct another full-scale cognitive intervention, you can often "plant seeds" for clients to take with them and consider after they have left treatment.

A brief session transcript illustrates how the treatment feedback might go.

THERAPIST: We are moving into the final stages of this treatment group, and I want to get a sense from you about what aspects of the group you found particularly useful, or those parts that didn't fit or seemed especially difficult for you. This is part of what I asked you to think about for homework last week. Who would like to begin?

DAVID: The part that grabbed me more than anything was the time we talked about being worth a damn, even though we have chronic pain.

THERAPIST: If I get what you are saying, David, this was when I asked you to consider your sense of yourself as a person in pain. I've noticed that you're not referring to yourself as a "chronic pain patient" these days. The goal is to move toward assuming the identity of a "well person with pain."

DAVID: Well, I'm not quite there yet either, but I don't feel like my only worth is whether I bring in a paycheck or not.

KIM: I was just blown away by the fears that I have that I didn't even know I had.

THERAPIST: It felt to me like you were really steering clear of emotions for a long time in this group—or you thought you were staying away from them

KIM: I was just denying that I had them. Now I can see them and tackle them

KRISTI: I'm still really having a hard time with the "asking for what you want" business. I just can't bring myself to do that. It's not what a "nice girl" is supposed to do!

THERAPIST: That sounds like an area that you could use more practice on, so that you get the idea that assertiveness does not mean being pushy or demanding, but just making a clear statement. I'd like to recommend a book for you to get after we finish today, if you're willing to work with this further.

KRISTI: I don't guess it could hurt.

THERAPIST: Okay, anyone else?

PAT: I know I didn't speak up much in here, but I was surprised to learn about how all these thoughts go racing through our minds without us even knowing it! I catch myself a lot now, and bang! I change it!

THERAPIST: It sounds like you've practiced the cognitive restructuring technique to the point that it's becoming automatic for you now. And you have the tools to go back and do it step-by-step when you run into a new situation, or a particularly stubborn thought. [The therapist should continue to elicit and respond to an example from every member of the group, if possible.] Since the group is ending, it will be important for you to become your own "leader" in continuing to practice these skills. One of the reasons I gave you the session-by-session outlines and worksheets, and the notebook to keep them in, is so that you'd have something to take away with you—something you could refer back to and work with.

MARTHA ANNE: Honestly, I'd like to go back through the entire group again, starting at the beginning. I'd think I'd get a lot more out of it the second time through.

THERAPIST: And using this notebook you've filled up as you went through the group, you *can* go through it again—and again, and again! Even though the group itself is ending, you've got a tool that works because you worked with it.

TONY: Yeah, but you gave the guidance and the feedback we needed so that we didn't get off track. I don't know that I trust myself to do this stuff without the group.

THERAPIST: This isn't magic—it's about working with some basic ideas, and working with them some more. I'm betting that if you look back on it, you may find that the weeks that you practiced the most, you got the most out of it. It turns out that this is a long-term project. Now I want to go back through the skills I've introduced and give you a final worksheet that can serve as a reminder to you, or a reference guide.

SESSION OBJECTIVE:
CONTINUE TO PRACTICE AND INCLUDE THESE TECHNIQUES IN EVERYDAY LIFE

The final aim of treatment is to promote continued practice and generalization outside of the therapeutic setting. Since clients have already been working with the material outside of the therapy sessions via their homework, working on their own is not a foreign concept to them. Nevertheless, *being* on their own is often anxiety-provoking for clients, particularly if they have valued the group process and the group leaders' expertise.

As in the transcript above, remind clients that the reason you provided the session-by-session outlines and worksheets, and the notebook to keep them all in, was so they would have a reference to go back to. Emphasize that the more they use they use these skills, the better they will get, and the more effortless using them will become. Having a set of materials in a notebook to refer back to is another way of encouraging clients to continue working on the concepts even after treatment per se has ended.

It will be also be important to get group members to think about potential roadblocks to practicing their newly acquired skills. Clients frequently share concerns that their pain will get worse or more debilitating. Remind clients that pain flare-ups are to be expected, rather than to be feared. Appraising a pain flare-up differently (i.e., as not life-threatening and not meaning a certain steady downward course), recognizing and challenging automatic thoughts about the flare-up, using coping self-statements and expressive writing, and assertively asking for help and support during a pain flare-up will make it a much less daunting situation.

HOMEWORK ASSIGNMENT

Of course, no "homework" is formally assigned at the end of the final session. However, I have found that clients appreciate an integrated list of options that they can refer to, in order to remind themselves about the tools they have learned and the basics involved in utilizing those tools. Such a "tip sheet" is included as Client Handout 10.3 (The Thoughts Toolbox) at the back of this module.

Once you have gone over The Thoughts Toolbox, ask clients to tell you how they will use it. The more specific you can get them to be, the better. Once again, reiterate that in the context of the actual treatment program, the techniques presented have only scratched the surface of introducing new skills to the clients. Treatment introduces the clients to the concepts, but long-term change is produced by practice. And changing the way we think is a long-term project! Also, as clients have already noted, when something is new, it feels awkward and unnatural. As it becomes more integrated into the clients' everyday repertoire, it begins to become more automatic and less effortful.

POSTSESSION PROCESS CHECK AND TERMINATION

At the very end of the session—after you have handed out the Postsession Process Check, had clients fill it in, and addressed any last-minute problems—make sure that you express appreciation to the group members for their work. Therapists always learn something from their clients, and telling them so helps them to feel even better about participating in the process. It is a *fact* that what you learn from individual patients, or pain management groups, can be directly utilized to better help the next group of patients.

Session 10 Outline for Therapists: Final Session

SESSION OBJECTIVES

- Review concepts taught and skills learned in this program.
- Provide feedback about helpful and challenging aspects of treatment.
- Continue to practice and include these techniques in everyday life.

NEEDED MATERIALS, HANDOUTS, AND WORKSHEETS

- Flipchart and markers
- Session 10 Outline for Therapists (this handout)
- Session 10 Summary for Clients (Client Handout 10.1)
- Presession Process Check (Appendix J)
- Important Concepts Learned in This Cognitive Program (Client Handout 10.2)
- The Thoughts Toolbox (Client Handout 10.3)
- Postsession Process Check (Appendix J)

PRESESSION PROCESS CHECK

- Hand out Presession Process Check and have clients fill it in.

REVIEW OF PREVIOUS WEEK'S SESSION

- Remind clients: "You have a right to express your wants and needs in a straightforward and unapologetic manner."
- "Assertive communication helps you to do so."
- "Assertive communication is not mean or selfish—it helps people to know exactly where you stand."
- "Your loved ones may not be used to assertive communication, but most people respond very well to it."
- "The Assertiveness Worksheet can be used to plan assertive communication."
- "Practicing assertive communication after you plan it is the way to get good at it."

HOMEWORK REVIEW

- Ask several clients: "What did you learn about *planning* an assertive communication?"
- "What did you learn about *carrying out* an assertive communication?"

(continued)

From *Cognitive Therapy for Chronic Pain* by Beverly E. Thorn. Copyright 2004 by The Guilford Press. Permission to photocopy this handout is granted to purchasers of this book for personal use only (see copyright page for details).

SESSION OBJECTIVE: REVIEW CONCEPTS TAUGHT AND SKILLS LEARNED IN THIS PROGRAM

- Give out copies of Client Handout 10.2 (Important Concepts Learned in This Cognitive Program) and go over the concepts:
  1. Pain is a stress-related phenomenon.
  2. Stress appraisals are important in our thoughts and emotions.
  3. Automatic thoughts, intermediate beliefs, and core beliefs all influence the way we cope with pain.
  4. Negatively distorted automatic thoughts are related to poor pain control and emotional upset.
  5. Cognitive restructuring is a tool that allows us to recognize negatively distorted thoughts, examine them for factual errors, challenge them, and construct more realistic alternative thoughts about our pain and associated stress.
  6. Our intermediate beliefs about our pain and how it should be treated can also be negatively distorted, and the cognitive restructuring exercise can help us examine these, challenge them, and create more realistic alternative beliefs.
  7. Our core beliefs about ourselves as persons in pain can have a powerful impact on how we cope. Moving from a core belief of "I am a disabled chronic pain patient" to a core belief of "I am a well person with pain" is an important ongoing goal.
  8. Strong emotions are part of coping with the ongoing stress associated with chronic pain, and expressive writing can serve as a way of recognizing, honoring, and understanding our strong emotions.
  9. Assertiveness is a tool for communicating our wants and needs in a direct, unapologetic, non-aggressive way, and helps us meet our interpersonal needs as well as improve our relationships.
  10. The skills learned in this group are new skills and must be practiced for us to get really good at them. The more we practice, the better we will be. The group is meant to get us started. Now the "real work" begins.

SESSION OBJECTIVE: PROVIDE FEEDBACK ABOUT HELPFUL AND CHALLENGING ASPECTS OF TREATMENT

- Ask clients: "What parts of the treatment program were most helpful?"
- "What parts of the treatment program did you struggle with?"
- "What parts of the program do you still have questions or concerns about?"

SESSION OBJECTIVE: CONTINUE TO PRACTICE AND INCLUDE THESE TECHNIQUES IN EVERYDAY LIFE

- Tell clients: "You now have the tools to be your own therapist."
- "Use your notebook to refer back to the concepts we learned."
- "The more you work with these skills, the better you will become—they will seem more a natural part of you, and require less effort."
- About expecting pain flare-ups, remind clients:
  - "Knowing that there are times when the pain will be worse is not the same as catastrophizing about it."
- About coping with pain flare-ups, remind clients:
  - "The most difficult time to use these skills is during episodes of increased pain."
  - "The most *important* time to use these skills is during episodes of increased pain."
  - "If you practice during the 'good times,' the skills are easier to use during pain flare-ups."
- Discuss with clients: "What roadblocks do you foresee in continuing to practice these skills?"

(continued)

225

HOMEWORK ASSIGNMENT

- Tell clients: "Your 'homework' involves using the tools in your toolbox on a daily basis!" (Give out Client Handout 10.3, The Thoughts Toolbox.)

POSTSESSION PROCESS CHECK AND TERMINATION

- Have clients fill out Postsession Process Check before they leave. Glance at responses and briefly troubleshoot if necessary.
- Remember to thank clients for their work, and for teaching you more about how to help others in chronic pain.

226

Session 10 Summary for Clients: Final Session

THE GOALS OF THIS SESSION

- To review concepts taught and skills learned in this program.
- To provide feedback about helpful and challenging aspects of treatment.
- To continue to practice and use these techniques in everyday life.

REVIEW OF PREVIOUS WEEK'S SESSION

- You have a right to express your wants and needs in a straightforward and unapologetic manner.
- Assertive communication helps you to do so.
- Assertive communication is not mean or selfish—it helps people to know exactly where you stand.
- Your loved ones may not be used to assertive communication, but most people respond very well to it.
- The Assertiveness Worksheet can be used to plan assertive communication.
- Practicing assertive communication after you plan it is the way to get good at it.

HOMEWORK REVIEW

- What did you learn about *planning* an assertive communication?
- What did you learn about *carrying out* an assertive communication?

REVIEWING CONCEPTS TAUGHT AND SKILLS LEARNED IN THIS PROGRAM

1. Pain is a stress-related phenomenon.
2. Stress appraisals are important in our thoughts and emotions.
3. Automatic thoughts, intermediate beliefs, and core beliefs all influence the way we cope with pain.
4. Negatively distorted automatic thoughts are related to poor pain control and emotional upset.
5. Cognitive restructuring is a tool that allows us to recognize negatively distorted thoughts, examine them for factual errors, challenge them, and construct more realistic alternative thoughts about our pain and associated stress.
6. Our intermediate beliefs about our pain and how it should be treated can also be negatively distorted, and the cognitive restructuring exercise can help us examine these, challenge them, and create more realistic alternative beliefs.
7. Our core beliefs about ourselves as persons in pain can have a powerful impact on how we cope. Moving from a core belief of "I am a disabled chronic pain patient" to a core belief of "I am a well person with pain" is an important ongoing goal.
8. Strong emotions are part of coping with the ongoing stress associated with chronic pain, and expressive writing can serve as a way of recognizing, honoring, and understanding our strong emotions.

(continued)

From *Cognitive Therapy for Chronic Pain* by Beverly E. Thorn. Copyright 2004 by The Guilford Press. Permission to photocopy this handout is granted to purchasers of this book for personal use only (see copyright page for details).

9. Assertiveness is a tool for communicating our wants and needs in a direct, unapologetic, nonaggressive way, and helps us meet our interpersonal needs as well as improve our relationships.
10. The skills learned in this group are new skills and must be practiced for us to get really good at them. The more we practice, the better we will be. The group is meant to get us started. Now the "real work" begins.

PROVIDING FEEDBACK ABOUT HELPFUL AND CHALLENGING ASPECTS OF TREATMENT

- What parts of the treatment program were most helpful?
- What parts of the treatment program did you struggle with?
- What parts of the program do you still have questions or concerns about?

CONTINUING TO PRACTICE AND INCLUDE THESE TECHNIQUES IN EVERYDAY LIFE

- You now have the tools to be your own therapist.
- Use your notebook to refer back to the concepts we learned.
- The more you work with these skills, the better you will become—they will seem more a natural part of you, and require less effort.
- About expecting pain flare-ups, remember:
  - Knowing that there are times when the pain will be worse is not the same as catastrophizing about it.
- About coping with pain flare-ups, remember:
  - The most difficult time to use these skills is during episodes of increased pain.
  - The most *important* time to use these skills is during episodes of increased pain.
  - If you practice during the "good times," the skills are easier to use during pain flare-ups.
- What roadblocks do you foresee in continuing to practice these skills?

HOMEWORK ASSIGNMENT

Your "homework" involves using the tools in The Thoughts Toolbox on a daily basis!

Important Concepts Learned in This Cognitive Program

1. Pain is a stress-related phenomenon.
2. Stress appraisals are important in your thoughts and emotions.
3. Automatic thoughts, intermediate beliefs, and core beliefs all influence the way you cope with pain.
4. Negatively distorted automatic thoughts are related to poor pain control and emotional upset.
5. Cognitive restructuring is a tool that allows you to recognize negatively distorted thoughts, examine them for factual errors, challenge them, and construct more realistic alternative thoughts about your pain and associated stress.
6. Your intermediate beliefs about your pain and how it should be treated can also be factually incorrect. The cognitive restructuring exercise can help you examine these, challenge them, and create more realistic alternative beliefs.
7. Your core beliefs about yourself as a person in pain can have a powerful impact on how you cope. Moving from a core belief of "I am a disabled chronic pain patient" to a core belief of "I am a well person with pain" is an important ongoing goal.
8. Recognizing, honoring, and understanding strong emotions are part of coping with the stress associated with chronic pain, and expressive writing can help you vent emotions without criticism.
9. Communicating your wants and needs in a direct, unapologetic, nonaggressive way is also part of coping with chronic pain. Assertive communication helps you meet your interpersonal needs as well as improve your relationships.
10. The skills learned in this group are new skills and must be practiced for you to get really good at them. The more you practice, the better you will be. The group is meant to get you started. Now your "real work" begins.

From *Cognitive Therapy for Chronic Pain* by Beverly E. Thorn. Copyright 2004 by The Guilford Press. Permission to photocopy this handout is granted to purchasers of this book for personal use only (see copyright page for details).

The Thoughts Toolbox

Remember the Stress–Appraisal–Coping Model of Pain: Pain is real, and it is stress-related. Your *thoughts* about pain and stress have an impact on your emotions, your other thoughts, how you cope, and even your physical well-being.

Tool 1: Stress Appraisal—When confronted with a stressful situation, are you judging it to be a threat, a loss, or a challenge? How does your judgment affect your thoughts and emotions, as well as your response to the stressor? Is there a way you can divide the stressor into more manageable pieces, some of which you could appraise as a challenge?

Tool 2: Automatic Thoughts—Automatic thoughts come up in response to stressful situations (including pain), and may be outside your immediate awareness. With practice, you can recognize automatic thoughts by asking yourself, "What just went through my mind?" when your emotions shift or you sense a change in your physical well-being. Automatic thoughts often contain some negative distortions, which make it harder to cope. With practice, you can examine your automatic thoughts for any negative distortions, challenge the distorted part, and construct more realistic alternative responses.

Tool 3: Intermediate Beliefs—Intermediate beliefs are the "rules" we all hold about ourselves, others, and the world around us. They are the "should," "must," and "ought to" ideas that you believe about yourself and others. Pain-related intermediate beliefs are ideas and attitudes about the pain, your ability to manage the pain, and your notions about how the pain should be treated. Intermediate beliefs are harder to challenge than automatic thoughts, but with practice you can learn to recognize negative distortions in these beliefs, or examine whether the beliefs are still serving you, and construct more realistic alternative intermediate beliefs.

Tool 4: Core Beliefs—Core beliefs are deeply held ideas we all have about ourselves and our competence or worth. Pain-related core beliefs are often associated with your notion of yourself as a "chronic pain patient" or "disabled" or "ill." Building a new core belief system takes time, but with diligence you can construct an alternative core belief about yourself as a "well person with pain." To do so, remember the "acting as if" exercise.

Tool 5: Coping Self-Statements—Coping self-statements are your emotional "cheerleaders." These positive self-statements are used to increase your sense of being in charge of at least some aspects of your pain experience, and to increase your sense of being able to do the tasks necessary to cope. Coping self-statements can be constructed in response to "frequent flyer" automatic thoughts. Coping cards can be made with coping self-statements on them and prominently displayed in places you are likely to notice them. Make sure you switch the cards occasionally—try different statements, different colors, and different places to display them.

Tool 6: Expressive Writing—Writing about your deepest thoughts and feelings regarding you pain situation can help you clarify and understand them. Particularly with emotions, writing about them can make them seem less scary and overwhelming. Expressive writing is also a way to get your feelings "off your chest" and be done with them for a time. Use this tool whenever you feel you need to vent, or whenever you are confused about your feelings or feel overwhelmed by your emotions. Remember to write only for yourself—don't censor what you have to say, and don't worry about spelling, grammar, or cross-outs.

(continued)

From *Cognitive Therapy for Chronic Pain* by Beverly E. Thorn. Copyright 2004 by The Guilford Press. Permission to photocopy this handout is granted to purchasers of this book for personal use only (see copyright page for details).

Tool 7: Assertive Communication—We all have wants and needs that we have a right to express directly without apology or excuses. Assertive communication is a great tool to use when you want to share your feelings about something, make a request, or say no. Practicing assertive communication by planning what you'd like to say ahead of time will increase the probability that you will get your wants and needs met. Assertive communication improves the quality of relationships, is respected by others, and helps you feel better about yourself. Remember to use "I" statements in assertive communication, and to avoid accusations. If there is a problem, describe it in simple terms to the person involved. Follow up with a direct request.

APPENDICES

Pathophysiology of Pain

Rather than negating the importance of pain physiology in proposing a stress-and-coping model of pain, I am advocating that we discontinue separating the "physical" from the "psychological" as if they were different entities. The fact is that psychological processes associated with pain have physiological manifestations, and biological concomitants of pain are made apparent by psychological mechanisms. In this appendix, I review the pathophysiology of pain.

In Chapter 1, I have traced the history of pain theories—from a fixed transmission system between stimulus and perception (traditional biomedical approach), to the more dynamic biopsychosocial model of pain. I have noted that according to the gate control theory of pain (Melzack & Wall, 1965, 1982), a gating mechanism in the spinal cord can widen or narrow as a result of descending signals from the brain, thus allowing relatively more or fewer pain signals to ultimately reach the brain.

In a reformulation of the gate control theory, Melzack has proposed a "neuromatrix" model (Melzack, 1990, 1999a, 1999b, 2001; Melzack, Coderre, Katz, & Vaccarino, 2001), which takes into account more recent information regarding neural networks. In the neuromatrix model, the metaphorical spinal gating mechanism previously hypothesized to modulate pain perception has been expanded to include a widespread network of neural loops (including such structures as the thalamus, limbic system, and cortex) to explain the experience of pain. The neuromatrix model also suggests that the processing of pain by the brain is genetically established, but modifiable by experience. In addition, Melzack has proposed that psychological factors can inhibit or enhance the sensory flow of pain signals, and thus can also influence the way the brain ultimately responds to nociceptive stimulation.

How do pain signals reach the brain, and what happens once they do? The next section reviews the basic neuroanatomy of pain transmission.

NEUROANATOMY OF PAIN TRANSMISSION

Pain sensations coming from skin, muscles, or internal organs are part of the somatosensory system. Pain receptors are called "nociceptors," and instead of being specialized sensory organs, they are free nerve endings. Free nerve endings are the receiving ends of nerve tissue in the skin, muscles, or viscera. Free nerve endings can be stimulated by a variety of means, including intense mechanical, thermal, or electrical stimulation. When tissues are damaged, free nerve endings are also chemically stimulated by the release of chemicals from injured cells. This chemical stimulation is a complex process, and the release of chemicals from injured cells in turn increases the sensitivity of free nerve endings to other chemicals (a process called "chemical sensitization").

Once free nerve endings are stimulated, the message travels to the spinal cord via transmission fibers called "axons." Whereas the free nerve endings are the receiving ends of nerve cells (or "neurons"), an axon is the part of a neuron that carries the message from one end of the cell to the other. At the level of the spinal cord, the first neuron in the message chain communicates with a second neuron via an electrochemical process that releases chemicals called "neurotransmitters." From the spinal cord, pain messages travel to the brain via several different potential pathways, and neurons along the way serve as relay stations in the transmission process. Some of the important pain pathways travel through areas of the brain that we already know to be important in emotion and cognition—for example, the thalamus and the limbic system. What we think of as the final destination of pain signals is the somatosensory cortex of the brain, where neurons are arranged into multiple maps of the body surface, each responding to a different kind of stimulation to a different part of the body (see Carlson, 1994, for a more detailed description).

We know that the process of pain perception is critically important to the survival of the organism. Pain motivates us to withdraw from potentially life-threatening stimuli (Iadarola & Caudle, 1997). People born with a congenital insensitivity to pain actually have a reduced life expectancy, due to their inability to perceive pain-related stimuli.

On the other hand, it is sometimes preferable to ignore pain to accomplish a task. There are myriad examples of this, ranging from athletes during fierce competition, to parents while rescuing a child in peril, to yogis during meditation. Although we are less clear about the brain processes involved in *reducing* pain perception than we are about the neuroanatomy of pain sensation, we are gaining such information at a rapid rate.

As early as the 1970s, researchers began to identify neural circuits that, when stimulated, produced "decreases" in pain perception. These circuits were called "descending pain inhibitory systems," because they were located in sections of the brain above the pain pathways ascending from the spinal cord. Both human and nonhuman animal research demonstrated that mild electrical currents administered via deep brain stimulators could eliminate the perception of pain, at least on a temporary basis. This phenomenon was called "stimulation-produced analgesia," and it was subsequently discovered that such brain stimulation results in the release of opiate-like substances produced within the brain ("endogenous opioids"). There has been a subsequent explosion of research investigating the endogenous opiate systems in the brain. Opiates, either released from within the brain (endogenous) or administered pharmaceutically (exogenous) appear to have their analgesic effect by inhibiting the transmission of pain signals at the level of the spinal cord.

We have also known for several decades that the emotional component of pain is processed in a different area of the brain than is the awareness of the pain stimulus (Price, 2000). For example, surgical removal of the thalamus (one of the pain relay stations in the brain) in an attempt to relieve the pain of patients with terminal cancer results in a continued *awareness* of the pain, but the pain is reported to be no longer bothersome (Mark, Ervin, & Yakovlev, 1962). In addition, individuals who report a greater sensitivity to pain show greater activation of the anterior cingulate cortex, which is part of the limbic system (another pain relay station in the brain) (Coghill, McHaffie, & Yen, 2003). And in a study using hypnosis to selectively alter the affective (emotional) component of pain, researchers were able to show direct changes in activity within the anterior cingulate cortex, although the somatosensory cortex activation remained unaltered (Rainville, Duncan, Price, Carrier, & Bushnell, 1997). Logic dictates that if activation of these relay stations involving pain affect can increase the overall experience of pain, *inhibition* of these areas can decrease the overall experience of pain. Our emotions and thoughts, then, can produce physical differences in the way the brain processes pain.

NEURONAL PLASTICITY AND ITS CONTRIBUTION TO CHRONIC PAIN

A more recently discovered phenomenon involves changes in the brain induced by the experience of pain itself. Recall that in the neuromatrix model, Melzack has hypothesized that although the processing of pain by the brain is genetically programmed, it is modifiable by experience. There is now substantial evidence that the experience of pain changes the brain. We call this phenomenon "neural plasticity"—the capacity of neurons to change their structure, their function, or even their chemical profile (Woolf & Salter, 2000). In the short term, brain-related pain processing can be altered (or "modulated") in a way that increases the sensitivity of neurons to even mild pain signals. As an example of short-term modulation of brain processes involved in pain perception, tissue injury causes the release of chemi-

(continued)

cals from injured cells, which in turn creates an increased sensitivity of the free nerve endings to other chemicals, thus creating a change in the way the nerve endings process a pain stimulus. Once the tissue is healed, the hypersensitivity *usually* returns to normal. Long-lasting alterations in neurons can also result from the experience of pain, and these changes are called "modifications." Modifications of the nervous system are more permanent; they include such structural changes as an increase in the number of pain receptors in the spinal cord following tissue damage and inflammation, and a reduction in brain inhibitory processes following nerve injury (Woolf & Salter, 2000).

Short- and long-term neural plasticity may lead to conditions that have previously gone unexplained. For example, "allodynia" is a condition in which nonpainful stimulation (e.g., light touch) produces pain; "hyperalgesia" is a situation where a mildly painful stimulus produces intense pain; and "referred pain" is the perception of pain spread to noninjured tissue (Covington, 2000; Iadarola & Caudle, 1997). Often these processes persist after healing of the damaged tissue. In addition, "neuropathic pain," or the sensation of pain long after injured nerve tissue has healed, is an illustration of pathological alteration of the nervous system via the experience of pain. A good example of neuropathic pain is the long-lasting exquisite pain experienced by some people after a herpes zoster ("shingles") outbreak.

This appendix provides only a brief overview of pain pathophysiology, and gives just a glimpse of the incredible complexity associated with brain processes and pain perception. The idea of a one-to-one correspondence between pain stimulus and pain perception has obviously been superseded by our current knowledge regarding pain physiology. The experience of pain is clearly not a simple awareness of the pain sensation; the brain is the physical processing unit for both the awareness of the sensation (previously referred to as "physical" pain) and the emotional/cognitive component of pain (the so-called "psychological" element). Furthermore, present information points to a dynamic and moldable brain system that not only processes pain, but is also sensitized by acute pain experiences. The evidence distinctly points to the idea that acute pain experiences can change the brain in a direction that facilitates chronic pain conditions. Over time, modifications of the nervous system may produce pain experiences quite independent of the tissue pathology that generated the initial perception of pain. It is not out of the realm of possibilities that adaptive cognitive and emotional processes could produce reparative modifications of the nervous system.

A Critique of the Current Diagnostic Systems and Procedural Terminology for Pain Disorders

DIAGNOSTIC ISSUES

As I have stated in Chapter 1, patients can currently receive pain-related diagnoses via the *International Classification of Diseases*, 10th revision (ICD-10; World Health Organization, 1992) or via the *Diagnostic and Statistical Manual of Mental Disorders*, 4th edition, text revision (DSM-IV-TR; American Psychiatric Association, 2000). The DSM and the ICD systems of diagnosing patients with pain have evolved somewhat to incorporate the biopsychosocial model, but in other ways our options for diagnosing such patients—particularly regarding the interaction of psychological factors and medical factors—remain inadequate. The ICD system used by physicians specifically separates pain disorders into those thought to be of psychogenic etiology and those thought to be of nonpsychogenic etiology. Pain disorders considered psychogenic are categorized within the mental disorders category of the ICD and classified as "psychalgias." The DSM system of diagnosing mental disorders lists pain disorder as a specific diagnosis under the broader category of "somatoform disorders." Both the ICD and the DSM systems of diagnosing pain disorders are based on the dualistic notion that pain is *either* pathophysiological *or* psychological. This distinction follows an outdated biomedical model, rather than the currently accepted biopsychosocial model. Although I do not discuss ICD terminology problems further here, the DSM diagnostic issues regarding pain disorder merit more exploration.

Within the DSM-IV-TR (American Psychiatric Association, 2000), making a diagnosis of pain disorder requires a clinical judgment that psychological issues play a significant role in the patient's pain. However, there are no criteria for determining when psychological factors have a significant impact on pain. In addition, a diagnosis of pain disorder is not given when the pain is better accounted for by another mental disorder, such as a mood, anxiety, or psychotic disorder. Yet there are no criteria for determining when psychological factors are sufficient to warrant a separate diagnosis (e.g., major depressive disorder). Since mood and anxiety disorders are often comorbid with pain disorder, this stipulation is particularly problematic. The major problem, however, is that patients receiving a DSM pain disorder diagnosis are, by definition, judged to be mentally ill.

Digging further, we find that the pain disorder diagnosis is located within the broader category of somatoform disorders in the DSM, as noted above. The hallmark of somatoform disorders is that patients experience physical symptoms with no known physiological basis. Furthermore, unconscious psychological factors are thought to drive the patients' illness. Although such patients are not thought to be consciously faking,[1] the implication is that individuals diagnosed with pain disorder are driven by *unconscious* needs to perceive pain, exaggerate pain, and/or become disabled by pain that has no physiological basis.

PROCEDURAL TERMINOLOGY

Until recently, mental health practitioners treating patients with pain (and patients with other medical diagnoses) were not reimbursed by third-party payers unless the patients received diagnoses of mental

---

[1]Individuals who are judged to be willfully feigning illness are either described as malingering (i.e., faking pain or illness in order to receive some external benefit, such as disability payments, or to get out of something, such as aversive family responsibilities), or diagnosed with factitious disorder (faking pain or illness in order to be in the sick role).

disorders. Procedural terminology amended by the American Medical Association in January 2002 now provides a means for mental health practitioners to work with patients who have physical health diagnoses, without the requirement that they have mental illness diagnoses. In such a case, a physician will have previously diagnosed a physical disease, illness, or health problem via the ICD diagnostic system. The six additional procedure codes, called Health and Behavior Codes, provide for assessment and intervention activities that include cognitive, behavioral, social, and psychophysiological procedures used for preventing, treating, or managing health problems (American Medical Association, 2004). Unlike the traditional psychotherapy codes, which are billed in hourly increments, the Health and Behavior Codes are billed in 15-minute increments. If a patient has both a physical illness and a mental illness diagnosis, the Health and Behavior Codes can only be used to address the individual's physical health problems, and mental health interventions cannot be billed on the same day.

The addition of the Health and Behavior Codes to the Current Procedural Terminology (CPT) system is a very exciting development for clinicians working with patients who have medical conditions, but not necessarily mental illnesses. An individual with a physical health problem may not meet the criteria for a psychiatric diagnosis, and these codes help avoid inappropriate labeling of such a patient as having a mental disorder. The codes also expand the types of assessments and interventions provided to individuals with health problems, thus increasing their quality of care. The Health and Behavior CPT codes can be used to accurately reflect the assessment and intervention procedures that are often used with patients coping with chronic painful conditions, including the assessment and treatment procedures suggested in this book. Unfortunately, these codes are not universally accepted by health insurance carriers (although, by law, Medicare must accept them), and many practitioners remain hesitant to use them for this reason. In addition, as with reimbursement for psychotherapy under the previous CPT coding system, licensed psychologists and psychiatrists are the most likely professionals to be reimbursed by third-party payers when filing insurance claims under these codes. The Health and Behavior Codes and a basic description of each procedure are listed in Table App. B.1. (See also American Medical Association, 2004, and *http://www.apa.org/practice/cpt_faq.html* for further information.)

TABLE APP. B.1. Health and Behavior Assessment and Intervention Reimbursement Codes under the Current Procedural Terminology (CPT) Coding System

- *96150*—Initial health and behavior assessment (e.g., clinical interview focusing on pain condition, associated distress, perceived disability; pain-specific questionnaires).
- *96151*—Reassessment of a previously assessed patient to determine the need for further treatment. May be conducted by a clinician other than the original assessor (e.g., interpretation of pain-related questionnaires and pain diaries, behavioral observations of patient–spouse or patient–partner interactions).
- *96152*—Individual intervention sessions (can be weekly) to modify psychological, behavioral, cognitive, and social factors affecting the patient's physical health (e.g., individual cognitive therapy to modify patient's motivation to engage in pain self-management behaviors).
- *96153*—Group intervention sessions (two or more patients) to address biopsychosocial issues associated with physical health (e.g., group cognitive therapy to modify patient's belief systems regarding the cause, appropriate treatment of, and ability to self-manage pain).
- *96154*—Intervention session with family and patient present (e.g., couple therapy to examine and change maladaptive interaction patterns promoting disability in the patient).
- *96155*—Intervention session with family of patient, without the patient present (e.g., cognitive therapy with family members of patient during an invasive procedure).

(continued)

Mental health practitioners now have the flexibility of treating patients with physical health diagnoses, and focusing on evidence-based means to prevent, treat, and manage physical health problems. In addition, mental health practitioners can continue to offer services to patients with a primary focus on mental health rather than physical health issues, when that approach seems to be most appropriate. Cognitive interventions can be implemented in either case, and are appropriate for patients with pain who may have very few issues affecting their mental health, as well as for patients with pain who have been affected significantly in terms of mental health.

In the section below, I have provided a sample health and behavior assessment summary. You will notice that the case illustration is the same one I have used in Chapter 4 (Martha Anne). To demonstrate how the assessment instruments covered in Chapter 4 can be used, I have provided a detailed account of my assessment findings regarding Martha Anne at the end of that chapter. The illustration below is a much more abbreviated version, and appropriate for the patient's chart as well as for the referring physician.

SUMMARY OF HEALTH AND BEHAVIOR ASSESSMENT FOR REFERRING PHYSICIAN

Patient name: Martha Anne Smith

Date: 4/30/03   *CPT code*: 96150

Patient's date of birth: 4/15/53

Age: 50   *Sex*: F   *Race*: W

Employer: None (disability)

Referral source: Gary Kilgo, MD

Physical condition being evaluated: Fibromyalgia, chronic fatigue syndrome

Date of diagnosis of physical illness: 11/5/02—Fibromyalgia
                                            2/3/03—Chronic fatigue syndrome

Rationale for assessment: Medical interventions have not successfully relieved the patient's pain or increased her functioning.

Relevant background information: Patient is divorced and relies on daughter for support in some activities of daily living (i.e., food preparation, household management).

Noteworthy medical history: Motor vehicle accident (MVA) 10/04/95, with multiple fractures of right shoulder, arm, and hand. Mild concussion with no residual brain-related impairment. Multiple sequential surgeries on shoulder, elbow, and wrist, with resulting impairment of 50% range of motion in her hand and arm.

Current medications[2]*—Brand (generic), dose, schedule*:

    Celebrex (Celecoxib), 200 mg, 1/day
    Fiorinal (butalbital), 40 mg, as needed
    Percodan (oxycodone/aspirin), 4.5 mg oxycodone/325 mg aspirin, as needed
    Anaprox (naproxen sodium), 550 mg, 1/day
    Effexor (venlafaxine HCl), 37.5 mg, 1/day
    Neurontin (gabapentin), 300 mg, 1/day
    Prozac (fluoxetine HCl), 20 mg, 4/day

---

[2]See *http://www.rxlist.com* for a good Internet reference guide to many common medications.

(continued)

Assessment results: Initial cognitive assessment of Ms. Smith indicates noteworthy pain-related anxiety, and beliefs regarding pain signals as potentially harmful—both of which promote avoidance of therapeutic activities and increasing disability. Ms. Smith's report of poor concentration ability may be related to her attentional focus on pain signals and her subsequent rumination about them. Ms. Smith has frequent thoughts of helplessness regarding her pain, has few adaptive cognitive coping strategies in her repertoire, and does not believe in her own ability to carry out pain self-management skills. All this—coupled with high dependency needs, and beliefs that others should be solicitous of her pain—will encourage further passivity and avoidance of therapeutic activities, as well as reliance on others, including the health care system. Further assessment may be indicated to explore interpersonal relationship factors that may be contributing to Ms. Smith's passivity and dysfunction. Ms. Smith also sees herself as disabled, and this self-concept further discourages active engagement in self-care behaviors. Thus successfully engaging her in a treatment requiring active patient involvement may be problematic. On the other hand, assessment has also revealed several good prognostic signs. Ms. Smith holds adaptive beliefs regarding the interaction of emotions and pain, and her history of engaging in psychotherapy indicates receptivity toward this type of intervention. In addition, she reports a good understanding of her pain problem, displays no indication that she is fixated on obtaining a physical diagnosis or "cure" for her pain, and does not demonstrate psychological dependence on pain medications.

Recommendations:

1. Since the assessment has indicated general themes of loss and guilt, it will be necessary to monitor Ms. Smith for the presence of mood disorders, although she does not have a history of major depressive disorder. Helping her resolve emotions (e.g., guilt) regarding her MVA may be beneficial. Expressive writing exercises may be particularly useful.
2. Since Ms. Smith is motivated to reduce her reliance on pain medications, facilitate this desire with her physician. Providing her with other coping strategies to replace her reliance on medications will be especially advantageous.
3. Because of her pain-related anxiety, passivity, and dependency, it will be necessary to proceed slowly, introducing small goals likely to produce success experiences. Gradual success experiences, coupled with coping self-statement exercises, may increase Ms. Smith's sense of ability to carry out pain self-management tasks.
4. Challenge catastrophic cognitions and erroneous beliefs, using cognitive restructuring exercises.
5. Consider conjoint sessions with daughter and Ms. Smith. Assertiveness exercises may be of particular relevance for Ms. Smith.

Name of clinician: Beverly E. Thorn, PhD, Licensed Psychologist

CC: Gary Kilgo, MD

Dysfunctional Attitude Scale–24 Items (DAS-24)

Attitudes	Totally Agree	Agree Very Much	Agree Slightly	Neutral	Disagree Slightly	Disagree Very Much	Totally Disagree
1. If I fail partly, it is as bad as being a complete failure.							
2. If others dislike you, you cannot be happy.							
3. I should be happy all the time.							
4. People will probably think less of me if I make a mistake.							
5. My happiness depends more on other people than it does on me.							
6. I should always have complete control over my feelings.							
7. My life is wasted unless I am a success.							
8. What other people think about me is very important.							
9. I ought to be able to solve my problems quickly and without a great deal of effort.							
10. If I don't set the highest standards for myself, I am likely to end up a second-rate person.							
11. I am nothing if a person I love doesn't love me.							
12. A person should be able to control what happens to him.							

(continued)

Copyright 1994 by Michael J. Power. Reprinted by permission in *Cognitive Therapy for Chronic Pain* by Beverly E. Thorn. Copyright 2004 by The Guilford Press. Permission to photocopy this appendix is granted to purchasers of this book for personal use only (see copyright page for details).

Attitudes	Totally Agree	Agree Very Much	Agree Slightly	Neutral	Disagree Slightly	Disagree Very Much	Totally Disagree
13. If I am to be a worthwhile person, I must be truly outstanding in at least one major respect.							
14. If you don't have other people to lean on, you are bound to be sad.							
15. It is possible for a person to be scolded and not get upset.							
16. I must be a useful, productive, creative person, or life has no purpose.							
17. I can find happiness without being loved by another person.							
18. A person should do well at everything he undertakes.							
19. If I do not do well all the time, people will not respect me.							
20. I do not need the approval of other people in order to be happy.							
21. If I try hard enough, I should be able to excel at anything I attempt.							
22. People who have good ideas are more worthy than those who do not.							
23. A person doesn't need to be well liked in order to be happy.							
24. Whenever I take a chance or risk, I am only looking for trouble.							

DAS-24 SCORING KEY

Every item on the DAS-24 is scored from 1 to 7. Depending on whether the particular item is scored in the forward direction or the backward direction, the actual score awarded for each item will vary from 1 to 7 for the two extremes of "Totally Agree" (+7) to "Totally Disagree" (+1).

The following items are scored in a forward direction: 17, 20, and 23. That is, Totally Agree = +1, Agree Very Much = +2, Agree Slightly = +3, Neutral = +4, Disagree Slightly = +5, Disagree Very Much = +6, Totally Disagree = +7. The rest of the items in the questionnaire are scored in the reverse direction. That is, Totally Agree = +7, Agree Very Much = +6, Agree Slightly = +5, Neutral = +4, Disagree Slightly = +3, Disagree Very Much = +2, Totally Disagree = +1.

The total DAS-24 score is obtained by summing the response value of all the items. The three subscale scores are obtained by summing all ratings provided for each scale and dividing by the number of items responded to within each scale.

Subscale items (asterisks indicate forward-score items):

Achievement: 1, 4, 7, 10, 13, 16, 19, 22
Dependency: 2, 5, 8, 11, 14, 17*, 20*, 23*
Self-Control: 3, 6, 9, 12, 15, 18, 21, 24

Scores of Formerly Depressed Psychiatric Patients and Undergraduates on the DAS-24

DAS-24 scale	Undergraduate sample	Psychiatric sample
Achievement	21.67 (9.38)	25.74 (11.01)
Dependency	27.48 (9.61)	30.41 (8.82)
Self-control	26.57 (7.91)	29.43 (8.32)
Total	75.71 (20.76)	85.59 (22.81)

Note. Data from Power et al. (1994).

Pain Appraisal Inventory (PAI)

We are interested in how you have been thinking about your pain. Please read each of these sentences. Think about whether you agree or disagree with the sentence. Circle the number that fits with your answer.

Strongly Disagree	Moderately Disagree	Slightly Disagree	Slightly Agree	Moderately Agree	Strongly Agree	
1	2	3	4	5	6	

1. I am concerned that the pain might mean something is wrong with me   1 2 3 4 5 6

2. I think the pain is a chance to prove myself   1 2 3 4 5 6

3. I am concerned that the pain might become more than I can manage   1 2 3 4 5 6

4. I think the pain is a test of my strength and ability   1 2 3 4 5 6

5. I think something good might come out of having the pain   1 2 3 4 5 6

6. I am worried about getting things done   1 2 3 4 5 6

7. I think the pain makes me a stronger person   1 2 3 4 5 6

8. I am concerned about how much more pain I can take   1 2 3 4 5 6

9. I think the pain is a chance to learn more about myself   1 2 3 4 5 6

10. The pain seems threatening   1 2 3 4 5 6

11. I think without pain, there is no gain   1 2 3 4 5 6

12. I am worried about being depressed or discouraged because of the pain   1 2 3 4 5 6

13. I think of this pain as a challenge   1 2 3 4 5 6

14. I feel controlled by the pain   1 2 3 4 5 6

15. I think the pain tests how well I can manage   1 2 3 4 5 6

16. I think of this pain as a threat   1 2 3 4 5 6

Copyright 1998 by Anita Unruh. Reprinted by permission in *Cognitive Therapy for Chronic Pain* by Beverly E. Thorn. Copyright 2004 by The Guilford Press. Permission to photocopy this appendix is granted to purchasers of this book for personal use only (see copyright page for details).

PAI SCORING KEY

Threat/loss: 1, 3, 6, 8, 10, 12, 14, 16
Challenge: 2, 4, 5, 7, 9, 11, 13, 15

Sum all ratings provided for each scale, and divide by the number of items responded to within each scale.

Pain Beliefs and Perceptions Inventory (PBPI)

Please indicate the degree to which you agree or disagree with each of the following statements. Simply circle the number that corresponds with your level of agreement.

	Strongly Disagree	Disagree	Agree	Strongly Agree
1. No one's been able to tell me exactly why I'm in pain.	−2	−1	1	2
2. I used to think my pain was curable, but now I'm not so sure.	−2	−1	1	2
3. There are times when I am pain-free.	−2	−1	1	2
4. My pain is confusing to me.	−2	−1	1	2
5. My pain is here to stay.	−2	−1	1	2
6. I am continuously in pain.	−2	−1	1	2
7. If I am in pain, it is my own fault.	−2	−1	1	2
8. I don't know enough about my pain.	−2	−1	1	2
9. My pain is a temporary problem in my life.	−2	−1	1	2
10. It seems like I wake up with pain and I go to sleep with pain.	−2	−1	1	2
11. I am the cause of my pain.	−2	−1	1	2
12. There is a cure for my pain.	−2	−1	1	2
13. I blame myself if I am in pain.	−2	−1	1	2
14. I can't figure out why I'm in pain.	−2	−1	1	2
15. Someday I'll be 100% pain-free again.	−2	−1	1	2
16. My pain varies in intensity but is always with me.	−2	−1	1	2

Copyright 1989 by David A. Williams. Reprinted by permission in *Cognitive Therapy for Chronic Pain* by Beverly E. Thorn. Copyright 2004 by The Guilford Press. Permission to photocopy this appendix is granted to purchasers of this book for personal use only (see copyright page for details).

PBPI SCORING KEY

Asterisks indicate reverse-scored items.

Pain as Mystery: 1, 2, 4, 14
Pain as Constant: 3,* 6, 10, 16*
Pain as Permanent: 5, 9,* 12,* 15*
Self-Blame: 7, 8, 11, 13

Sum all ratings provided for each scale (transform reverse-scored items before summing with other ratings), and divide by the number of items responded to within each scale.

Survey of Pain Attitudes—Revised (SOPA-R)

Please indicate how much you agree with each of the following statements about your pain problem by using the response key below.

Response key: 0 = This is very untrue for me.
1 = This is somewhat untrue for me.
2 = This is neither true nor untrue for me (or it does not apply to me).
3 = This is somewhat true for me.
4 = This is very true for me.

1. The pain I feel is a sign that damage is being done	0 1 2 3 4
2. I will probably always have to take pain medications	0 1 2 3 4
3. When I hurt, I want my family to treat me better	0 1 2 3 4
4. If my pain continues at its present level, I will be unable to work	0 1 2 3 4
5. The amount of pain I feel is out of my control	0 1 2 3 4
6. I do not expect a medical cure for my pain	0 1 2 3 4
7. Pain does not have to mean that my body is being harmed	0 1 2 3 4
8. I have had the most relief from pain with the use of medications	0 1 2 3 4
9. Anxiety increases the pain I feel	0 1 2 3 4
10. There is little that I can do to ease my pain	0 1 2 3 4
11. When I am hurting, I deserve to be treated with care and concern	0 1 2 3 4
12. I pay doctors so they will cure me of my pain	0 1 2 3 4
13. My pain problem does not need to interfere with my activity level	0 1 2 3 4
14. It is the responsibility of my family to help me when I feel pain	0 1 2 3 4
15. Stress in my life increases the pain I feel	0 1 2 3 4
16. Exercise and movement are good for my pain problem	0 1 2 3 4
17. Medicine is one of the best treatments for chronic pain	0 1 2 3 4
18. My family needs to learn how to take better care of me when I am in pain	0 1 2 3 4
19. Depression increases the pain I feel	0 1 2 3 4
20. If I exercise, I could make my pain problem much worse	0 1 2 3 4
21. I can control my pain by changing my thoughts	0 1 2 3 4
22. I need more tender loving care than I am now getting when I am in pain	0 1 2 3 4
23. I consider myself to be disabled	0 1 2 3 4
24. I have learned to control my pain	0 1 2 3 4
25. I trust that doctors can cure my pain	0 1 2 3 4

(continued)

Copyright 1994 by Mark P. Jensen and Paul Karoly. Reprinted by permission in *Cognitive Therapy for Chronic Pain* by Beverly E. Thorn. Copyright 2004 by The Guilford Press. Permission to photocopy this appendix is granted to purchasers of this book for personal use only (see copyright page for details).

26. My pain does not stop me from leading a physically active life   0   1   2   3   4

27. My physical pain will never be cured   0   1   2   3   4

28. There is a strong connection between my emotions and my pain level   0   1   2   3   4

29. I am not in control of my pain   0   1   2   3   4

30. No matter how I feel emotionally, my pain stays the same   0   1   2   3   4

31. When I find the right doctor, he or she will know how to reduce my pain   0   1   2   3   4

32. If my doctor prescribed pain medications for me, I would throw them away   0   1   2   3   4

33. I will never take pain medications again   0   1   2   3   4

34. Exercise can decrease the amount of pain I experience   0   1   2   3   4

35. My pain would stop anyone from leading an active life   0   1   2   3   4

SOPA-R SCORING KEY

Asterisks indicate reverse-scored items.

Control: 5,* 10,* 21, 24, 29*
Disability: 4, 13,* 23, 26,* 35
Harm: 1, 7,* 16,* 20, 34*
Emotion: 9, 15, 19, 28, 30*
Medication: 2, 8, 17, 32,* 33*
Solicitude: 3, 11, 14, 18, 22
Medical Cure: 6,* 12, 25, 27,* 31

Sum all ratings provided for each scale (transform reverse-scored items—i.e., 4 minus rating given—before summing with other ratings), and divide by the number of items responded to within each scale.

Pain Catastrophizing Scale (PCS)

Everyone experiences painful situations at some point in their lives. Such experiences may include headaches, tooth pain, joint pain, or muscle pain. People are often exposed to situations that may cause pain such as illness, injury, dental procedures, or surgery.

We are interested in the types of thoughts and feelings that you have when you are in pain. Listed below are thirteen statements describing different thoughts and feelings that may be associated with pain. Using the following scale, please indicate the degree to which you have these thoughts and feelings when you are experiencing pain.

0—not at all	1—to a slight degree	2—to a moderate degree	3—to a great degree	4—all the time

When I'm in pain . . .

1. ☐ I worry all the time about whether the pain will end.

2. ☐ I feel I can't go on.

3. ☐ It's terrible and I think it's never going to get any better.

4. ☐ It's awful and I feel that it overwhelms me.

5. ☐ I feel I can't stand it any more.

6. ☐ I become afraid that the pain will get worse.

7. ☐ I keep thinking of other painful events.

8. ☐ I anxiously want the pain to go away.

9. ☐ I can't seem to keep it out of my mind.

10. ☐ I keep thinking about how much it hurts.

11. ☐ I keep thinking about how badly I want the pain to stop.

12. ☐ There's nothing I can do to reduce the intensity of the pain.

13. ☐ I wonder whether something serious may happen.

. . . Total

Copyright 1995 by Michael J. Sullivan. Reprinted by permission in *Cognitive Therapy for Chronic Pain* by Beverly E. Thorn. Copyright 2004 by The Guilford Press. Permission to photocopy this appendix is granted to purchasers of this book for personal use only (see copyright page for details).

PCS SCORING KEY

Rumination: 8, 9, 10, 11
Magnification: 6, 7, 13
Helplessness: 1, 2, 3, 4, 5, 12

Sum all ratings provided for each scale, and divide by the number of items responded to within each scale.

Means and Standard Deviations of PCS Scores for Patients Undergoing Evaluation and Treatment at a Multidisciplinary Pain Clinic

Total	Rumination	Magnification	Helplessness
28.2 (12.3)	10.1 (4.3)	4.8 (2.8)	13.3 (6.1)

Note: Data from Sullivan, Stanish, Waite, Sullivan, and Tripp (1998). Based on these data, it has been suggested that patients obtaining a total score above 38 (80th percentile) are particularly likely to experience adjustment difficulties and to progress poorly in rehabilitation programs.

Cognitive Coping Strategies Inventory—Revised (CCSI-R)

Instructions: The following statements describe different thoughts and behaviors that people engage in when they experience pain. For each statement you are to indicate whether it is never, some of the time, one-half of the time, most of the time, or all of the time true about the way in which you deal with your pain. You may find it helpful to think back to the most recent time you were in some degree of pain and imagine as if you were answering these questions while in pain. If the individual *content* of a test item is not similar, but the *style* in which you deal with the pain is similar to the item, you should mark the item in the true categories. Make only one response per item and try and answer each item.

1	2	3	4	5
Never True	Some of the Time True	One-Half of the Time True	Most of the Time True	All of the Time True

1. _____ I use my imagination to change the situation or place where I am experiencing pain in order to try and make the pain more bearable.
2. _____ I think of photographs or paintings that I have seen in the past.
3. _____ I feel like I just want to get up and run away.
4. _____ I imagine the pain becoming even more intense and hurtful.
5. _____ I begin thinking of all the possible bad things that could go wrong in association with the pain.
6. _____ I "psych" myself up to deal with the pain, perhaps by telling myself that it won't last much longer.
7. _____ I picture in my "mind's eye" a lush, green forest or other similar peaceful scene.
8. _____ I try and imagine that for some reason it is important for me to endure the pain.
9. _____ I tell myself that I don't think I can bear the pain any longer.
10. _____ I use my imagination to develop pictures which help distract me.
11. _____ I imagine that the pain is really not as severe as it seems to feel.
12. _____ In general, my ability to see things visually in my "mind's eye" or imagination is quite good.
13. _____ I develop images or pictures in my mind to try and ignore the pain.
14. _____ I might concentrate on how attractive certain colors are in the room or place that I am experiencing pain.
15. _____ I find myself worrying about possibly dying.
16. _____ I take myself very far away from the pain by using my imagination.
17. _____ I find myself expecting the worst.
18. _____ I try and pretend that I am on the beach, or somewhere else enjoying a summer day.

Copyright of original CCSI 1985 by Robert W. Butler. Copyright of CCSI-R 2003 by Beverly E. Thorn, L. Charles Ward, and Kristi L. Clements. Reprinted by permission in *Cognitive Therapy for Chronic Pain* by Beverly E. Thorn. Copyright 2004 by The Guilford Press. Permission to photocopy this appendix is granted to purchasers of this book for personal use only (see copyright page for details).

1	2	3	4	5
Never True	Some of the Time True	One-Half of the Time True	Most of the Time True	All of the Time True

19. _____ I tell myself that I can cope with the pain without imagining or pretending anything.

20. _____ I concentrate on making the pain feel as if it hurts less.

21. _____ I tend to think that my pain is pretty awful.

22. _____ I concentrate on convincing myself that I will deal with the pain and that it will get better in the near future.

23. _____ I think of myself as being interested in pain and wanting to describe it to myself in detail.

24. _____ I think of and picture myself being with my spouse/boyfriend/girlfriend.

25. _____ I might try and think that I'm overreacting and that my pain is really not as severe as it seems.

26. _____ I might begin making plans for a future event, such as a vacation, to distract me from thinking about the pain.

27. _____ I can't help but concentrate on how bad the pain actually feels.

28. _____ I work at talking myself into believing that the pain is really not all that bad and that there are others who are much worse off than me.

29. _____ I might pretend that my pain was similar to pain I have felt after a good session of exercise.

30. _____ I try and preoccupy my mind by daydreaming about various pleasant things such as clouds or sailboats.

31. _____ I find it virtually impossible to keep my mind off my pain and how bad it hurts.

32. _____ I begin to worry that something might be seriously wrong with me.

CCSI-R SCORING KEY

Distraction: 1, 2, 7, 10, 12, 13, 14, 16, 18, 24, 26, 30
Catastrophizing: 3, 4, 5, 9, 15, 17, 21, 27, 31, 32
Coping Self-Statements/Cognitive Minimization of Stimulus: 6, 8, 11, 19, 20, 22, 23, 25, 28, 29

Sum all ratings provided for each scale, and divide by the number of items responded to within each scale.

Coping Strategies Questionnaire—Revised (CSQ-R)

Individuals who experience pain have developed a number of ways to cope with, or deal with, their pain. These include saying things to themselves when they experience pain, or engaging in different activities. Below are a list of things that patients have reported doing when they feel pain. For each activity, I want you to indicate, using the scale below, how much you engage in that activity when you feel pain, where a 0 indicates you never do that when you experience pain, a 3 indicates you sometimes do that when you experience pain, and a 6 indicates you always do it when you are experiencing pain. Remember, you can use any point along the scale.

0	1	2	3	4	5	6
Never do that			Sometimes do that			Always do that

When I feel pain . . .

_____ 1. I try to feel distant from the pain, almost as if the pain was in somebody else's body.

_____ 2. I try to think of something pleasant.

_____ 3. It's terrible and I feel it's never going to get any better.

_____ 4. I tell myself to be brave and carry on despite the pain.

_____ 5. I tell myself that I can overcome the pain.

_____ 6. It's awful and I feel that it overwhelms me.

_____ 7. I feel my life isn't worth living.

_____ 8. I pray to God it won't last long.

_____ 9. I try not to think of it as my body, but rather as something separate from me.

_____ 10. I don't think about the pain.

_____ 11. I tell myself I can't let the pain stand in the way of what I have to do.

_____ 12. I don't pay any attention to it.

_____ 13. I pretend it's not there.

_____ 14. I worry all the time about whether it will end.

_____ 15. I replay in my mind pleasant experiences in the past.

_____ 16. I think of people I enjoy doing things with.

_____ 17. I pray for the pain to stop.

_____ 18. I imagine that the pain is outside of my body.

_____ 19. I just go on as if nothing happened.

_____ 20. Although it hurts, I just keep on going.

_____ 21. I feel I can't stand it any more.

_____ 22. I ignore it.

_____ 23. I rely on my faith in God.

_____ 24. I feel like I can't go on.

_____ 25. I think of things I enjoy doing.

_____ 26. I do something I enjoy, such as watching TV or listening to music.

_____ 27. I pretend it's not a part of me.

Copyright of original CSQ 1983 by Anne K. Rosenstiel Gross. Copyright of revised CSQ 1997 by Joseph L. Riley and Michael E. Robinson. Reprinted by permission in *Cognitive Therapy for Chronic Pain* by Beverly E. Thorn. Copyright 2004 by The Guilford Press. Permission to photocopy this appendix is granted to purchasers of this book for personal use only (see copyright page for details).

CSQ-R SCORING KEY

Distraction: 2, 15, 16, 25, 26
Catastrophizing: 3, 6, 7, 14, 21, 24
Ignoring Pain: 10, 12, 13, 19, 22
Distancing from the Pain: 1, 9, 18, 27
Coping Self-Statements: 4, 5, 11, 20
Praying: 8, 17, 23

Sum all ratings provided for each scale, and divide by the number of items responded to within each scale. You may also contact Michael Robinson (*merobin@nersp.nerdc.ufl.edu*) for a computerized version of the scoring program.

Pre- and Postsession Process Check

PRESESSION PROCESS CHECK

1. List the main point of last week's session.

2. List one thing you did or thought differently following last week's session.

3. Was there anything said during last week's session that confused or troubled you?

4. Do you have any questions from last week's session?

(continued)

From *Cognitive Therapy for Chronic Pain* by Beverly E. Thorn. Copyright 2004 by The Guilford Press. Permission to photocopy this handout is granted to purchasers of this book for personal use only (see copyright page for details).

POSTSESSION PROCESS CHECK

1. List the main point of this week's session.

2. List one thing you can do or think differently during the next week as a result of this week's session.

3. Was there anything said during this week's session that confused or troubled you?

4. Do you have any questions from this week's session?

From *Cognitive Therapy for Chronic Pain* by Beverly E. Thorn. Copyright 2004 by The Guilford Press. Permission to photocopy this handout is granted to purchasers of this book for personal use only (see copyright page for details).

REFERENCES

Affleck, G., Urrows, S., Tennen, H., & Higgins, P. (1992). Daily coping with pain from rheumatoid arthritis: Patterns and correlates. *Pain, 51,* 221–229.

Ajzen, I., & Fishbein, M. (1977). Attitude–behavior relations: A theoretical analysis and review of empirical research. *Psychological Bulletin, 84,* 888–918.

American Medical Association. (2004). *Current procedural terminology.* Chicago: Author.

American Psychiatric Association. (2000). *Diagnostic and statistical manual of mental disorders* (4th ed., text rev.). Washington, DC: Author.

Arathuzik, M. D. (1991). The appraisal of pain and coping in cancer patients. *Western Journal of Nursing Research, 13,* 714–731.

Asmundson, G. J. G., Kuperos, J. L., & Norton, G. R. (1997). Do patients with chronic pain selectively attend to pain-related information?: Preliminary evidence for the mediating role of fear. *Pain, 72,* 27–32.

Bandura, A. (1986). *Social foundations of thought and action.* Englewood Cliffs, NJ: Prentice-Hall.

Beck, A. T. (1976). *Cognitive therapy and the emotional disorders.* New York: International Universities Press.

Beck, A. T., Steer, R. A., & Brown, G. K. (1996). *Beck Depression Inventory—Second Edition: Manual.* San Antonio, TX: Psychological Corp.

Beck, J. S. (1995). *Cognitive therapy: Basics and beyond.* New York: Guilford Press.

Beecher, H. K. (1959). *Measurement of subjective responses.* New York: Oxford University Press.

Binzer, M., Almay, B., & Eisemann, M. (2003). Chronic pain disorder associated with psychogenic versus somatic factors: A comparative study. *Nordic Journal of Psychiatry, 57,* 61–66.

Blazer, D. (1994). Epidemiology of late-life depression. In L. Schneider, C. F. Reynolds, B. Lebowitz, & A. Friedhoff (Eds.), *Diagnosis and treatment of depression in late life* (pp. 9–19). Washington, DC: American Psychiatric Press.

Boothby, J. L., & Thorn, B. E. (2002). Evaluating pain patients involved in personal injury litigation. *Innovations in Clinical Practice: A Source Book, 20,* 167–182.

Boothby, J. L., Thorn, B. E., Stroud, M., & Jensen, M. (1999). Coping with pain. In R. J. Gatchel & D. J. Turk (Eds.), *Psychosocial factors in pain: Critical perspectives* (pp. 343–359). New York: Guilford Press.

Boothby, J. L., Thorn, B. E., Ward, L. C., & Overduin, L. Y. (2004). Catastrophizing and perceived partner responses to pain. *Pain, 109,* 500–506.

Bradley, L. A., & McKendree-Smith, N. L. (2001). Assessment of psychological status using interviews and self-report instruments. In D. C. Turk & R. Melzack (Eds.), *Handbook of pain assessment* (2nd ed., pp. 292–319). New York: Guilford Press.

Brooks, G. R., & Richardson, F. C. (1980). Emotional skills training: A treatment program for duodenal ulcer. *Behavior Therapy, 11*, 198–207.

Brown, G., & Nicassio, P. (1987). The development of a questionnaire for the assessment of active and passive coping strategies in chronic pain patients. *Pain, 31*, 53–65.

Burns, D. D. (1980). *Feeling good: The new mood therapy.* New York: Morrow.

Burns, J. W., Kubilus, A., Bruehl, S., Harden, R. N., & Lofland, K. (2003). Do changes in cognitive factors influence outcome following multidisciplinary treatment for chronic pain?: A cross-lagged panel analysis. *Journal of Consulting and Clinical Psychology, 71*, 81–91.

Burton, A. K., Tillotson, K. M., Main, C. J., & Hollis, S. (1995). Psychosocial predictors of outcome in acute and sub acute low back trouble. *Spine, 20*, 722–728.

Butler, R. W., Damarin, F. L., Beaulieu, C. L., Schwebel, A. I., & Thorn, B. E. (1989). Assessing cognitive coping strategies for acute pain. *Psychological Assessment: A Journal of Consulting and Clinical Psychology, 1*(1), 41–45.

Carlson, N. R. (1994). Audition, the body senses, and the chemical senses. In N. R. Carlson, *Physiology and behavior* (pp. 180–224). Needham Heights, MA: Allyn & Bacon.

Caudill, M. (2002). *Managing pain before it manages you* (rev. ed.). New York: Guilford Press.

Charmaz, K. (1999). From the "sick role" to stories of self: understanding the self in illness. In R. J. Contrada & R. D. Ashmore (Eds.), *Self, social identity, and physical health* (pp. 209–239). Oxford: Oxford University Press.

Chaves, J. F., & Brown, J. M. (1987). Spontaneous cognitive strategies for the control of clinical pain and stress. *Journal of Behavioral Medicine, 10*, 263–276.

Coghill, R. C., McHaffie, J. G., & Yen, Y. F. (2003). Neural correlates of interindividual differences in the subjective experience of pain. *Proceedings of the National Academy of Sciences USA, 100*, 8538–8542.

Covington, E. C. (2000). The biological basis of pain. *International Review of Psychiatry, 12*, 128–148.

Crombez, G., Eccleston, C., Van den Broek, A., Van Doudenhove, B., & Goubert, L. (2002). The effects of catastrophic thinking about pain on attentional interference by pain: No mediation of negative affectivity in healthy volunteers and in patients with low back pain. *Pain Research and Management, 7*, 31–33.

Crombez, G., Vervaet, L., Lysens, R., Baeyens, F., & Eelen, P. (1998). Avoidance and confrontation of painful back straining movement in chronic back pain patients. *Behavior Modification, 22*, 62–77.

Cutler, R. B., Fishbein, D. A., Rosomoff, H. L., Abdel-Moty, E., Khalil, T. M., & Rosomoff, R. S. (1994). Does nonsurgical pain center treatment of chronic pain return patient to work?: A review and meta-analysis of the literature. *Spine, 19*, 643–652.

DeGood, D. E., & Tait, R. C. (2001). Assessment of pain beliefs and pain coping. In D. C. Turk & R. Melzack (Eds.), *Handbook of pain assessment* (2nd ed., pp. 320–345). New York: Guilford Press.

DeRubeis, R. J., & Feeley, M. (1990). Determinants of change in cognitive therapy for depression. *Cognitive Therapy and Research, 14*, 469–482.

Dozois, D. J. A., Dobson, K. S., Wong, M., Hughes, D., & Long, A. (1996). Predictive utility of the CSQ in low back pain: Individual vs. composite measures. *Pain, 66*, 251–259.

D'Souza, P., Lumley, M., Kraft, C., Dooley, J., Roberson, T., Stanislawski, B., & Romos, M. (2003). Emotional disclosure and relaxation training for migraine and tension headaches: A randomized trial. *Psychosomatic Medicine, 65*, A-6.

Dyck, M. J., & Agar-Wilson, J. (1997). Cognitive vulnerabilities predict medical outcome in a sample of pain patients. *Psychology, Health and Medicine, 2*, 41–50.

Engel, G. L. (1977). The need for a new medical model: A challenge for biomedicine. *Science, 196*, 129–136.

Fearon, I., McGrath, P. J., & Achat, H. (1996). "Booboos": The study of everyday pain among young children. *Pain, 68*, 55–62.

Fedoravicius, A. S., & Klein, B. J. (1986). Social skills training in an outpatient medical setting. In A. D. Holzman & D. C. Turk (Eds.), *Pain management: A handbook of psychological treatment approaches* (pp. 86–99). Elmsford, NY: Pergamon Press.

Feeley, M., DeRubeis, R. J., & Gelfand, L. A. (1999). The temporal relation of adherence and alliance to symptom change in cognitive therapy for depression. *Journal of Consulting and Clinical Psychology, 67*, 578–582.

Fernandez, E., & Turk, D. C. (1989). The utility of cognitive coping strategies for altering pain perception: A meta-analysis. *Pain, 38*, 125–135.

Fillingim, R. B. (Ed.). (2001). *Sex, gender, and pain*. Seattle, WA: IASP Press.

Fishbein, M., & Ajzen, I. (1975). *Belief, attitude, intention and behavior. An introduction to theory and research*. Reading, MA: Addison-Wesley.

Flor, H., Behle, D. J., & Birbaumer, N. (1993). Assessment of pain-related cognitions in chronic pain patients. *Behaviour Research and Therapy, 31*, 63–73.

Flor, H., Breitenstein, C., Birbaumer, N., & Fuerst, M. (1995). A psychophysiological analysis of spouse solicitousness towards pain behaviors, spouse interaction, and pain perception. *Behavior Therapy, 26*, 255–272.

Flor, H., Kerns, R. D., & Turk, D. C. (1987). The role of spouse reinforcement, perceived pain, and activity levels of chronic pain patients. *Journal of Psychosomatic Research, 31*, 251–259.

Flor, H., & Turk, D. C. (1988). Chronic back pain and rheumatoid arthritis: Predicting pain and disability from cognitive variables. *Journal of Behavioral Medicine, 11*, 251–265.

Flor, H., Turk, D. C., & Scholz, O. B. (1988). Impact of chronic pain on the spouse: Marital, emotional and physical consequences. *Journal of Psychosomatic Research, 31*, 63–71.

Fordyce, W. E. (1976). *Behavioral methods for chronic pain and illness*. St. Louis, MO: Mosby.

Fordyce, W. E. (1998). Environmental issues in disability status. *Canadian Journal of Rehabilitation, 11*, 170–171.

Fordyce, W. E., Fowler, R., & DeLateur, B. (1968). An application of behaviour modification technique to a problem of chronic pain. *Behaviour Research and Therapy, 6*, 105–107.

Geisser, M. E., Robinson, M. E., & Henson, C. D. (1994). The Coping Strategies Questionnaire and chronic pain adjustments: A conceptual and empirical reanalysis. *Clinical Journal of Pain, 10*, 98–106.

Geisser, M. E., Robinson, M. E, Keefe, F. J., & Weiner, M. L. (1994). Catastrophizing, depression and the sensory, affective and evaluative aspects of chronic pain. *Pain, 59*, 79–83.

Geisser, M. E., Robinson, M. E., & Riley, J. L. (1999). Pain beliefs, coping, and adjustment to chronic pain: Let's focus more on the negative. *Pain Forum, 8*, 161–168.

Gil, K. M., Abrams, M. R., Phillips, G., & Keefe, F. J. (1989). Sickle cell disease pain: Relation of coping strategies to adjustment. *Journal of Consulting and Clinical Psychology, 57*, 725–731.

Gil, K. M., Thompson, R. J., Keith, B. R., Tota-Faucette, M., Noll, S., & Kinney, T. R. (1993). Sickle cell disease pain in children and adolescents: Change in pain frequency and coping strategies over time. *Journal of Pediatric Psychology, 18*, 621–637.

Gil, K. M., Williams, D. A., Keefe, F. J., & Beckham, J. C. (1990). The relationship of negative thoughts to pain and psychological distress. *Behavior Therapy, 21*, 349–362.

Gil, K. M., Wilson, J. J., Edens, J. L., Webster, D. A., Abrams, M. A., Orringer, E., et al. (1996). The effects of cognitive coping skills training on coping strategies and experimental pain sensitivity in African American adults with sickle cell disease. *Health Psychology, 15*, 3–10.

Gillis, M., Lumley, M. Koch, H., Mosley-Williams, A., Leisen, J., & Roehrs, T. (2003). Written emotional disclosure in fibromyalgia syndrome. *Psychosomatic Medicine, 65*, A-12.

Haaga, D. A., Dyck, M. I., & Ernst, D. (1991). Empirical status of cognitive therapy of depression. *Psychological Bulletin, 110*, 215–236.

Hadjstavropoulous, H. D., Hadjstavropoulous, T., & Quine, A. (2000). Health anxiety moderates the effects of distraction versus attention to pain. *Behaviour Research and Therapy, 38*, 425–438.

Harkapaa, K. (1991). Relationships of psychological distress and health locus of control beliefs with the use of cognitive and behavioral coping strategies in low back pain patients. *Clinical Journal of Pain, 7,* 275–282.

Harkapaa, K., Jarvikoski, A., Mellin, G., Hurri, H., & Luoma, J. (1991). Health locus of control beliefs and psychological distress as predictors for treatment outcome in low-back pain patients: Results of a 3–month follow-up of a controlled intervention study. *Pain, 46,* 35–41.

Hasvold, T., & Johnson, R. (1993). Headache and neck and shoulder pain: Frequent and disabling complaints in the general population. *Scandinavian Journal of Primary Health Care, 11,* 21–224.

Hathaway, S. R., McKinley, J. C., Butcher, J. N., Dahlstrom, W. G., Graham, J. R., Tellegen, A., et al. (1989). *Minnesota Multiphasic Personality Inventory–2: Manual for administration.* Minneapolis: University of Minnesota Press.

Henriques, G., & Leitenberg, H. (2002). An experimental analysis of the role of cognitive errors in the development of depressed mood following negative social feedback. *Cognitive Therapy and Research, 26,* 245–260.

Hewson, D. (1997). Coping with loss of ability: "Good grief" or episodic stress response. *Social Science and Medicine, 44,* 1129–1139.

Heyneman, N. E., Fremouw, W. J., Gano, D., Kirkland, F., & Heiden, L. (1990). Individual differences and the effectiveness of different coping strategies for pain. *Cognitive Therapy and Research, 14,* 63–77.

Hill, A. (1993). The use of pain coping strategies by patients with phantom limb pain. *Pain, 55,* 347–353.

Hochstetler, S. A., Rejeski, W. J., & Best, D. L. (1985). The influence of sex-role orientation on ratings of perceived exertion. *Sex Roles, 12,* 825–835.

Holroyd, K. A., Andrasik, F., & Westbrook, T. (1977). Cognitive control of tension headache. *Cognitive Therapy and Research, 1,* 121–133.

Holroyd, K. A., Penzien, D. B., Hursey, K. G., Tobin, D. L., Rogers, L., Holm, J. E., et al. (1984). Change mechanisms in EMG biofeedback training: Cognitive changes underlying improvements in tension headache. *Journal of Consulting and Clinical Psychology, 52,* 1039–1053.

Humphrey, J. H. (Ed.). (1984). *Human stress: Current selected research* (Vol. 1). New York: AMS Press.

Iadarola, M. J., & Caudle, R. M. (1997). Good pain, bad pain. *Science, 278,* 239–240.

Jacob, M. C., & Kerns, R. D. (2001). Assessment of the psychosocial context of the experience of chronic pain. In D. C. Turk & R. Melzack (Eds.), *Handbook of pain assessment* (2nd ed., pp. 362–384). New York: Guilford Press.

Jacobsen, P. B., & Butler, R. W. (1996). Relation of cognitive coping and catastrophizing to acute pain and analgesic use following breast cancer surgery. *Journal of Behavioral Medicine, 19,* 17–29.

Jacobson, N. S., Dobson, K. S., Truax, P. A., Addis, M. E., Kowerner, K. Gollan, J. K., et al. (1996). A component analysis of cognitive behavioral treatment for depression. *Journal of Consulting and Clinical Psychology, 64,* 295–304.

James, L. D., Thorn, B. E., & Williams, D. A. (1993). Goal specification in cognitive behavioral therapy for chronic headache pain. *Behavior Therapy, 24,* 305–320.

Jensen, I., Nygren, A., Gamberale, R., Goldie, I., & Westerholm, P. (1994). Coping with long-term musculoskeletal pain and its consequences: Is gender a factor? *Pain, 57,* 167–172.

Jensen, M. C., Brant-Zawadzki, M. N., Obuchowski, N., Modic, M. T., Malkasian, D., & Ross, J. S. (1994). Magnetic resonance imaging of the lumbar spine in people without back pain. *New England Journal of Medicine, 331,* 69–73.

Jensen, M. P., & Karoly, P. (1991). Control beliefs, coping efforts, and adjustment to chronic pain. *Journal of Consulting and Clinical Psychology, 59,* 431–438.

Jensen, M. P., Karoly, P., & Huger, R. (1987). The development and preliminary validation of an instrument to assess patients' attitudes toward pain. *Journal of Psychosomatic Research, 31,* 393–400.

Jensen, M. P., Nielson, W. R., & Kerns, R. D. (2003). Toward the development of a motivational model of pain self-management. *Journal of Pain, 4,* 477–492.

Jensen, M. P., Turner, J. A., & Romano, J. M. (1991). Self-efficacy and outcome expectancies: Relationship to chronic pain coping strategies and adjustment. *Pain, 44,* 263–270.

Jensen, M. P., Turner, J. A., & Romano, J. M. (2000). Pain belief assessment: A comparison of short and long versions of the Survey of Pain Attitudes. *Journal of Pain, 1,* 138–150.

Jensen, M. P., Turner, J. A., Romano, J. M., & Karoly, P. (1991). Coping with chronic pain: A critical review of the literature. *Pain, 47,* 249–283.

Jensen, M. P., Turner, J. A., Romano, J. M., & Lawler, B. K. (1994). Relationship of pain-specific beliefs to chronic pain adjustment. *Pain, 57,* 301–109.

Jensen, M. P., Turner, J. A., Romano, J. M., & Strom, S. E. (1995). The Chronic Pain Coping Inventory: Development and preliminary validation. *Pain, 60,* 203–216.

Johansson, C., Dahl, J., Jannert, M., Melin, L., & Andersson, G. (1998). Effects of a cognitive-behavioural pain-management program. *Behaviour Research and Therapy, 36,* 915–930.

Johnson, P. R., & Thorn, B. E. (1989). Cognitive behavioral treatment of chronic headache: Group versus individual treatment format. *Headache, 29,* 358–365.

Judge, T. A., Erez, A., Bono, J. E., & Thoresen, C. J. (2002). Are measures of self-esteem, neuroticism, locus of control, and generalized self-efficacy indicators of a common core construct? *Journal of Personality and Social Psychology, 83,* 693–710.

Kahneman, D. (1973). *Attention and effort.* Englewood Cliffs, NJ: Prentice-Hall.

Keefe, F. J., Beaupre, P. M., & Gil, K. M. (2002). Group therapy for patients with chronic pain. In D. C. Turk & R. J. Gatchel (Eds.), *Psychological approaches to pain management: A practitioner's handbook* (2nd ed., pp. 234–255). New York: Guilford Press.

Keefe, F. J., Brown, G. K., Wallston, K. A., & Caldwell, D. S. (1989). Coping with rheumatoid arthritis: catastrophizing as a maladaptive strategy. *Pain, 37,* 51–56.

Keefe, F. J., Lefebvre, J. C., Egert, J. R., Affleck, G., Sullivan, M. J. L., & Caldwell, D. S. (2000). The relationship of gender to pain, pain behavior, and disability in osteoarthritis patients: The role of catastrophizing. *Pain, 87,* 325–334.

Keefe, F. J., Lefebvre, J. C., & Smith, S. J. (1999). Catastrophizing research: Avoiding conceptual errors and maintaining a balanced perspective. *Pain Forum, 8,* 176–180.

Keefe, F. J., Lipkus, I., Lefebvre, J. C., Hurwitz, H., Cliff, E., & Porter, L. (2003). The social context of gastrointestinal cancer pain: A preliminary study examining the relation of patient pain catastrophizing to patient perceptions of social support. *Pain, 103,* 151–156.

Keogh, E., & Herdenfeldt, M. (2002). Gender, coping and the perception of pain. *Pain, 97,* 195–201.

Keller, M. B., McCullough, J. P., & Klein, D. N. (2000). A comparison of nefazodone, the cognitive behavioral-analysis system of psychotherapy, and their combination for the treatment of chronic depression. *New England Journal of Medicine, 342,* 1462–1470.

Kelley, J. E., Lumley, M. A., & Leisen, J. C. C. (1997). Health effects of emotional disclosure in rheumatoid arthritis patients. *Health Psychology, 16,* 331–340.

Kerns, R. D., Rosenberg, R., Jamison, R. N., Caudill, M. A., & Haythornthwaite, J. (1997). Readiness to adopt a self-management approach to chronic pain: The Pain Stages of Change Questionnaire (PSOCQ). *Pain, 72,* 227–234.

Kerns, R. D., Turk, D. C., Holzman, A. D., & Rudy, T. E. (1986). Comparison of cognitive-behavioral and behavioral approaches to the outpatient treatment of chronic pain. *Clinical Journal of Pain, 1,* 195–203.

Kerns, R. D., Turk, D. C., & Rudy, T. E. (1985). The West Haven–Yale Multidimensional Pain Inventory (WHYMPI). *Pain, 23,* 345–356.

Knapp, T. W., & Florin, I. (1981). The treatment of migraine headache by training in vasoconstriction of the temporal artery and a cognitive stress-coping training. *Behavior Analysis and Modification, 4,* 267–274.

Kohn, P. M. (1996). On coping adaptively with daily hassles. In M. Zeidner & N. S. Endler (Eds.), *Handbook of coping: Theory, research, applications* (pp. 181–201). New York: Wiley.

Kosambi, D. D. (1967). Living prehistory in India. *Scientific American, 216,* 105–114.

Kropp, P., Gerber, W., Keinath-Specht, A., Kopal, T., & Niederberger, U. (1997). Behavioral treatment in migraine. Cognitive-behavioral therapy and blood-volume-pulse biofeedback: A cross-over study with a two-year follow up. *Functional Neurology: New Trends in Adaptive and Behavioral Disorders, 12,* 17–24.

Kuhajda, M. C., & Thorn, B. E. (2002). *Cognitive group therapy for chronic pain patients: Development of treatment manual.* Unpublished manuscript.

Kuhajda, M. C., Thorn, B. E., & Klinger, M. R. (1998). The effect of pain on memory for affective words. *Annals of Behavioral Medicine, 20,* 1–5.

Kuhajda, M. C., Thorn, B. E., Klinger, M. R., & Rubin, N. J. (2002). The effect of headache pain on attention (encoding) and memory (recognition). *Pain, 97,* 213–221.

Lautenbacher, S., & Rollman, G. B. (1993). Gender differences in response to pain and non-painful stimuli are dependent upon stimulation method. *Pain, 53,* 255–164.

Lazarus, R. S., & Folkman, S. (1984). *Stress, appraisal, and coping.* New York: Springer.

Lefebre, M. F. (1981). Cognitive distortion and cognitive errors in depressed psychiatric and low back pain patients. *Journal of Consulting and Clinical Psychology, 49,* 517–525.

Levin, F. M., & DeSimone, L. L. (1991). The effects of experimenter gender on pain report in male and female subjects. *Pain, 44,* 69–72.

Lipchik, G. L., Milles, K., & Covington, E. C. (1993). The effects of multidisciplinary pain management treatment on locus of control and pain beliefs in chronic non-terminal pain. *Clinical Journal of Pain, 9,* 49–57.

Lousberg, R., Schmidt, A. J., & Groenman, N. H. (1993). The relationship between spouse solicitousness and pain behavior: Searching for more experimental evidence. *Pain, 51,* 75–79.

Lumley, M. A. (in press). Alexithymia, emotional disclosure, and health: A program of research. *Journal of Personality.*

Mark, V. H., Ervin, F. R., & Yakovlev, P. I. (1962). The treatment of pain by stereotaxic methods. *Confina Neurologica, 22,* 238–245.

Martin, M. Y., Bradley, L. A., Alexander, R. W., Alarcon, G. S., Triana-Alexander, M., Aaron, L. A., et al. (1996). Coping strategies predict disability in patients with primary fibromyalgia. *Pain, 68,* 45–53.

McCracken, L. M. (1997). "Attention" to pain in persons with chronic pain. *Behavior Therapy, 28,* 283–289.

McCracken, L. M. (1998). Learning to live with pain: Acceptance of pain predicts adjustment in persons with chronic pain. *Pain, 74,* 21–27.

Melzack, R. (1990). Phantom limbs and the concept of a neuromatrix. *Trends in Neurosciences, 13,* 88–92.

Melzack, R. (1999a). From the gate to the neuromatrix. *Pain* (Suppl. 6), S121–S126.

Melzack, R. (1999b). Pain and stress: A new perspective. In R. J. Gatchel & D. C. Turk (Eds.), *Psychosocial factors in pain: Critical perspectives* (pp. 89–106). New York: Guilford Press.

Melzack, R. (2001). Pain and the neuromatrix in the brain. *Journal of Dental Education, 65,* 1378–1382.

Melzack, R. Coderre, T. J., Katz, J., & Vaccarino, A. L. (2001). Central neuroplasticitiy and pathological pain. *Annals of the New York Academy of Sciences, 933,* 157–174.

Melzack, R., & Wall, P. D. (1965). Pain mechanisms: A new theory. *Science, 150,* 971–979.

Melzack, R., & Wall, P. D. (1982). *The challenge of pain.* New York: Basic Books.

Merskey, H. (1986). Classification of chronic pain. Descriptions of chronic pain syndromes and definitions. *Pain* (Suppl. 3), 345–356.

Merskey, H., & Bogduk, N. (Eds.). (1994). *Classification of chronic pain: Descriptions of chronic pain syndromes and definitions of pain terms* (2nd ed.). Seattle, WA: IASP Press.

Miller, A. (1997). *Ingenious pain.* New York: Harcourt Brace.

Mitchell, K. R., & White, R. G. (1977). Behavioral self-management: An application to the problem of migraine headaches. *Behavior Therapy, 8,* 213–221.

Moos, R. H., & Schaefer, J. A. (1993). Coping resources and processes: Current concepts and measures. In L. Goldberger & S. Breznitz (Eds.), *Handbook of stress: Theoretical and clinical aspects* (2nd ed., pp. 234–257). New York: Free Press.

Morley, S., Eccleston, C., & Williams, A. (1999). Systematic review and meta-analysis of randomized controlled trials of cognitive behavior therapy for chronic pain in adults, excluding headache. *Pain, 80,* 1–13.

Morley, S., Shapiro, D. A., & Biggs, J. (2004). Manualizing attention control training in the cognitive behavioral treatment of chronic pain: Development of a prototype manual. *Cognitive Behaviour Therapy, 33,* 1–11.

Nielson, W. R., Jensen, M. P., & Kerns, R. D. (2003). Initial development and validation of a Multidimensional Pain Readiness to Change Questionnaire (MPRCQ). *Journal of Pain, 4,* 148–158.

Nielson, W. R., Maleus, L. S., Jensen, M. P., & Kerns, R. D. (2004, May). *Further development of the Multidimensional Pain Readiness to Change Questionnaire.* Paper presented at the annual meeting of the American Pain Society.

Normon, S. A., Lumley, M. A., Dooley, J. A., & Diamond, M. P. (2004). For whom does it work? Moderators of the effects of written emotional disclosure in a randomized trial among women with chronic pelvic pain. *Psychosomatic Medicine, 66,* 174–183.

Osman, A., Barrios, F. X., Gutierrez, P. M., Kopper, B. A., Merrifield, T., & Grittmann, L. (2000). The Pain Catastrophizing Scale: Further psychometric evaluation with adult samples. *Journal of Behavioral Medicine, 23,* 351–365.

Osman, A., Bunger, S., Osman, J. R., & Fisher, L. (1993). The Inventory of Negative Thoughts in Response to Pain: Factor structure and psychometric properties in a college sample. *Journal of Behavioral Medicine, 16,* 219–225.

Otto, M. W., & Dougher, M. J. (1985). Sex differences and personality factors in responsivity to pain. *Perceptual and Motor Skills, 61,* 383–390.

Pennebaker, J. W., & Beall, S. K. (1986). Confronting a traumatic event: Toward an understanding of inhibition and disease. *Journal of Abnormal Psychology, 95,* 74–281.

Pennebaker, J. W., Mayne, T. J., & Francis, M. E. (1997). Linguistic predictors of adaptive bereavement. *Journal of Personality and Social Psychology, 72,* 864–871.

Ploghaus, A., Tracey, I., Gati, J. S., Clare, S., Menon, R. S., Matthews, P. M., et al. (1999). Dissociating pain from its anticipation in the human brain. *Science, 284,* 1979–1981.

Power, M. J., Katz, R., McGuffin, P., Duggan, C. F., Lam, D., & Beck, A. T. (1994). The Dysfunctional Attitude Scale (DAS): A comparison of Forms A and B and proposal for a new subscaled version. *Journal of Research in Personality, 28,* 263–276.

Price, D. D. (2000). Psychological and neural mechanisms of the affective dimension of pain. *Science, 288,* 1769–1772.

Prkachin, K. M. (1986). Pain behavior is not unitary. *Behavioral and Brain Sciences, 9,* 754–755.

Prochaska, J. O., & DiClemente, C. C. (1984). *The transtheoretical approach: Crossing traditional boundaries of change.* Homewood, IL: Dow Jones/Irwin.

Rainville, P., Duncan, G. H., Price, D. D., Carrier, B., & Bushnell, M. C. (1997). Pain affect encoded in human anterior cingulate but not somatosensory cortex. *Science, 277,* 968–971.

Ranjan, R. (2001). *Social relations and chronic pain.* Dordrecht, The Netherlands: Kluwer Academic.

Regan, C. A., Lorig, K., & Thoresen, K. (1988). Arthritis appraisal and ways of coping: scale development. *Arthritis Care and Research, 3,* 139–150.

Rhodes, L. A., McPhillips-Tangum, C. A., Markham, C., & Klenk, R. (1999). The power of the visible: The meaning of diagnostic tests in chronic back pain. *Social Science and Medicine, 48,* 1189–1203.

Riley, J. L., & Robinson, M. E. (1997). The Coping Strategies Questionnaire: Five factors or fiction? *Clinical Journal of Pain, 13,* 156–162.

Riley, J. L., Robinson, M. E., & Geisser, M. E. (1999). Empirical subgroups of the Coping Strategies Questionnaire—Revised: A multi-sample study. *Clinical Journal of Pain, 15,* 111–116.

Robinson, M. E., Riley, J. L., Myers, C. D., Sadler, I. J., Kvaal, S. A., Geisser, M. E., et al. (1997). The Coping Strategies Questionnaire: A large sample, item level factor analysis. *Clinical Journal of Pain, 13,* 43–49.

Rokke, P. D., al Absi, M., Lal, R., & Klein, O. (1991). When does a choice of coping strategies help? The interaction of choice and locus of control. *Journal of Behavioral Medicine, 14,* 491–504.

Romano, J. M., Jensen, M. P., Turner, J. A., Good, A. B., & Hops, H. (2001). Chronic pain patient–partner interactions: Further support for a behavioral model of chronic pain. *Behavior Therapy, 31,* 415–550.

Romano, J. M., Turner, J. A., Friedman, L. S., Bulcroft, R. A., Jensen, M. P., & Hops, H. (1992). Sequential analysis of chronic pain behaviors and spouse responses. *Journal of Consulting and Clinical Psychology, 60,* 777–782.

Rosenstiel, A. K., & Keefe, F. J. (1983). The use of coping strategies in chronic low back pain patients: Relationship to patient characteristics and current adjustment. *Pain, 17,* 33–44.

Rudy, T. E. (1989). *Multiaxial assessment of pain: Multidimensional Pain Inventory. Computer Program user's manual. Version 2.1.* Pittsburgh, PA: Pain Evaluation and Treatment Institute.

Sanders, S. H. (1983) Component analysis of a behavioral treatment program for chronic low-back pain. *Behavior Therapy, 14,* 697–705.

Sanford, S. D., Kersh, B. C., Thorn, B. E., Rich, M. A., & Ward, L. C. (2002). Psychosocial mediators of sex differences in pain responsivity. *Journal of Pain, 3,* 58–64.

Schwartz, G. E., & Kline, J. P. (1995) Repression, emotional disclosure, and health: Theoretical, empirical, and clinical considerations. In J. W. Pennebaker (Ed.), *Emotion, disclosure, and health* (pp. 177–193). Washington, DC: American Psychological Association.

Scott, D. S., & Barber, T. X. (1977). Cognitive control of pain: Effects of multiple cognitive strategies. *Psychological Reports, 37,* 122–129.

Smith, C. A., & Wallston, K. A. (1992). Adaptation in patients with chronic rheumatoid arthritis: Application of a general model. *Health Psychology, 11,* 151–162.

Smith, T. W., Christensen, A. J., Peck, J. R., & Ward, J. R. (1994). Cognitive distortion, helplessness, and depressed mood in rheumatoid arthritis: A four-year longitudinal analysis. *Health Psychology, 13,* 213–217.

Smith, T. W., Follick, M. J., Ahern, B. K., & Adams, A. V. (1986). Cognitive distortion and disability in chronic low back pain. *Cognitive Therapy and Research, 10,* 201–210.

Smith, T. W., Peck, J. R. Milano, R. A., & Ward, J. R. (1988). Cognitive distortion in rheumatoid arthritis: relation to depression and disability. *Journal of Consulting and Clinical Psychology, 56,* 412–416.

Smyth, J. M. (1998). Written emotional expression: Effect sizes, outcome types, and moderating variables. *Journal of Consulting and Clinical Psychology, 66,* 174–184.

Smyth, J. M., Stone, A. A., Hurewitz, A., & Kaell, A. (1999). Effects of writing about stressful experiences on symptom reduction in patients with asthma or rheumatoid arthritis: A randomized trial. *Journal of the American Medical Association, 281,* 1304–1309.

Spanos, N. P., Radtke-Bodorik, H. L., Ferguson, J. D., & Jones, B. (1979). The effects of hypnotic susceptibility, suggestions for analgesia, and utilization of cognitive strategies on the reduction of pain. *Journal of Abnormal Psychology, 88,* 282–292.

Stanton, A. L., Danoff-Burg, S., Sworowski, L. A., Collins, C. A., Branstetter, A. D., Rodriguez-Hanley, A., et al. (2002). Randomized, controlled trial of written emotional expression and benefit finding in breast cancer patients. *Journal of Clinical Oncology, 20,* 4160–4168.

Stewart, M. W., Harvey, S. T., & Evans, I. M. (2001). Coping and catastrophizing in chronic pain: A psychometric analysis and comparison of two measures. *Journal of Clinical Psychology, 57,* 131–138.

Sullivan, M. J. L., Adams, H., & Sullivan, M. (2004). Communicative dimensions of pain catastrophizing: Social cueing effects on pain behavior. *Pain, 107,* 220–226.

Sullivan, M. J. L., Bishop, S., & Pivik, J. (1995). The Pain Catastrophizing Scale: Development and validation. *Psychological Assessment, 7,* 524–532.

Sullivan, M. J. L., & D'Eon, J. L. (1990). Relation between catastrophizing and depression in chronic pain patients. *Journal of Abnormal Psychology, 99,* 260–263.

Sullivan, M. J. L., & Neish, N. (1998). Catastrophizing, anxiety and pain during dental hygiene treatment. *Community Dental Oral Epidemiology, 37,* 243–250.

Sullivan, M. J. L., & Neish, N. (1999). The effects of disclosure on pain during dental hygiene treatment: The moderating role of catastrophizing. *Pain, 79,* 155–163.

Sullivan, M. J. L., Rouse, D., Bishop, S., & Johnson, S. (1997). Thought suppression, catastrophizing, and pain. *Cognitive Therapy and Research, 21,* 555–568.

Sullivan, M. J. L., Stanish, W., Sullivan, M. E., & Tripp, D. (2001). Differential predictors of pain and disability following whiplash injury. *Pain Research and Management, 7,* 68–74.

Sullivan, M. J. L., Stanish, W., Waite, H., Sullivan, M. E., & Tripp, D. (1998). Catastrophizing, pain, and disability following soft tissue injuries. *Pain, 77,* 253–260.

Sullivan, M. J. L., Thorn, B. E., Haythornthwaite, J., Keefe, F., Martin, M., Bradley, L., et al. (2001)

Theoretical perspectives on the relation between catastrophizing and pain. *Clinical Journal of Pain, 17,* 52–64.

Sullivan, M. J. L., Thorn, B. E., Rogers, W. A., & Ward, L. C. (2004). Path model of psychological antecedents to pain experience: Experimental and clinical findings. *Clinical Journal of Pain, 20,* 164–173.

Sullivan, M. J. L., Tripp, D. A., Rodgers, W., & Stanish, W. (2000). Catastrophizing and pain perception in sports participants. *Journal of Applied Sport Psychology, 12,* 151–167.

Sullivan, M. J. L., Tripp, D. A., & Santor, D. (2000). Gender differences in pain and pain behavior: The role of catastrophizing. *Cognitive Therapy and Research, 24,* 121–134.

Suls, J., & Fletcher, B. (1985). The relative efficacy of avoidant and nonavoidant coping strategies: A meta-analysis. *Health Psychology, 4,* 249–288.

Swartzman, L. C., Gwadry, F. G., Shapiro, A. P., & Teasell, R. W. (1994). The factor structure of the Coping Strategies Questionnaire. *Pain, 57,* 311–316.

Szpalski, M., Nordin, M., Skovron, M. L., Melot, C., & Cukier, D. (1995). Health care utilization for low back pain in Belgium: Influence of sociocultural factors and health beliefs. *Spine, 20,* 431–442.

Tan, T. Z., & DeRubeis, R. J. (1999). Reconsidering rapid early response in cognitive behavioral therapy for depression. *Clinical Psychology: Science and Practice, 6,* 283–288.

Taylor, H., & Curran, N. M. (1985). *The Nuprin pain report.* New York: Louis Harris.

Thorn, B. E. (2001). *Comparison of cognitive treatments for headache pain* (Grant No. 1R15NS041323-01). Available: *http://crisp.cit.nih.gov*

Thorn, B. E., Clements, K. L., Ward, L. C., Dixon, K. E., Kersh, B. C., Boothby, J. L., et al. (in press). Personality factors in the explanation of sex differences in pain catastrophizing and response to experimental pain. *Clinical Journal of Pain.*

Thorn, B. E., Rich, M. A., & Boothby, J. L. (1999) Pain beliefs and coping attempts. *Pain Forum, 8*(4), 169–171.

Thorn, B. E., Ward, L. C., & Clements, K. L. (2003, March). *The Cognitive Coping Strategy Inventory: Factor structure and relationships with other indices and predictors of pain behavior.* Poster presented at the annual meeting of the American Pain Society, Toronto.

Thorn, B. E., Ward, L. C., Sullivan, M. J. L., & Boothby, J. L. (2003). Communal coping model of catastrophizing; conceptual model building. *Pain, 106,* 1–2.

Tobin, D. L., Holroyd, K. A., Baker, A., Reynolds, R. V., & Holm, J. E. (1988). Development and clinical trial of a minimal contact, cognitive-behavioral treatment of tension headache. *Cognitive Therapy and Research, 12,* 325–339.

Tunks, E., & Bellissimo, A. (1988). Coping with the coping concept: A brief comment. *Pain, 34,* 171–174.

Turk, D. C. (2001). Treatment of chronic pain: Clinical outcomes, cost-effectiveness, and cost benefits. *Drug Benefit Trends, 13,* 36–38.

Turk, D. C. (2002a). Clinical effectiveness and cost-effectiveness of treatments for patients with chronic pain. *Clinical Journal of Pain. 18,* 355–365.

Turk, D. C. (2002b). A diathesis–stress model of chronic pain and disability following traumatic injury. *Pain Research and Management, 7,* 9–19.

Turk, D. C., & Holzman, A. D. (1986). Commonalities among psychological approaches in the treatment of chronic pain: Specifying the meta-contracts. In A. D. Holzman & D. C. Turk (Eds.), *Pain management: A handbook of psychological treatment approaches* (pp. 257–267). New York: Pergamon Press.

Turk, D. C., Meichenbaum, D. H., & Genest, M. (1983). *Pain and behavioral medicine: A cognitive-behavioral perspective.* New York: Guilford Press.

Turk, D. C., & Melzack, R. (Eds.). (2001). *Handbook of pain assessment* (2nd ed.). New York: Guilford Press.

Turk, D. C., & Okifuji, A. (1996). A perception of traumatic onset, compensation status, and physical findings: Impact on pain severity, emotional distress, and disability in chronic pain patients. *Journal of Behavioral Medicine, 19,* 435–453.

Turk, D. C., & Okifuji, A. (2001). Pain terms and taxonomies of pain. In J. D. Loeser, S. H. Butler, C. R.

Chapman, & D. C. Turk (Eds.), *Bonica's management of pain* (3rd ed., pp. 17–25). Philadelphia: Lippincott, Williams and Wilkins.

Turk, D. C., Okifuji, A., Starz, T. W., & Sinclair, J. D. (1996). Effects of type of symptom onset on psychological distress and disability in fibromyalgia syndrome patients. *Pain, 68*, 423–440.

Turk, D. C., & Rudy, T. E. (1990). The robustness of an empirically derived taxonomy of chronic pain patients. *Pain, 43*, 27–36.

Turk, D. C., & Rudy, T. E. (1992a). Classification logic and strategies in chronic pain. In D.C. Turk & R. Melzack (Eds.), *Handbook of pain assessment* (pp. 409–428). New York: Guilford Press.

Turk, D. C., & Rudy, T. E. (1992b). Cognitive factors and persistent pain: A glimpse into Pandora's box. *Cognitive Therapy and Research, 16*, 99–122.

Turner, J. A., & Clancy, S. (1986). Strategies for coping with chronic low back pain: Relationship to pain and disability. *Pain, 24*, 355–364.

Turner, J. A., Clancy, S., & Vitaliano, P. P. (1987). Relationships of stress appraisals of coping to chronic low back pain. *Behaviour Research and Therapy, 25*, 281–288.

Turner, J. A., & Jensen, M. P. (1993). Efficacy of cognitive therapy for chronic low back pain. *Pain, 52*, 169–177.

Tuttle, D. H., Shutty, M. S., & DeGood, D. E. (1991). Empirical dimensions of coping in chronic pain patients: A factorial analysis. *Rehabilitation Psychology, 36*, 179–188.

Unruh, A. M. (1996). Gender variations in clinical pain experience. *Pain, 65*, 123–167.

Unruh, A. M., & Ritchie, J. A. (1998). Development of the Pain Appraisal Inventory: Psychometric properties. *Pain Research and Medicine, 3*, 105–110.

Van Lankveld, W., Van't Pad Bosch, P., Van De Putte, L., Naring, G., & Van Der Straak, C. (1994). Disease-specific stressors in rheumatoid arthritis: Coping and well-being. *British Journal of Rheumatology, 33*, 1067–1073.

Vendrig, A. A. (2000). The Minnesota Multiphasic Personality Inventory and chronic pain: A conceptual analysis of a long-standing but complicated relationship. *Clinical Psychology Review, 20*, 533–559.

Verbrugge, L. M. (1990). The twain meet: Empirical explanations of sex differences in health and mortality. In M. G. Ory & H. R. Warner (Eds.), *Gender, health, and longevity: Multidisciplinary perspectives* (pp. 159–199). New York: Springer.

Viennau, T. L., Clark, A. J., Lynch, M. E., & Sullivan, M. J. L. (1999). Catastrophizing, functional disability, and pain reports in adults with chronic low back pain. *Pain Research and Management, 4*, 93–96.

Vlaeyen, J. W. S., & Linton, S. J. (2000). Fear-avoidance and its consequences in chronic musculoskeletal pain: A state of the art. *Pain, 85*, 331–332.

Walker, J., Holloway, I., & Sofaer, B. (1999). In the system: The lived experience of chronic back pain from the perspectives of those seeking help from pain clinics. *Pain, 80*, 621–628.

Weir, R., Browne, G., Roberts, J., Tunks, E., & Gafni, A. (1994). The Meaning of Illness Questionnaire: Further evidence for its reliability and validity. *Pain, 58*, 377–386.

Weissman, A. N. (1979). The Dysfunctional Attitude Scale: A validation study. *Dissertation Abstracts International, 40*(3-B), 1389–1390.

Weissman, A. N., & Beck, A. T. (1978). *Development and Validation of the Dysfunctional Attitude Scale: A preliminary investigation*. Paper presented at the annual meeting of the American Educational Research Association, Toronto.

Williams, D. A., & Thorn, B. E. (1989). An empirical assessment of pain beliefs. *Pain, 36*, 351–358.

Williamson, D., Robinson, M. E., & Melamed, B. (1997). Pain behavior, spouse responsiveness, and marital satisfaction in patients with rheumatoid arthritis. *Behavior Modification, 21*, 97–118.

Woolf, C. J., & Salter, M. W. (2000). Neuronal plasticity: Increasing the gain in pain. *Science, 288*, 1765–1772.

World Health Organization. (1992). *International statistical classification of diseases and related health problems* (10th rev.). Geneva: Author.

Wrubel, J., Benner, P., & Lazarus, R. S. (1981). Social competence from the perspective of stress and coping. In J. Wine & M. Smye (Eds.), *Social competence* (pp. 61–99). New York: Guilford Press.

INDEX

Page numbers followed by an *f* indicate figure, *n* indicate note, and *t* indicate table; all therapist and client handouts appear in **bold**.